METHODOLOGICAL CHALLENGES IN BIOMEDICAL HIV PREVENTION TRIALS

Committee on the Methodological Challenges in HIV Prevention Trials

Board on Global Health

Stephen W. Lagakos and Alicia R. Gable, *Editors*

INSTITUTE OF MEDICINE
OF THE NATIONAL ACADEMIES

THE NATIONAL ACADEMIES PRESS
Washington, D.C.
www.nap.edu

THE NATIONAL ACADEMIES PRESS **500 Fifth Street, N.W. Washington, DC 20001**

NOTICE: The project that is the subject of this report was approved by the Governing Board of the National Research Council, whose members are drawn from the councils of the National Academy of Sciences, the National Academy of Engineering, and the Institute of Medicine. The members of the committee responsible for the report were chosen for their special competences and with regard for appropriate balance.

This study was supported by Contract No. 43580 between the National Academy of Sciences and the Bill & Melinda Gates Foundation. Any opinions, findings, conclusions, or recommendations expressed in this publication are those of the author(s) and do not necessarily reflect the view of the organizations or agencies that provided support for this project.

International Standard Book Number-13: 978-0-309-11430-1
International Standard Book Number-10: 0-309-11430-6

Additional copies of this report are available from the National Academies Press, 500 Fifth Street, N.W., Lockbox 285, Washington, DC 20055; (800) 624-6242 or (202) 334-3313 (in the Washington metropolitan area); Internet, http://www.nap.edu.

For more information about the Institute of Medicine, visit the IOM home page at: **www.iom.edu.**

Printed in the United States of America

The serpent has been a symbol of long life, healing, and knowledge among almost all cultures and religions since the beginning of recorded history. The serpent adopted as a logotype by the Institute of Medicine is a relief carving from ancient Greece, now held by the Staatliche Museen in Berlin.

Suggested citation: IOM (Institute of Medicine). 2008. *Methodological challenges in biomedical HIV prevention trials.* Washington, DC: The National Academies Press.

"Knowing is not enough; we must apply.
Willing is not enough; we must do."
—Goethe

INSTITUTE OF MEDICINE
OF THE NATIONAL ACADEMIES

Advising the Nation. Improving Health.

THE NATIONAL ACADEMIES

Advisers to the Nation on Science, Engineering, and Medicine

The **National Academy of Sciences** is a private, nonprofit, self-perpetuating society of distinguished scholars engaged in scientific and engineering research, dedicated to the furtherance of science and technology and to their use for the general welfare. Upon the authority of the charter granted to it by the Congress in 1863, the Academy has a mandate that requires it to advise the federal government on scientific and technical matters. Dr. Ralph J. Cicerone is president of the National Academy of Sciences.

The **National Academy of Engineering** was established in 1964, under the charter of the National Academy of Sciences, as a parallel organization of outstanding engineers. It is autonomous in its administration and in the selection of its members, sharing with the National Academy of Sciences the responsibility for advising the federal government. The National Academy of Engineering also sponsors engineering programs aimed at meeting national needs, encourages education and research, and recognizes the superior achievements of engineers. Dr. Charles M. Vest is president of the National Academy of Engineering.

The **Institute of Medicine** was established in 1970 by the National Academy of Sciences to secure the services of eminent members of appropriate professions in the examination of policy matters pertaining to the health of the public. The Institute acts under the responsibility given to the National Academy of Sciences by its congressional charter to be an adviser to the federal government and, upon its own initiative, to identify issues of medical care, research, and education. Dr. Harvey V. Fineberg is president of the Institute of Medicine.

The **National Research Council** was organized by the National Academy of Sciences in 1916 to associate the broad community of science and technology with the Academy's purposes of furthering knowledge and advising the federal government. Functioning in accordance with general policies determined by the Academy, the Council has become the principal operating agency of both the National Academy of Sciences and the National Academy of Engineering in providing services to the government, the public, and the scientific and engineering communities. The Council is administered jointly by both Academies and the Institute of Medicine. Dr. Ralph J. Cicerone and Dr. Charles M. Vest are chair and vice chair, respectively, of the National Research Council.

www.national-academies.org

COMMITTEE ON THE METHODOLOGICAL CHALLENGES IN HIV PREVENTION TRIALS

STEPHEN W. LAGAKOS (*Chair*), Professor of Biostatistics, Department of Biostatistics, Harvard School of Public Health, Boston
HARVEY J. ALTER, Chief, Infectious Diseases Section, Department of Transfusion Medicine, Warren G. Magnuson Clinical Center, National Institutes of Health, Bethesda
RONALD BAYER, Professor, Department of Sociomedical Sciences, Mailman School of Public Health, Columbia University, New York
SOLOMON R. BENATAR, Professor of Medicine; Director, Bioethics Centre, Department of Medicine, University of Cape Town, South Africa
RONALD S. BROOKMEYER, Professor of Biostatistics, Department of Biostatistics; Chair of the Master of Public Health Program, Johns Hopkins Bloomberg School of Public Health, Baltimore
CARLOS DEL RIO, Professor of Medicine (Infectious Diseases); Vice Chair for Grady Affairs, Department of Medicine; Director for Clinical Sciences and International Research, Center for AIDS Research; Director of AIDS International Training and Research Program, Emory University School of Medicine, Atlanta
DAVID W. FEIGAL, Senior Vice President of Global Regulatory Affairs and Global Safety Surveillance, Élan Pharmaceuticals, San Francisco
ELS GOETGHEBEUR, Associate Professor, Department of Applied Mathematics and Computer Science; Chair, Center for Statistics, Ghent University, Belgium
LAURA A. GUAY, Associate Professor, Department of Pathology, Johns Hopkins School of Medicine, Balitimore
SALLY L. HODDER, Director, HIV Program; Executive Vice Chair, Department of Medicine, University of Medicine and Dentistry of New Jersey, Newark
SHABBAR JAFFAR, Reader in Epidemiology, London School of Hygiene and Tropical Medicine, London, UK
EDWARD K. KIRUMIRA, Professor of Sociology; Dean, Faculty of Social Sciences, Makerere University, Kampala, Uganda
GEORGE W. RUTHERFORD, Salvatore Pablo Lucia Professor and Vice Chair, Department of Epidemiology and Biostatistics; Director, Institute for Global Health, University of California, San Francisco
OLIVE SHISANA, President and CEO, South African Human Sciences Research Council, Cape Town, South Africa
GINA WINGOOD, Associate Professor, Emory University, Rollins School of Public Health, Atlanta

Staff

ALICIA R. GABLE, Study Director
SARAH SCHEENING, Senior Program Associate
KIM LUNDBERG, Research Associate (through August 2007)
RACHEL PASSMAN, Senior Program Assistant
PATRICK KELLEY, Board Director

Consultants

SANDRA HACKMAN, Editor

Reviewers

This report has been reviewed in draft form by individuals chosen for their diverse perspectives and technical expertise, in accordance with procedures approved by the National Research Council's (NRC's) Report Review Committee. The purpose of this independent review is to provide candid and critical comments that will assist the institution in making its published report as sound as possible and to ensure that the report meets institutional standards for objectivity, evidence, and responsiveness to the study charge. The review comments and draft manuscript remain confidential to protect the integrity of the deliberative process. We wish to thank the following individuals for their review of this report:

Zvavahera Michael Chirenje, Department of Obstetrics and Gynaecology, University of Zimbabwe
Thomas J. Coates, UCLA AIDS Institute and Division of Infectious Diseases at the David Geffen School of Medicine, University of California, Los Angeles
Myron Cohen, Division of Infectious Diseases, University of North Carolina
François Dabis, Université Victor Segalen, Bordeaux, France
Susan Ellenberg, Center for Clinical Epidemiology and Biostatistics, University of Pennsylvania School of Medicine
David Holtgrave, Department of Health, Behavior and Society, Johns Hopkins Bloomberg School of Public Health
Jeffrey Kahn, Center for Bioethics, University of Minnesota

Veronica Miller, Forum for Collaborative HIV Research, Department of Prevention & Community Health, George Washington University
Steve Morin, Center for AIDS Prevention Studies, Division of Prevention Science, Department of Medicine, University of California, San Francisco
James D. Neaton, Division of Biostatistics, School of Public Health, University of Minnesota
Suniti Solomon, Voluntary Health Services, Y.R. Gaitonde Centre for AIDS Research and Education, Chennai, India
Steffanie A. Strathdee, Division of International Health & Cross-Cultural Medicine, School of Medicine, University of California, San Diego
Jeremy Sugarman, Berman Institute of Bioethics and Department of Medicine, Johns Hopkins University
Scott Zeger, Department of Biostatistics, Johns Hopkins Bloomberg School of Public Health

Although the reviewers listed above have provided many constructive comments and suggestions, they were not asked to endorse the conclusions or recommendations nor did they see the final draft of the report before its release. The review of this report was overseen by **Dr. Kristine M. Gebbie,** Columbia University School of Nursing, and **Dr. Paul A. Volberding,** San Francisco VA Medical Center and Department of Medicine, University of California, San Francisco. Appointed by the NRC and the Institute of Medicine, they were responsible for making certain that an independent examination of this report was carried out in accordance with institutional procedures and that all review comments were carefully considered. Responsibility for the final content of this report rests entirely with the authoring committee and the institution.

Contents

APPENDIXES

Summary

ABSTRACT: *This IOM committee was formed at the request of the Bill & Melinda Gates Foundation and charged with addressing methodological challenges in late-stage nonvaccine biomedical HIV prevention trials with a specific focus on microbicide and pre-exposure prophylaxis trials.*

A near-perfect biomedical intervention for preventing HIV infection is unlikely to be available in the near future. This underscores the need for late-stage clinical trials of biomedical interventions that can detect and quantify modest intervention effects on HIV infection, and adequately evaluate product safety.

The committee's key recommendations for pretrial research and planning include the following. Estimating HIV incidence is critical to determining the size and duration of a late-stage trial and should be based on direct longitudinal follow-up of individuals in the planned trial site(s), and corroborated by at least one other source. Investigators should also undertake pretrial assessments of a product's potential effects on pregnant women and their fetuses to determine circumstances in which women who become pregnant during a trial might continue to use the study product. Investigators should place a high priority on developing effective strategies to achieve accrual targets, retain participants, and improve adherence to study products. The committee underscores the need for sponsors to adequately invest in trial site capacity (human, physical, and regulatory) and develop sustainability plans so that a trial site can continue to contribute to the community and other research studies after the trial is completed.

Late-stage trials designed to evaluate biomedical interventions should incorporate randomized comparisons of behavioral interventions when pos-

sible. Other important design recommendations include: using endpoint-driven trials; considering inclusion of both blinded and unblinded control arms in future trials; collecting information for evaluating the effects of biomedical interventions on women who become pregnant during a trial and their fetuses; and selecting methods for evaluating product adherence and risk-taking behavior.

Key recommendations for conducting late-stage HIV prevention trials include monitoring the evolving results of a trial to ensure that it is maintaining the best interests of participants, adjusting the trial to improve adherence or other aspects of the study protocol, and using safety information that may become available from external sources.

Recommendations for analyzing trial results include using participant adherence in evaluating the relationship between interventions and HIV risk; the practice of excluding results from participants judged to have been already infected at the time of enrollment, and accounting for product discontinuation due to pregnancy in the analysis of the risk of HIV infection.

Finally, in order to enable more efficient evaluations of biomedical interventions, the committee recommends that researchers give priority to developing biomarkers of recent HIV infection which can be used in cross-sectional samples to estimate HIV incidence rates, identifying surrogate markers for HIV infection and product activity that investigators can reliably use as intermediate trial endpoints, and exploring alternative trial designs that might answer important research questions more efficiently than the traditional two-arm superiority design.

In the more than 25 years of the human immunodeficiency (HIV) epidemic, significant strides have been made in identifying effective HIV prevention interventions. Early successes included biomedical interventions, most notably those that led to dramatic increases in safety of the blood supply (IOM, 1995) and the prevention of mother-to-child transmission (The International Perinatal HIV Group, 1999; Bulterys et al., 2004). Some behavioral interventions and voluntary testing and counseling interventions have also been shown to reduce reported sexual and injecting risk behaviors and non-HIV sexually transmitted infections (STIs), although none has been shown to reduce HIV infection (Auerbach et al., 2006). Treatment for injecting drug users and programs providing access to sterile injecting equipment can also decrease the risk of HIV infection in drug users (IOM, 2007). Condoms remain a vital prevention technology. When used correctly and consistently, condoms can reduce HIV infection risk by 80–90 percent (Weller and Davis, 2002; Kajubi et al., 2005), though in practice they are often not used to their potential. Most recently, three

BOX S-1
Biomedical Approaches to HIV Prevention Tested in Late-Stage Efficacy Trials

Male circumcision, or removal of the penile foreskin, has been shown to reduce the risk of HIV infection in men.
Microbicides are topical substances applied to the vagina or rectum that can potentially prevent HIV.
Pre-exposure prophylaxis (PrEP), employing antiretroviral drugs used for HIV treatment, may help prevent HIV infection.
Cervical barriers were hypothesized to protect women from HIV by covering the cervix and blocking the upper genital tract, which is more vulnerable to HIV infection.
Suppression of HSV-2, the primary cause of genital herpes, may help reduce sexual acquisition and transmission of HIV.
Vaccines may enhance the body's immune defenses to prevent HIV infection.

SOURCE: Global HIV Prevention Working Group, 2006.

randomized, controlled trials found that male circumcision reduced the risk of heterosexually acquired HIV infection among men (Auvert et al., 2005; Bailey et al., 2007; Gray et al., 2007).

Yet the epidemic continues to take a terrible toll. With an estimated 2.5 million new HIV infections occurring globally each year (UNAIDS, 2007), efforts are urgently needed to better utilize existing effective HIV prevention strategies and to identify new ones. Because of the large number of women who become infected under circumstances not under their control, the need for additional women-controlled methods of prevention is vital.

Researchers are currently testing or have recently evaluated a variety of biomedical HIV prevention interventions in late-stage clinical trials.[1] These interventions include vaginal microbicides, pre-exposure prophylaxis (PrEP) using antiretroviral drugs, suppression of genital herpes (HSV-2) with acyclovir, cervical barriers, male circumcision, and vaccines[2] (see Box S-1). These strategies primarily target sexual transmission of HIV, which accounts for the vast majority of new infections, although PrEP and vaccines may also help prevent HIV infection in populations at risk through other avenues, such as injecting drug use.

Yet many recent trials have had disappointing results. Late-stage trials

[1]Late stage trials of behavioral interventions are also underway but are not the focus of this report.

[2]Vaccine trials are not covered in this report.

have failed to demonstrate a benefit in reducing HIV infection risk, including a phase 3 trial of the diaphragm and Replens gel (Padian, 2007) and two phase 3 trials of HSV-2 suppression with acyclovir (Watson-Jones et al., 2007; Celum et al., 2008). Two vaginal microbicide trials (of N-9 and cellulose sulfate [CS]) were halted because of evidence that they may have a harmful effect (Van Damme et al., 2002; Van Damme, 2007), and a separate trial of CS was stopped as a precautionary measure based on evidence from the other CS trial (Cates, 2007). Several PrEP trials were prematurely closed or canceled because of ethical concerns raised by advocates, governments, and community members. One PrEP trial and two microbicide trials in (Savvy in Ghana and Nigeria) did not have sufficient power to determine efficacy of the intervention (Peterson et al., 2007a,b). In addition, two trials of an HIV vaccine were recently stopped based on a lack of evidence of benefit and concerns that the vaccine might also increase HIV infection risk.[3]

It was in this context that the Bill & Melinda Gates Foundation asked the Institute of Medicine (IOM) in November 2006 to convene a committee to examine the methodological challenges facing late-stage biomedical HIV prevention trials (see Box S-2 for the Statement of Task). The sponsor clarified that the committee's review should cover late-stage nonvaccine biomedical HIV prevention trials, with a focus on microbicide and PrEP trials. The committee did not review vaccine or mother-to-child transmission trials. However, the committee did consider the role of risk reduction counseling in biomedical prevention trials (see Chapter 3).

This report recommends a number of ways to improve the design, monitoring, and analysis of late-stage randomized clinical trials that evaluate nonvaccine biomedical interventions to prevent HIV infection. The goals are to increase the chances that these trials will detect a beneficial intervention effect and better quantify the effect size, to more fully assess the effects of using an intervention on behavior and how this and product adherence might influence effectiveness in preventing HIV infection, and to reduce biases that can lead to false positive trial results. Another goal is to allow early termination of these trials, if warranted by their interim results or external information.

Below the committee highlights its key recommendations (see Box S-3 at the end of the chapter for a complete list). Where possible, the committee recommends investigators consider alternative trial designs which

[3]The STEP study was discontinued based on recommendations made by a Data and Safety Monitoring Board, which concluded that the vaccine neither prevented HIV infection nor reduced the amount of virus in those who became infected with HIV (http://www.avac.org/pdf/STEP_data_release.7Nov.pdf), and possibly might have increased the risk of HIV infection. Based on review of the STEP data, the Phambili study in South Africa was also stopped (http://www.hvtn.org/media/pr/PhambiliSAAVIstatement.pdf).

BOX S-2
Statement of Task

The Institute of Medicine (IOM) will convene a committee to examine methodological challenges in HIV prevention trials. The committee will prepare a report to improve the methodology, design, and conduct of HIV prevention trials, focusing on microbicide and pre-exposure prophylaxis (PrEP) trials, in order to increase their likelihood of success and to enable donors to optimally invest resources. The committee will undertake a study with the following tasks:

1. The committee will review select phase 2 and 3 HIV prevention trials in order to provide an assessment of best practices for site preparedness and estimation of incidence.
2. The committee will make recommendations regarding methodological best practices for microbicide and PrEP efficacy trials. Issues to be addressed include but are not limited to: loss of study power through lower-than-expected incidence and high pregnancy rates; other design considerations such as choice of endpoints and control groups; methods for monitoring the interim results of trials (including adjustments to trial size/duration); pooling of data from trials testing the same product; methods for improving adherence to study regimens and the quality of self-reported behavioral data; and optimizing retention of trial participants. The committee will also consider the ethical issues directly related to methodological issues under study, such as those that might arise during interim monitoring of trials.

This study will not address broader ethical issues such as adequacy of informed consent, compensation for trial-related adverse events, access to HIV treatment for seroconverters, and best practices for engaging community members.

could offer potential advantages over the traditional two-arm superiority design.

EFFICACY VERSUS EFFECTIVENESS TRIALS AND LACK OF A RELIABLE SURROGATE MARKER

An initial consideration when designing a clinical trial is whether the goal is to assess efficacy—whether a product works in a tightly controlled setting—or effectiveness: whether a product works in the real world. For HIV prevention trials, in which investigators can only partially control participants' adherence to the product regimen and risk-taking behavior, this distinction between efficacy and effectiveness can be substantial (Chapter 2).

Effectiveness trials have historically measured disease outcomes, such as clinical improvement or survival. In contrast, efficacy trials often use intermediate, or "surrogate," endpoints rather than clinical outcomes—if those surrogates are sufficiently predictive of the clinical endpoint, and if the effect of the interventions on the surrogate predicts its effect on the clinical response (see, for example, Prentice, 1989). This allows investigators to assess interventions in much less time and/or with fewer subjects. For example, HIV treatment trials use viral suppression as a surrogate marker for clinical progression.

Both efficacy and effectiveness trials for biomedical prevention interventions must use HIV infection as the primary endpoint, as no reliable marker is available to serve as a surrogate endpoint. This slows research considerably. Moreover, because HIV infection is a relatively uncommon event (compared with other disease outcomes), even in areas with high HIV incidence rates, short-term HIV prevention efficacy trials often need to enroll large numbers of subjects, just as longer-term effectiveness trials do.

Late-stage effectiveness trials that evaluate HIV infection offer the opportunity to evaluate potential surrogate markers for HIV infection, and the committee believes that this is a worthwhile secondary goal for these studies. The choice of candidate surrogates must be securely anchored in the knowledge of the pathophysiology of infection, and how the surrogate marker relates biologically to HIV infection.

In addition to increasing the time and resources needed to evaluate a new nonvaccine HIV intervention, the lack of a surrogate marker raises another complication. If an efficacy trial demonstrates a reduction in the short-term risk of becoming HIV infected, it may be difficult to ethically justify conducting a subsequent longer-term effectiveness trial that uses a placebo group, even if there remain uncertainties about the ability of the intervention to confer a longer-term protective effect. Similar ethical concerns may affect Phase 2B trials, which follow subjects for similar durations as phase 3 effectiveness trials, but aim to save funds by enrolling fewer subjects, and then conducting a longer trial only if the Phase 2B trial results are sufficiently promising.

This situation has led the committee to recommend the following:

- Although such research is challenging, priority should be given to identifying and validating surrogate endpoints for HIV infection for use in late-stage trials of nonvaccine biomedical interventions.
- Until a surrogate endpoint is identified, modified trial designs should be used to provide information on both the short- and longer-term benefits of an intervention. In particular, investigators should consider greater use

of two modified designs—an efficacy study with extended follow-up and a phase 3 trial with stopping rules for futility.

The first modified trial design can allow investigators to obtain some information on longer-term effectiveness in an efficacy trial whose main goal is to assess short-term efficacy. The second modified trial design can allow investigators to terminate a longer-term effectiveness trial if an interim analysis shows insufficient evidence of short-term efficacy. The rationale behind these designs is that an HIV prevention product that has efficacy might not be effective in a real-world setting, and that a product that does not have efficacy would likely not be effective in a real-world setting (Chapter 2).

ESTIMATING POWER AND SAMPLE SIZE

Several factors can adversely affect a trial's power if investigators do not adequately account for them when calculating a trial's sample size and duration before the study starts. These include HIV incidence, participant attrition, and the number of participants who discontinue using the study product because of pregnancy or other reasons. Although the committee emphasizes the need for accurate *a priori* estimates of these factors in calculating the required sample size for a late-stage trial, the committee also realizes that such estimates can be imprecise for a variety of reasons, including both random sampling error and systematic sources of bias. As a guard against inaccurate estimates, the committee recommends the use of "events-driven" trial designs, which follow participants until a prespecified number of subjects become HIV infected, rather than for a prespecified period of time (Chapter 2).

CHOICE OF CONTROL GROUP

In most randomized trials that test whether a new intervention is superior to the current standard, a double-blind design is highly desirable to help ensure an unbiased evaluation of the relative effect of the intervention. However, the use of a blinded control group in late-stage HIV prevention trials of a biomedical intervention can be disadvantageous if a participant's knowledge of his/her intervention would affect that person's risk-taking behavior. In that case, the relative effectiveness observed in the trial might not reflect that seen when the intervention is introduced into the community. Trials that include unblinded arms that more closely mimic the real world could potentially provide more useful results. The committee believes that both blinded and unblinded control arms can provide useful information on the effects of an intervention on risk-taking behavior and the risk of

HIV infection. Investigators and donors should consider conducting trials that include both control groups (Chapter 2).

In some instances, there can be value in identifying alternative interventions that are believed to have similar effectiveness to more standard interventions (such as risk reduction counseling and condom use), but which have other advantages. These advantages could include reduced cost, fewer side effects, or the personal preference of the user. For example, women who find negotiating condom use difficult might prefer microbicides or PrEP. For these settings, noninferiority (or "equivalence") designs, which aim to identify interventions of similar efficacy rather than aiming to show that one is superior, could be useful (Chapter 10).

EVALUATING AND INTEGRATING BEHAVIORAL RISK-REDUCTION STRATEGIES INTO BIOMEDICAL PREVENTION TRIALS

In discussions over the past decade about the ethics of vaccine trials, researchers, community representatives, human rights advocates, and ethicists reached broad agreement—based on several ethical principles, including beneficence, autonomy, and justice—that participants in clinical trials of HIV prevention interventions should receive risk-reduction counseling, and access to condoms and other means to reduce their risk of becoming infected with HIV (UNAIDS, 2000).

Despite this widespread agreement, considerable uncertainty remains about what the nature and intensity of such interventions should be. Uncertainty about the appropriate prevention standard in biomedical HIV prevention trials stems in part from ethical considerations. For example, should the standard risk-reduction intervention be the one shown to be most effective, regardless of cost or sustainability? The ethical uncertainties are compounded by the lack of definitive findings on the effectiveness of behavioral risk-reduction interventions in many of the resource-poor settings where biomedical HIV prevention trials are conducted. That knowledge gap reflects the fact that studies of behavioral risk-reduction interventions have largely been conducted in the United States, and from the difficulty of extrapolating behavioral risk-reduction interventions shown to be efficacious in one setting and population to settings with different populations, risk behaviors, and sociocultural norms. Finally, although some behavioral risk-reduction interventions have been shown to decrease self-reported risk behaviors, and a few have shown decreases in STIs, none to date have been shown to significantly reduce HIV infection rates.

Effective behavioral interventions increase the effectiveness of biomedical interventions and are valuable in their own right. Thus, in light of the uncertainties about the effectiveness of behavioral risk reduction interventions in settings where many biomedical trials are being planned, the committee believes that investigators designing biomedical intervention trials should also incorporate randomized comparisons of behavioral interventions into the trials whenever possible (Chapter 3). While doing so would increase the logistical complexity of a site's responsibilities, finding improved behavioral interventions for reducing HIV risk would provide lasting benefits to the community. One methodological approach to achieving this is to use a partially blinded factorial design (see Chapter 10). Such a design can assess both the relative efficacy of a new biomedical intervention and the comparative effectiveness of different behavioral interventions without an increase in sample size.

Other types of trial designs can also make an important impact on the HIV epidemic by attempting to identify ways of using a variety of partially effective interventions more efficiently. These include noninferiority trials, trials utilizing HIV discordant couples, and dynamic designs (which aim to evaluate strategies for using and modifying different combinations of behavioral and biomedical interventions over time) (see Chapter 10).

In addition, investigators should involve behavioral and social scientists, the community, and other stakeholders, in the early planning stages of a trial, to identify the most appropriate and sustainable behavioral risk-reduction interventions for use in that community, and to most efficiently plan their implementation. If a trial will adapt specific interventions shown to be effective in other settings, investigators should field-test the strategies during the planning of the trial, to ensure that they can be implemented as envisioned.

PREGNANCY

Many late-stage biomedical HIV prevention trials are conducted among sexually active women of reproductive age in areas with high fertility rates. Despite intensive counseling on family planning, and provision of or access to contraceptives, a large percentage of women enrolled in biomedical HIV prevention trials become pregnant. Trials testing new products and devices (or new indications of existing drugs) typically restrict pregnant women from enrolling and take women who become pregnant during the trial off the product, either permanently or for the duration of their pregnancy, based on concerns about its potential effect on the pregnant woman and the fetus. If a study discontinues product use among participants who become pregnant and no longer follows them for HIV infection, it can lose statistical power. That is, it will be less able to detect any effect of the biomedical intervention, because of the reduced number of women-years of observation. Failing to follow a woman who becomes pregnant for HIV infection can also bias the analyses of a trial's results. Thus the committee emphasizes the importance of continuing to follow pregnant women for HIV infection regardless of whether they discontinue use of the product, and using this information in the analysis of trial results. This will minimize bias, yet such discontinuations will reduce study power. Thus, the committee also recommends ways of calculating the required sample size and duration of a trial to adjust for the anticipated loss of power when an intervention will be discontinued upon pregnancy.

An even greater concern is that trials that discontinue product use in women who become pregnant typically do not provide any information about the safety and efficacy of the product for pregnant women and their fetuses. This is important because if the intervention were introduced into the community, many women would continue to use it after becoming pregnant, despite any cautions about its unknown effects on pregnancy. Assessing safety and efficacy in pregnant women after completing a trial is challenging. Because pregnancy is a common occurrence among women who would use a biomedical HIV intervention, it is critical that an overall product evaluation plan include specific and realistic plans for assessing the intervention's impact on pregnant women and their fetuses.

Because of the difficulty of obtaining such information after a successful trial, the committee finds that the current "one size fits all" policy of discontinuing product use upon pregnancy is unnecessary and potentially counterproductive. The committee suggests specific circumstances in which it might be ethical to allow trial participants who become pregnant to continue to use the study product.

The committee also recommends that trials collect and analyze information on pregnancy outcomes on all women who become pregnant during a trial, regardless of their study arm or whether they discontinue product use, as this will provide preliminary information on the possible effects of the product on the fetus.

The committee further recommends that investigators specify in advance of a late-stage clinical trial how they will establish product safety and efficacy for pregnant women and their fetuses, based on information collected before, during, and after the trial. Investigators should complete reproductive toxicity and pharmacokinetic studies in animals—ideally before the start of phase 2 clinical trials, but no later than the start of phase 2B/3 trials. The study protocol should specify how investigators will collect and monitor information on pregnancy outcomes during the trial, and indicate activities that they will undertake if the trial demonstrates that the product is effective in preventing HIV infection (Chapter 4).

PRODUCT ADHERENCE AND RISK-TAKING BEHAVIOR

The ultimate effectiveness of a biomedical intervention is mediated by how well participants adhere to the regimen for using it, and by their risk-taking behavior during the trial. For example, if a trial shows that a product provides an overall benefit, being able to relate the level of protection to the level of adherence could be very useful in interpreting the results. Similarly, if a trial fails to show a protective effect, it would be valuable to distinguish the extent to which the product was not biologically efficacious, participants did not use it as directed, or they engaged in more risky behavior because they thought the product was protecting them.

Although researchers agree on the importance of product adherence in both research and real-world settings, there is less agreement on how to define, measure, improve, and analyze it. Clinical trials often report adherence by a single number, such as the percentage of coital acts in which participants use a gel, or the percentage of pills they take over a given time period (Chesney, 2006). While simple, use of such measures to define adherence may mask crucial insights into adherence problems, product acceptability, and potential areas for intervention (Kerr et al., 2005; Berg and Arnsten, 2006). Because understanding these patterns can be critical to identifying and ameliorating problems with product use, investigators should develop, evaluate, and use adherence measures that can capture different adherence patterns over time.

Investigators can gather information on product adherence and risk behavior through a variety of measures. Indirect measures include self-reports, pill counts, electronic product monitoring, pharmacy refills, and biomarkers of product exposure and risk behavior. Direct measures of product adherence include pharmacokinetic studies (which measure drug levels or metabolites in subjects' blood or bodily fluids), and directly observed therapy. These measures vary substantially in expense, the effort required of participants and their partners, their perceived invasiveness, and their accuracy and reliability (Berg and Arnsten, 2006).

Several studies have found that using multiple measures to "triangulate" adherence levels and risk behaviors is helpful in reducing the error introduced by any particular method (Liu et al., 2001; Pool, 2006). The committee endorses this approach. Rather than collecting detailed information on all participants, investigators could collect such information on a well-chosen random sample, and collect less detailed information on other participants. While directly observed therapy (DOT) or modified DOT could be very useful for proof-of-concept trials, investigators should not use these approaches in effectiveness trials if that approach will not work in real-world practice because the trial results may be poor predictors of the effectiveness of an intervention.

Little empirical evidence exists on the effectiveness of strategies to improve adherence to nonvaccine biomedical HIV prevention interventions. Methods to improve the adherence of HIV-infected patients to antiretroviral therapy (ART) can inform efforts to enhance adherence in biomedical HIV prevention trials. Experience with ART may have particular relevance for medication-based HIV prevention strategies, such as PrEP or acyclovir for HSV-2 suppression. Recent meta-analyses of strategies to improve ART adherence found that such interventions can have a positive impact on adherence, but these analyses offer few prescriptive guidelines about the specific intervention components that are most effective for which populations in which circumstances. Thus the committee recommends that investigators undertake empirical evaluations of strategies to increase adherence during and after HIV prevention trials. These evaluations should be adequately powered, methodologically rigorous, socially and culturally relevant, and grounded in behavioral and social theories. Additional evidence is needed in particular about the effectiveness of adherence strategies in resource-poor areas where many biomedical HIV prevention trials are conducted. Investigators should analyze adherence and behavior as both outcomes in an HIV prevention trial and modifiers of the effect of the biomedical intervention on HIV infection risk. Investigators should also specify in the protocols how they plan to measure, monitor, improve, and analyze adherence (Chapter 5).

The availability of reliable information on product adherence and sexual behavior is critical to developing "dynamic" HIV intervention strategies consisting of decision rules for how to vary interventions for individuals over time according to measurements of adherence and behavior for each individual (Chapter 10). The committee believes that collecting reliable information on adherence and risk-taking behavior is critical to understanding how best to utilize biomedical HIV interventions.

RECRUITMENT AND RETENTION

Late-stage biomedical HIV prevention trials typically require investigators to enroll 1,000–4,000 participants at one or multiple sites, and to follow them for several years. A lower-than-expected rate of enrollment can result in an underpowered trial that fails to reveal an effective intervention, or delay the public health impact of a positive trial. Retention is equally critical because loss of trial participants to follow-up reduces study power and can lead to biased results. Despite the critical threat that inadequate recruitment and retention pose to trial validity, there is very little empirical evidence about the effectiveness of alternative recruitment and retention strategies (Lovato et al., 1997; Robinson et al., 2007; Villacorta et al.,

2007). Most of the strategies identified in the literature are based on practical "lessons learned" from investigators in the field.

Investigators and sponsors should anticipate that maintaining timely accrual and high retention rates will be labor intensive and costly throughout a trial. However, these investments are necessary to maintain internal and external validity. Successful recruitment and retention will require the use of multiple strategies and incentives, the ability to rapidly change procedures when they are not working, and persistence and innovation among staff.

Because of the loss in study power that can result from inadequate accrual and because the potential biases resulting from losses to follow-up cannot be avoided simply by increasing sample size, investigators should place a high priority on developing effective strategies to achieve accrual rate goals and to minimize losses to follow-up. To this end, the committee recommends that investigators conduct pretrial research to assess the community's and individuals' interest in the trial (including motivations and barriers to participating), to pilot test recruitment and retention strategies and procedures, and to set realistic timeline and resource needs for the enrollment period and retention. The committee also recommends that investigators develop a detailed and multifaceted plan for retaining enrolled participants before beginning a study, for monitoring retention during the conduct of the trial if retention rates are lower than anticipated. Investigators should collect detailed tracking information on all participants early in the process and should develop strategies to engage, train, and reward staff for building trust and accountability with participants and within the community and for meeting recruitment and retention targets.

SITE PREPAREDNESS

The HIV prevention research agenda requires access to large study populations in settings with the capacity to conduct a wide range of clinical trials. The regions with the greatest need for HIV prevention efforts are often those with limited medical and research infrastructure. When developing the research protocol for a late-stage trial, and when selecting and preparing a trial site, external investigators should develop equal partnerships with local investigators and to involve community representatives in developing the protocol and throughout the trial. Investigators also may need to conduct extensive pretrial research at the study sites, with populations similar to those that the main trial will enroll, to ensure that the interventions are culturally relevant, and to estimate the anticipated rates of HIV infection, attrition, pregnancy, and adherence for the trial site. Donors need to invest adequate resources to developing the infrastructure for trial sites, especially in terms of human resources (Chapter 7).

The time and resources required to build a relationship with local investigators and local communities, conduct pretrial research, and establish the infrastructure needed to conduct a late-stage trial are considerable. However, such efforts are critical to ensuring high-quality research and the ultimate value to the community of trial results. Investigators and donors establishing new research sites should work with the community to create a sustainability plan that will allow a site to continue to perform research after a trial closes, to enable the community to reap long-term benefit.

ESTIMATING HIV INCIDENCE

One of the most important aspects of planning a late-stage HIV prevention trial is accurately estimating the HIV incidence rate in the trial population. Because studies are powered based on the number of HIV infections investigators expect to occur among participants during the trial, modest overestimates of HIV incidence can substantially reduce the power of a trial to detect an important intervention effect. Overestimates of HIV incidence have led to premature closure of several recent trials.

Three general approaches are available for estimating HIV incidence, each with its strengths and weaknesses: longitudinal cohort studies, laboratory biomarkers to identify recent infections, and mathematical modeling of serial prevalence data (Chapter 8). The committee finds that direct longitudinal follow-up of individuals, through cohort studies, provides the most unbiased estimate of HIV incidence, compared with the indirect approaches currently available. However, longitudinal cohort studies have several drawbacks including the time and expense to conduct them, and the lack of precision in the resulting estimates of HIV incidence rates.

Thus the committee recommends that investigators rely on at least one direct longitudinal follow-up study of individuals in the trial setting to estimate HIV incidence, and that they use at least one other independent source to corroborate that estimate. The committee further emphasizes that the development of a reliable, accurate biomarker-based test for recent HIV infection that can be run with blood from a single draw would be a major advance in estimating incidence. Donors and appropriate U.S. and international agencies should make such research a high priority. While current approaches, based on the Serologic Testing Algorithm for Determining HIV Seroconversion (STAHRS) or BED capture enzyme immunoassay (BED-CEIA), are promising, further validation studies are needed to address concerns that these tests may produce biased estimates of HIV incidence. As a result, the committee recommends that investigators should not now rely solely on these biomarker assays of recent infection to estimate HIV incidence for the purpose of designing a prevention trial.

INTERIM MONITORING AND ANALYSIS OF TRIAL RESULTS

Because late-stage HIV prevention trials can require several years to complete, it is ethically important and scientifically valuable to monitor a trial's evolving results. An independent data monitoring committee (DMC) typically performs such monitoring. The DMC evaluates (1) whether the key assumptions underlying the trial's size and duration are consistent with the evolving data, (2) whether interim results on the efficacy of the intervention warrant early termination of the trial, (3) whether any unanticipated safety concerns have arisen, and (4) whether the emergence of any external information requires modifying or terminating the trial.

The committee makes several recommendations regarding the role of DMCs in HIV prevention trials (Chapter 5). First, because of differing social and cultural norms, it is important that the composition of DMCs include appropriate expertise and representation from participating countries and regions, and that they meet often enough to ensure that the trial is maintaining the best interests of the participants. Second, DMCs should always have the option of unblinding the interim results of a trial if, for any reason, the DMC believes that doing so is in the best interests of the trial participants. Third, in addition to criteria for a DMC recommendation to terminate a trial based on safety concerns or early indications that the intervention is effective, late-stage HIV prevention trials should include criteria for termination owing to futility—that is, on the grounds that, if continued, there would be a very small chance of demonstrating benefit.

Finally, the committee believes that researchers should develop methodologies to enable DMCs of simultaneous HIV prevention trials with common intervention arms—that is, those that evaluate the same intervention—to share information on safety. Although concurrent trials provide a valuable opportunity to learn more about a product's safety, the valid and effective use of such information poses a number of challenges.

The committee discusses methods used to analyze the results of prevention trials using HIV infection as the primary efficacy endpoint, along with their limitations. A complication in such trials results from the fact that HIV infection is a silent event: at best, investigators can determine only a time interval in which an individual's infection occurred. The tests used to diagnose HIV infection are also imperfect, leading to the possibility that trials might unknowingly enroll individuals already infected and might not detect enrollees who become infected during the trial.

These features have implications for the analysis of trial results. These include the post hoc exclusion of enrollees who are suspected of having been HIV infected at enrollment, the importance of designing follow-up so infected subjects in each study arm have equal likelihood of being detected at each clinic visit, and the potential biases from censoring analyses of time to HIV infection upon product discontinuation owing to pregnancy or other reasons (Chapter 9).

In sum, the committee concludes that alternative trial designs, more extensive site preparation, and careful monitoring and analysis of trial results are key to evaluating prevention interventions and determining which of them can exert the greatest possible long-term impact on the HIV epidemic.

BOX S-3
Findings and Recommendations

Chapter 2
Basic Design Features: Size, Duration, and Type of Trials, and Choice of Control Group

Recommendation 2-1: Investigators should take steps to develop accurate a priori estimates of rates of participant accrual, HIV incidence, product discontinuation, and participant retention, and incorporate those into the sample size calculations. As a guard against inaccurate estimates, investigators should consider using an "events-driven" approach, by analyzing study results when the prespecified number of enrolled subjects has become HIV infected, rather than at prespecified calendar times.

Recommendation 2-2: Until validated surrogate endpoint(s) for HIV infection or product activity is (are) identified, investigators should use modified trial designs that can provide information on both the short- and long-term benefits of an intervention.

Recommendation 2-3: Sponsors, investigators, and regulatory agencies should consider using both blinded and unblinded control groups in future trials to more fully understand the effects of the intervention on HIV infection risk and behavior.

Chapter 3
Design Considerations: Risk-Reduction Counseling

Recommendation 3-1: Given the lack of evidence on the effectiveness of behavioral risk-reduction interventions in settings where many HIV biomedical trials are planned, investigators planning such trials should incorporate randomized comparisons of behavioral risk-reduction interventions into their designs whenever possible.

Recommendation 3-2: Donors and investigators should involve behavioral and social scientists in the early planning stages of a trial, to identify the most appropriate behavioral risk reduction interventions, and to efficiently plan their implementation during the trial.

Recommendation 3-3: Investigators planning to test behavioral risk-reduction interventions as part of a late-stage biomedical HIV prevention trial should consult with the community, governments, donors, and other stakeholders about the cost and sustainability of those interventions in the community.

Recommendation 3-4: If a trial will adapt specific behavioral interventions shown to be effective in other settings, investigators should field-test the strategies during the planning of the trial, to ensure that they can be implemented as envisioned.

Continued

BOX S-3 Continued

Chapter 4
Design Considerations: Pregnancy

Recommendation 4-1: Investigators should take several steps to minimize the loss of study power and potential biases in results that can occur when women become pregnant during a trial:

- Before the start of the trial, investigators should attempt to accurately estimate the rate of pregnancy that will occur during participant follow-up, and use these estimates in calculating sample size and trial duration.
- Data monitoring committees should monitor actual pregnancy rates during the trial, and recommend appropriate adjustments to sample size and trial duration if these rates exceed expectations.
- Investigators should continue to follow all women who become pregnant for HIV infection, regardless of whether they discontinue the study product.

Recommendation 4-2: Although the current policy of excluding pregnant women from biomedical HIV prevention and other trials stems from an historically protectionist orientation adopted by regulators, the principles of research ethics neither mandate nor preclude use of the product by pregnant women. Because any approved product subsequently would likely be used by many women who become pregnant, sponsors and investigators of a biomedical intervention should specify in advance of any late-stage trial how they will establish its safety and efficacy for pregnant women and their fetuses, based on information collected both during and after clinical trials. At a minimum, investigators should take the following steps to collect such information.

- Investigators should conduct appropriate preclinical tests in animals, including reproductive toxicity and pharmacokinetic studies, to allow a more informed decision on whether to continue product use in pregnant women participating in late-stage trials. These tests would ideally be completed before the product or device enters phase 2 testing, but should be completed no later than phase 3 testing.
- Investigators should routinely collect and analyze information about birth outcomes from women who become pregnant during a trial, regardless of whether a product is discontinued upon detection of pregnancy.
- In trials that discontinue the use of a product by women who become pregnant, investigators should allow women who are no longer pregnant to have the choice of resuming the study medication.
- Investigators should conduct observational or randomized studies in pregnant women in the postapproval, premarketing, and posttrial periods, to provide additional information on the safety and efficacy of biomedical HIV prevention interventions for pregnant women.

Recommendation 4-3: Regulators, sponsors, and investigators should evaluate the strength of the evidence on the beneficial and harmful effects to both a preg-

BOX S-3 Continued

nant woman and her fetus on a product-by-product basis, and evaluate whether there are circumstances in which women who become pregnant can continue to receive the study product, based on what is known about its benefits and risks.

Recommendation 4-4: Trials using products with favorable risk-benefit profiles, but which are nonetheless discontinued upon pregnancy, should monitor pregnancy outcomes during the interim analysis of trial results, as this information might alter the risk-benefit profile to allow continuation of the product during pregnancy. Such trials might be modified to thereafter allow women who become pregnant to remain on product or offer them the opportunity to be randomized to remain on product versus to discontinue product.

Recommendation 4-5: Regulatory agencies and institutional review boards (IRBs) should receive periodic safety updates during a trial that include experience with the product during pregnancy. When interim analyses provide evidence of fetal safety and potential benefit to women, regulators and IRBs should consider allowing women to stay on product while pregnant.

Chapter 5
Design Considerations: Adherence

Recommendation 5-1: Because simple measures of adherence can mask substantially different underlying adherence problems, investigators should develop and use adherence measures that can capture different adherence patterns over time.

Recommendation 5-2: In light of the uncertainty about the accuracy of various methods for collecting data on adherence and risk behavior, investigators of biomedical HIV prevention trials should strive to use multiple types of measures to triangulate adherence estimates. Rather than collecting detailed information on all participants, investigators could collect more detailed information on a well-chosen random sample, and collect less detailed information on all participants.

Recommendation 5-3: Although directly observed therapy (DOT) or modified DOT could be very useful in proof-of-concept trials, investigators should not use these methods in effectiveness trials if that approach will not be used in real-world practice, because the trial results may then be poor predictors of the effectiveness of the interventions.

Recommendation 5-4: Donors should fund and investigators should undertake empirical evaluations of strategies to increase adherence to biomedical HIV prevention products during and after a clinical trial. These evaluations should be adequately powered, methodologically rigorous, socially and culturally relevant, grounded in behavioral and social science theories, and conducted in the regions where the strategies will be utilized.

Continued

BOX S-3 Continued

Recommendation 5-5: Investigators should specify in the study protocol detailed plans for monitoring, measuring, and analyzing adherence data, and steps they will take to improve adherence if it is poorer than anticipated.

Recommendation 5-6: Investigators should provide data on product adherence and risk behavior results to the data monitoring committee, as this information may influence the committee's views of the relative efficacy and safety of the study arms, and the feasibility of the study.

Recommendation 5-7: Investigators should analyze adherence and behavior as both outcomes in an HIV prevention trial and modifiers of the effect of the biomedical intervention on HIV infection risk.

Recommendation 5-8: Investigators should analyze the potential impact of adherence by doing the following:

- Perform a stratified analysis when adherence appears similar between study arms. Such analyses aim to provide unbiased comparisons of subpopulations across study arms.
- Postulate causal models and performing randomization-based analyses.
- Perform matched case-control adherence analyses involving subjects who become HIV infected.

Chapter 6
Design Considerations: Recruitment and Retention

Recommendation 6-1: Investigators should conduct pretrial research to assess the community and individuals' interest in the trial, to pilot test recruitment and retention strategies, and to set a realistic timeline and resource needs for the enrollment period and for retention.

Recommendation 6-2: Because of the loss in study power that can result from inadequate accrual and because the potential biases resulting from losses to follow-up cannot be avoided simply by increasing sample size, investigators should place a high priority on developing effective strategies to achieve accrual rate goals and to minimize losses to follow-up. Specifically, investigators should do the following:

- Develop a detailed and multifaceted plan for retaining enrolled participants before beginning a study for systematically and frequently monitoring the results, and for modifying the plan if strategies are not working.
- Collect as much detailed tracking information as possible on participants.
- Develop systems to engage, train, and reward staff for building trust and accountability with participants and within the community, and for meeting recruitment and retention targets.

Recommendation 6-3: Funders and investigators should include evaluations of the effectiveness of recruitment and retention strategies in future research plans.

BOX S-3 Continued

Chapter 7
Site Preparedness

Recommendation 7-1: Donors and investigators should invest in the human capacity and physical infrastructure needed to ensure successful HIV prevention trials in resource-poor settings. These efforts should include a comprehensive and realistic assessment of how to prepare a site, a training plan for staff, and a mentoring plan for inexperienced investigators.

Recommendation 7-2: If the regulatory infrastructure of a planned study site is insufficient, study sponsors, funding agencies, research organizations, and other stakeholders should assist local IRBs in developing the ability to provide comprehensive and timely oversight of clinical trials according to international standards.

Recommendation 7-3: Sponsors and investigators from outside the trial region should solicit meaningful input from local investigators and community representatives as they develop the study protocol, and throughout the trial. The trial should itself promote equal partnerships between outside and local investigators.

Recommendation 7-4: Donors should fund and investigators should undertake extensive pretrial research to develop accurate estimates of HIV incidence, participant accrual, retention, and pregnancy rates, and to develop and evaluate logistical and regulatory processes to be used during the trial.

Recommendation 7-5: When considering a new trial site that requires extensive preparation, investigators, sponsors, and community leaders should discuss and carefully consider how the site could be sustained after completion of the trial.

Recommendation 7-6: Given limited funding and the extensive investment required to prepare research sites, donors and investigators should explore creative and flexible collaborations with HIV and non-HIV trial networks, health organizations, and local research units that have access to suitable study populations or existing research infrastructure, with cost sharing benefiting both partners.

Chapter 8
Estimating HIV Incidence

Recommendation 8-1: Investigators should base their estimate of HIV incidence on at least one source of data from the direct longitudinal follow-up of individuals in the trial setting. Given the importance of accurate estimates and the inherent uncertainties of any single approach, the direct estimate of HIV incidence should be corroborated by at least one other source.

Recommendation 8-2: Donors and appropriate U.S. and international agencies should make development of a reliable, accurate biomarker-based test for recent

Continued

BOX S-3 Continued

HIV infection that can be run with blood from a single draw a high priority. They should provide the necessary funding and laboratory resources to conduct a substantial cross-sectional screening program. This will require recruiting subjects from countries with low-level, concentrated, and generalized epidemics during the preseroconversion period and following them for several years.

Recommendation 8-3: Although further validation studies are being conducted to examine concerns that the STAHRS and BED tests may produce biased estimates of HIV incidence, investigators should not rely solely at this time on these or other biomarker assays of recent infection to estimate HIV incidence for the specific purpose of designing a prevention trial.

Chapter 9
Performing Interim Monitoring and Analyzing Trial Results

Recommendation 9-1: The data monitoring committees of trials with sponsors and scientific leaders from outside the host countries should include multiple representatives from those countries. These members—who should compose at least one-third of the committee—should include scientists, ethicists, and lay people familiar with the community and local norms.

Recommendation 9-2: The data monitoring committees for HIV prevention trials should always have the option of unblinding interim results if they believe that doing so might lead them to recommend that the trial be modified or terminated, or lead to other actions that are in the best interests of the trial participants. In particular, when the efficacy data show nonsignificant trends favoring one of the blinded arms, a DMC should unblind itself as this might reflect an intervention that may be harming patients.

Recommendation 9-3: Investigators should clearly describe in the study protocol the basis and criteria for any recommendation by the data monitoring committee to modify a trial's size or duration. If such changes are implemented, the protocol should also specify how investigators should evaluate the trial results.

Recommendation 9-4: For effectiveness trials, guidelines for stopping HIV prevention trials based on positive interim results should require evidence of a sustained impact on cumulative HIV incidence.

Recommendation 9-5: Investigators, donors, and regulatory agencies should encourage research on how to combine safety information from concurrent trials of similar products, including the scientific advantages and disadvantages of sharing information, the timing and logistics of doing so, ethical concerns (such as how such information might affect the informed-consent process), and how to report the results from such trials.

BOX S-3 Continued

Recommendation 9-6: Investigators should base their primary analysis of the efficacy of an intervention on all randomized subjects. Secondary sensitivity analyses that exclude subjects believed to have been HIV infected when they were randomized can be useful. However, investigators should not substitute such analyses for the primary analysis, unless such exclusions (and nonexclusions) can confidently be made without error.

Recommendation 9-7: Investigators of trials evaluating an intervention that is believed to have a delayed impact may find it efficient to exclude people found to be HIV infected after randomization but before a given follow-up time. If so, the trial protocol should specify and justify such an approach, and investigators should use it only if follow-up of subjects and assessment and confirmation of HIV infection during this period is identical in all study arms. Investigators should undertake secondary analyses based on all randomized subjects.

Recommendation 9-8: In all trials, investigators should continue to follow women who become pregnant for HIV infection, regardless of whether they discontinue their study intervention. In addition, intention-to-treat analyses should be the primary basis for comparing intervention groups with respect to HIV infection and other efficacy endpoints. Investigators can include as-treated analyses as secondary analyses, but should interpret them cautiously, because of the possibility that such discontinuations represent a type of informative censoring.

Chapter 10
Alternative Trial Designs

Recommendation 10-1: Investigators planning late-stage randomized trials of biomedical interventions are encouraged to utilize partially blinded factorial designs in order to also evaluate the relative effectiveness of different behavioral intervention strategies. Factorial designs can provide valuable information about both types of interventions with the same sample size as a trial evaluating only the biomedical intervention.

Recommendation 10-2: When feasible and consistent with the scientific goals of a late-stage HIV prevention trial, investigators are encouraged to consider discordant couple designs because of their advantages over designs in which the actual HIV exposures of participants are unknown.

Recommendation 10-3: Investigators should consider the potential merits of using noninferiority, cluster randomization, and dynamic designs in future biomedical HIV prevention trials.

REFERENCES

Auerbach, J. D., R. J. Hayes, and S. M. Kandathil. 2006. Overview of effective and promising interventions to prevent HIV infection. *World Health Organization Technical Report Series* 938:43-78; discussion 317-341.

Auvert, B., D. Taljaard, E. Lagarde, J. Sobngwi-Tambekou, R. Sitta, and A. Puren. 2005. Randomized, controlled intervention trial of male circumcision for reduction of HIV infection risk: The ANRS1265 trial. *PLoS Medicine* 2(11):e298.

Bailey, R. C., S. Moses, C. B. Parker, K. Agot, I. Maclean, J. N. Krieger, C. F. Williams, R. T. Campbell, and J. O. Ndinya-Achola. 2007. Male circumcision for HIV prevention in young men in Kisumu, Kenya: A randomised controlled trial. *Lancet* 369(9562):643-656.

Berg, K. M., and J. H. Arnsten. 2006. Practical and conceptual challenges in measuring antiretroviral adherence. *Journal of Acquired Immune Deficiency Syndromes* 43(Suppl 1): S79-S87.

Bulterys, M., M. G. Fowler, K. K. Van Rompay, and A. P. Kourtis. 2004. Prevention of mother-to-child transmission of HIV-1 through breast-feeding: Past, present, and future. *Journal of Infectious Diseases* 189(12):2149-2153.

Cates, W. 2007. *HIV prevention research: The optimist's view.* Paper presented at the Fourth International AIDS Society Conference on HIV Pathogenesis, Treatment, and Prevention, Sydney, Australia.

Celum, C., A. Wald, J. Hughes, J. Sanchez, S. Reid, S. Delaney-Moretlwe, F. M. Cowan, J. Fuchs, B. Koblin, L. Corey, and HPTN-039. 2008. *HSV-2 suppressive therapy for prevention of HIV acquisition: Results of HPTN 039.* Paper presented at Conference on Retroviruses and Opportunistic Infections, Boston, Massachusetts.

Chesney, M. A. 2006. The elusive gold standard. Future perspectives for HIV adherence assessment and intervention. *Journal of Acquired Immune Deficiency Syndromes* 43(Suppl 1):S149-S155.

Chesney, M. A., D. B. Chambers, and J. O. Kahn. 1997. Risk behavior for HIV infection in participants in preventive HIV vaccine trials: A cautionary note. *Journal of Acquired Immune Deficiency Syndromes and Human Retrovirology* 16(4):266-271.

Global HIV Prevention Working Group. 2006. *New approaches to HIV prevention: Accelerating research and ensuring future access.* Prepared for the Bill & Melinda Gates Foundation and the Kaiser Family Foundation.

Gray, R. H., G. Kigozi, D. Serwadda, F. Makumbi, S. Watya, F. Nalugoda, N. Kiwanuka, L. H. Moulton, M. A. Chaudhary, M. Z. Chen, N. K. Sewankambo, F. Wabwire-Mangen, M. C. Bacon, C. F. Williams, P. Opendi, S. J. Reynolds, O. Laeyendecker, T. C. Quinn, and M. J. Wawer. 2007. Male circumcision for HIV prevention in men in Rakai, Uganda: A randomised trial. *Lancet* 369(9562):657-666.

International Perinatal HIV Group. 1999. The mode of delivery and the risk of vertical transmission of human immunodeficiency virus type 1—a meta-analysis of 15 prospective cohort studies. *New England Journal of Medicine* 340(13):977-987.

IOM (Institute of Medicine). 1995. *HIV and the blood supply.* Washington, DC: National Academy Press.

IOM (Institute of Medicine). 2007. *Preventing HIV infection among injecting drug users in high-risk countries: An assessment of the evidence.* Washington, DC: The National Academies Press.

Kajubi, P., M. R. Kamya, S. Kamya, S. Chen, W. McFarland, and N. Hearst. 2005. Increasing condom use without reducing HIV risk: Results of a controlled community trial in Uganda. *Journal of Acquired Immune Deficiency Syndromes* 40(1):77-82.

Kerr, T., J. Walsh, E. Lloyd-Smith, and E. Wood. 2005. Measuring adherence to highly active antiretroviral therapy: Implications for research and practice. *Current HIV/AIDS Reports* 2(4):200-205.

Liu, H., C. E. Golin, L. G. Miller, R. D. Hays, C. K. Beck, S. Sanandaji, J. Christian, T. Maldonado, D. Duran, A. H. Kaplan, and N. S. Wenger. 2001. A comparison study of multiple measures of adherence to HIV protease inhibitors. *Annals of Internal Medicine* 134(10):968-977.

Lovato, L. C., K. Hill, S. Hertert, D. B. Hunninghake, and J. L. Probstfield. 1997. Recruitment for controlled clinical trials: Literature summary and annotated bibliography. *Controlled Clinical Trials* 18(4):328-352.

McKenzie, M., J. P. Tulsky, H. L. Long, M. Chesney and A. Moss. 1999. Tracking and follow-up of marginalized populations: A review. *Journal of Health Care for the Poor and Underserved* 10(4):409-429.

Peterson, L., D. Taylor, R. Roddy, G. Belai, P. Phillips, K. Nanda, R. Grant, E. E. K. Clarke, A. S. Doh, R. Ridzon, H. S. Jaffe, and W. Cates. 2007a. Tenofovir disoproxil fumarate for prevention of HIV infection in women: A phase 2, double-blind, randomized, placebo-controlled trial. *PLoS Clinical Trials* 2(5).

Peterson, L., K. Nanda, B. K. Opoku, W. K. Ampofo, M. Owusu-Amoako, A. Y. Boakye, W. Rountree, A. Troxler, R. Dominik, R. Roddy, and L. Dorflinger. 2007b. Savvy(R) (C31g) gel for prevention of HIV infection in women: A phase 3, double-blind, randomized, placebo-controlled trial in Ghana. *PLoS ONE* 2(12):e1312.

Pool, R. 2006. *PC64 Innovative uses of multi-method triangulation to increase the accuracy of adherence and sexual behaviour data in the MDP301 trial.* Paper presented at the Microbicides 2006 conference, Cape Town, South Africa.

Prentice, R. L. 1989. Surrogate endpoints in clinical trials: Definition and operational criteria. *Statistics in Medicine* 8(4):431-440.

Robinson, K. A., C. R. Dennison, D. M. Wayman, P. J. Pronovost, and D. M. Needham. 2007. Systematic review identifies number of strategies important for retaining study participants. *Journal of Clinical Epidemiology* 60(8):757-765.

UNAIDS. 2000. *Ethical considerations in HIV preventive vaccine research.* Geneva, Switzerland: UNAIDS.

UNAIDS. 2007. *2007 AIDS Epidemic Update.* Geneva, Switzerland: UNAIDS.

Van Damme, L. 2007. *Phase 3 trial of 6% cellulose sulfate (CS) gel for the prevention of HIV transmission.* Paper read at the Fourth International AIDS Society Conference on HIV Pathogenesis, Treatment and Prevention, Sydney, Australia.

Van Damme, L., G. Ramjee, M. Alary, B. Vuylsteke, V. Chandeying, H. Rees, P. Sirivongrangson, L. Mukenge-Tshibaka, V. Ettiegne-Traore, C. Uaheowitchai, S. S. Karim, B. Masse, J. Perriens, and M. Laga. 2002. Effectiveness of col-1492, a nonoxynol-9 vaginal gel, on HIV-1 transmission in female sex workers: A randomised controlled trial. *Lancet* 360(9338):971-977.

Villacorta, V., S. Kegeles, J. Galea, K. A. Konda, J. P. Cuba, C. F. Palacios, and T. J. Coates. 2007. Innovative approaches to cohort retention in a community-based HIV/STI prevention trial for socially marginalized Peruvian young adults. *Clinical Trials* 4(1):32-41.

Watson-Jones, D., M. Rusizoka, H. Weiss, K. Mugeye, K. Baisley, J. Changalucha, D. Everett, C. Tanton, T. Clayton, D. Ross, and R. Hayes. 2007. *Impact of HSV-2 suppressive therapy on HIV incidence in HSV-2 seropositive women: A randomised controlled trial in Tanzania.* Paper read at Fourth International AIDS Society Conference on HIV Pathogenesis, Treatment and Prevention, Sydney, Australia.

Weller, S., and K. Davis. 2002. Condom effectiveness in reducing heterosexual HIV transmission. *Cochrane Database System Review* (1):CD003255.

Introduction

If the world is to successfully address the HIV epidemic, preventing new infections will be as important as treating those who are infected (see Box I-1). However, in the foreseeable future, there will be no single prevention product ("magic bullet") that will prevent the spread of HIV. Thus the need to identify a range of effective, practical, and affordable preventive strategies, and to determine how best to combine them, is critical. A number of promising new HIV prevention strategies and products are currently being tested in late-stage clinical trials. Yet HIV prevention trials face a myriad of methodological challenges which slow the pace of research and limit the ability to identify and fully evaluate effective biomedical interventions.

Key methodological challenges include the lack of a surrogate marker for HIV infection, the choice of a control group and type of trial design, the loss of study power due to lower than expected incidence rates and higher than expected pregnancy rates, high rates of participant attrition, suboptimal adherence among participants to the product being tested, and challenges in measuring participants' adherence to the product and risk behavior.

Although not discussed in this report, trials also face major ethical and regulatory challenges. Key ethical concerns include ensuring access to antiretroviral treatment for individuals who become infected during a trial, adequate informed consent, and compensation to participants for adverse medical events related to the trial. Another important concern is ensuring adequate engagement of community members prior to, during, and after the trial. Regulatory hurdles—such as the limited capacity of developing

BOX I-1
The Global HIV Epidemic

In 2007, an estimated 2.5 million people became infected with HIV, 33.2 million individuals were living with HIV, and 2.1 million people died from AIDS (UNAIDS, 2007). Sub-Saharan Africa continues to bear the largest burden of the HIV epidemic, accounting for an estimated 68 percent of new infections, 68 percent of adults and 90 percent of children living with HIV worldwide, and 76 percent of all deaths from AIDS (UNAIDS, 2007).

Unprotected vaginal intercourse accounts for the vast majority of new infections worldwide (UNAIDS, 2006). The HIV epidemic in many parts of Asia and Eastern Europe, which is also growing rapidly in some countries, is spreading from more isolated drug user networks and female sex workers to their sexual partners and the broader population (UNAIDS, 2006). Latin and North American countries have recorded high levels of HIV infection among men who have sex with men (UNAIDS, 2006).

In many countries, women—especially young women—are disproportionately affected by HIV. The problem is particularly acute in some parts of sub-Saharan Africa, where women ages 15-24 are up to three times more likely to be infected than men of the same age (UNAIDS, 2006). UNAIDS estimates that women account for about half of the people living with HIV worldwide, and 60 percent of those living with HIV in Africa (UNAIDS, 2007).

Several factors contribute to this disparity. Women are more physiologically vulnerable to acquisition of HIV infection than men. Women also face numerous social, economic, and legal disadvantages that interfere with their ability to protect themselves against HIV infection. And because of gender norms and power imbalances, women are often unable to negotiate the use of condoms with their male partners (UNAIDS, 2006). Women who have had violent or controlling male partners also may be at increased risk for infection (Maman et al., 2000; Dunkle et al., 2004; Jewkes et al., 2006). Thus, the need for female-controlled methods of preventing HIV infection is urgent.

countries to approve products, and complex requirements for licensing products with multiple active compounds—further complicate biomedical prevention trials.

These challenges underscore the need for well-conceived and conducted late-stage intervention trials of biomedical HIV preventive interventions, using the best available methodologies, that can identify different (combinations of) interventions for different populations.

CHARGE TO THE COMMITTEE

The Bill & Melinda Gates Foundation requested in November 2006 that the Institute of Medicine (IOM) convene a committee to examine the methodological challenges entailed in HIV prevention trials. The committee was asked to report on how to improve the methodology, design, and conduct of biomedical HIV prevention trials—focusing on those involving microbicides and PrEP—to increase the likelihood of success, and to enable donors to invest their resources optimally. The foundation's charge to the committee included several specific tasks:

1. The committee will review select phase 2 and 3 HIV prevention trials in order to provide an assessment of best practices for site preparedness and estimation of incidence.
2. The committee will make recommendations regarding methodological best practices for microbicide and PrEP efficacy trials. Issues to be addressed include but are not limited to

- loss of study power through lower-than-expected incidence and high pregnancy rates,
- other design considerations such as choice of endpoints and control groups,
- methods for monitoring the interim results of trials (including adjustments to trial size and duration),
- pooling of data from trials testing the same product,
- methods for improving adherence to study regimens and the quality of self-reported behavioral data, and
- optimizing retention of trial participants.

The Gates Foundation also asked the committee to consider the ethical challenges directly related to these methodological issues, such as those that might arise during interim monitoring of trials. These challenges include whether to modify or stop a trial if information from another trial shows that the intervention is either working or not working. Other ethical concerns—including the adequacy of informed consent, compensation for participants who experience trial-related adverse events, access to treatment for people who become HIV infected during the trial, and best practices for fully engaging community members in trials conducted in their areas—were explicitly excluded from the committee's statement of task (Box I-2).

SCOPE OF WORK

This report recommends ways to improve the design, monitoring, and analysis of clinical trials evaluating nonvaccine biomedical interventions to prevent HIV infection, so that these trials can increase the chances of detecting and quantifying a beneficial intervention effect, more fully assess the efficacy and effectiveness of interventions, reduce biases that can lead

BOX I-2
Statement of Task

The Institute of Medicine (IOM) will convene a committee to examine methodological challenges in HIV prevention trials. The committee will prepare a report to improve the methodology, design, and conduct of HIV prevention trials, focusing on microbicide and pre-exposure prophylaxis (PrEP) trials, in order to increase their likelihood of success and to enable donors to optimally invest resources. The committee will undertake a study with the following tasks:

1. The committee will review select phase 2 and 3 HIV prevention trials in order to provide an assessment of best practices for site preparedness and estimation of incidence.
2. The committee will make recommendations regarding methodological best practices for microbicide and PrEP efficacy trials. Issues to be addressed include but are not limited to loss of study power through lower-than-expected incidence and high pregnancy rates, other design considerations such as choice of endpoints and control groups, methods for monitoring the interim results of trials (including adjustments to trial size/duration), pooling of data from trials testing the same product, methods for improving adherence to study regimens and the quality of self-reported behavioral data, and optimizing retention of trial participants. The committee will also consider the ethical issues directly related to methodological issues under study, such as those that might arise during interim monitoring of trials.

This study will not address broader ethical issues such as adequacy of informed consent, compensation for trial-related adverse events, access to HIV treatment for seroconverters, and best practices for engaging community members.

to false positive trial results, and be terminated early if warranted by their interim results or external information.

At the committee's first workshop, the Gates Foundation clarified that its review should focus on late-stage microbicide and PrEP trials, although where appropriate, the committee could consider lessons that might be learned from other late-stage biomedical trials. Given the broad scope of research on HIV vaccines and the limited time available, the sponsor specified that the committee's review should not include vaccine trials.

The committee's charge assumes that funders and investigators have made a decision to plan and undertake a late-stage randomized HIV prevention trial of a biomedical intervention. The charge therefore focuses on the methodological challenges that arise in planning, conducting, and analyzing such a trial.

The committee affirms the central role of randomized controlled trials in evaluating the effectiveness of HIV prevention interventions. However, less rigorous quasi-experimental and observational studies can provide evidence to motivate more definitive randomized trials. For example, three recent randomized, controlled trials of male circumcision (Auvert et al., 2005; Bailey et al., 2007; Gray et al., 2007) were motivated by earlier observational studies that circumcised men had lower rates of HIV infection. Quasi-experimental and observational studies have also been used as evidence to support implementation of prevention interventions, such as needle and syringe exchange and post-exposure prophylaxis (PEP) when randomized, controlled trials were not considered ethical.

The committee recognizes that a number of issues can arise prior to, during, and following the planning and conduct of randomized, controlled trials that are critical to HIV prevention research but outside the committee's charge. One such issue is ensuring that the early process for developing biomedical HIV interventions, before late-stage trials begin, is thorough and effective. Another concern is ensuring a sound system for prioritizing the most promising candidate interventions in the face of uncertainties about safety and efficacy, to allow those interventions to move to large, late-stage randomized trials.

Biological plausibility is central to ensuring effective preclinical testing and sound prioritization of interventions. Ideally, substantial evidence from basic research and animal models on an intervention's potential for preventing HIV transmission would be available before initiation of late-stage clinical trials. Although the committee did not assess the biological plausibility or implausibility of various biomedical prevention interventions, it believes that funders and investigators need to carefully consider biological plausibility during preclinical testing and when prioritizing interventions.

Other critical issues surrounding late-stage trials include regulatory concerns and the impact of a trial on the community. For example, the conduct of a PrEP trial in areas where access to antiretroviral therapy is limited, and thus rationed, may raise concerns about fairness or the possible spread of resistant strains of HIV from trial participants to other members of the community. While this report emphasizes the importance of community involvement in the planning of a late-stage trial, the committee does not assess best practices for how to engage communities. Finally, a late-stage trial that shows that an intervention is effective in reducing the risk of HIV infection raises a number of key policy issues about how to implement that intervention on a wider scale.

Although all these issues are outside its charge, the committee wishes to underscore their critical importance in efforts to identify effective prevention interventions.

STUDY PROCESS

The committee convened a public workshop in Washington, DC, in February 2007 to gather information on methodological challenges in HIV prevention trials. The committee heard from principal investigators of late-stage microbicide and PrEP trials and other experts in HIV prevention. The committee then held a second public workshop in London in April 2007, to gather additional information on issues in trial design and implementation, as well as other recent late-stage biomedical HIV prevention trials, including male circumcision, suppression of genital herpes (HSV-2), and cervical barriers. The committee held 2-day closed meetings immediately after each workshop. (See Appendix A for workshop agendas.) The committee also reviewed the literature on methodological issues arising in HIV prevention trials.

Several committee members and IOM staff conducted site visits to Uganda (April 2007) and South Africa (July 2007) to meet with principal investigators, staff, and participants of several prevention trials, as well as community, government, and research stakeholders. The purpose of these visits was to learn from those with experience on the ground, thus helping to inform the committee's recommendations.

The committee then assessed the evidence it had gathered and reviewed drafts of this report during two closed meetings, one in Woods Hole, Massachusetts, in July 2007, and the other in Washington, DC, in September 2007.

STUDY CONSIDERATIONS

Several considerations strongly affected the committee's thinking on methodological challenges arising in HIV prevention trials:

- A biomedical intervention with near-perfect protective efficacy that can be fully delivered as intended is unlikely to be available in the near future. Until then, ultimate effectiveness of any biomedical intervention will be closely tied to individual behavior and the multiple factors that shape it. This underscores the need for multidisciplinary research expertise, including a strong behavioral and social science component, in designing, conducting, and analyzing clinical trials, to ensure that they are feasible, ethical, relevant, and efficient.
- Although biomedical HIV prevention trials must provide risk reduction counseling to all participants, these trials are typically not designed to evaluate the effectiveness of the behavioral risk reduction intervention(s) they employ.
- Pregnancy is a common event in many biomedical HIV prevention

trials and reflects the high background pregnancy rate in the target population for these interventions. Because an approved prevention product will, on introduction into a community, likely be used by many women even after they become pregnant, it is critical that an overall product evaluation plan include specific and realistic plans for assessing the intervention's impact on pregnant women and their fetuses.

- Researchers conducting HIV prevention trials need to develop a deep understanding of and close collaboration with the communities in which trials are conducted, and where the results will ultimately be applied to ensure the interventions are relevant to and sustainable in the community and that efforts to promote recruitment, retention, product adherence, and risk reduction behaviors are based on an understanding of community norms and behaviors.
- Most late-stage biomedical HIV prevention trials have used a two-arm superiority design, which compares a new biomedical intervention, such as a PrEP or a microbicide gel, to a control arm—often a placebo. Such trials aim to assess whether the new intervention is superior to a standard prevention method, in which case it would become the new standard. However, other designs can sometimes have advantages over this approach by addressing different scientific goals or by allowing investigators to study multiple prevention methods that can be used in combination.
- Finally, although this report focuses specifically on non-vaccine biomedical HIV prevention interventions, a comprehensive approach to prevention is needed to control the HIV pandemic. Components of such an approach include effective behavioral and biomedical HIV prevention interventions, widespread access to treatment, destigmatization of HIV, care for vulnerable populations, policy environments supportive of change, and structural interventions targeting poverty, gender equity, nutritional status, living conditions, education, and health care infrastructure in developing countries. Achieving success in fighting the pandemic will require the cooperation and collaboration of multiple stakeholders, including national and local governments, private and public health care institutions, communities, researchers, donors, civil society, employers and business, and the media.

REPORT STRUCTURE

Chapter 1 provides an overview of the status of biomedical HIV prevention trials and highlights the methodological challenges that commonly occur in these trials. The chapter also highlights the influence of behavioral and sociocultural factors on biomedical trials and calls for investigators to integrate behavioral and social science research into such trials.

Chapter 2 examines the choices available to investigators regarding the size and duration of a randomized phase 3 trial to achieve a desired power to detect an intervention effect. The chapter also shows how inaccuracies in the assumed HIV incidence rates, intervention effect size, and participant adherence and attrition rates used to determine the size and duration of the trial can seriously undermine the power of the study. The chapter then examines two other design considerations: whether to undertake an efficacy trial, a phase 2B trial, or an effectiveness trial; and the choices and consequences of using different types of control groups. Chapters 3 through 6 review specific design considerations, including risk-reduction counseling (as a cointervention in a biomedical HIV prevention trial), pregnancy, adherence, and retention.

Chapters 7 and 8 address issues in site preparedness. In Chapter 7, the committee highlights the important concerns for investigators and sponsors to consider when developing the research protocol and human and physical infrastructure for late-stage trials. In Chapter 8, the committee recommends best practices for estimating HIV incidence prior to the trial start.

Chapter 9 discusses the importance of interim monitoring of trial results and best practices for analyzing interim and well as final results. In conclusion, Chapter 10 proposes alternative study designs that can sometimes offer advantages over the current two-arm superiority design used in most biomedical HIV prevention trials.

Appendixes A–E include agendas for the committee's public meetings, a list of acronyms used in the report, supporting materials for Chapter 2, details on methods for analyzing adherence data, and committee member biographies.

REFERENCES

Auvert, B., D. Taljaard, E. Lagarde, J. Sobngwi-Tambekou, R. Sitta, and A. Puren. 2005. Randomized, controlled intervention trial of male circumcision for reduction of HIV infection risk: The ANRS 1265 trial. *PLoS Medicine* 2(11):e298.

Bailey, R. C., S. Moses, C. B. Parker, K. Agot, I. Maclean, J. N. Krieger, C. F. Williams, R. T. Campbell, and J. O. Ndinya-Achola. 2007. Male circumcision for HIV prevention in young men in Kisumu, Kenya: A randomised controlled trial. *Lancet* 369(9562): 643-656.

Dunkle, K. L., R. K. Jewkes, H. C. Brown, G. E. Gray, J. A. McIntryre, and S. D. Harlow. 2004. Gender-based violence, relationship power, and risk of HIV infection in women attending antenatal clinics in South Africa. *Lancet* 363(9419):1415-1421.

Gray, R. H., G. Kigozi, D. Serwadda, F. Makumbi, S. Watya, F. Nalugoda, N. Kiwanuka, L. H. Moulton, M. A. Chaudhary, M. Z. Chen, N. K. Sewankambo, F. Wabwire-Mangen, M. C. Bacon, C. F. Williams, P. Opendi, S. J. Reynolds, O. Laeyendecker, T. C. Quinn, and M. J. Wawer. 2007. Male circumcision for HIV prevention in men in Rakai, Uganda: A randomised trial. *Lancet* 369(9562):657-666.

Jewkes, R., K. Dunkle, M. Nduna, J. Levin, N. Jama, N. Khuzwayo, M. Koss, A. Puren, and N. Duvvury. 2006. Factors associated with HIV sero-status in young rural South African women: Connections between intimate partner violence and HIV. *International Journal of Epidemiology* 35(6):1461-1468.

Maman, S., J. Campbell, M. D. Sweat, and A. C. Gielen. 2000. The intersections of HIV and violence: Directions for future research and interventions. *Social Science and Medicine* 50(4):459-478.
UNAIDS. 2006. *Report on the global epidemic: A UNAIDS 10th anniversary special edition.* Geneva, Switzerland: UNAIDS.
UNAIDS. 2007. *2007 AIDS Epidemic Update.* Geneva, Switzerland: UNAIDS.

1

The Status and Challenges of Biomedical HIV Prevention Trials

A series of spectacular successes in biomedical prevention of HIV transmission occurred in the 1980s and 1990s. Beginning with protection of the blood, organ, and tissue supply with tests for antibodies and later antigens of HIV (see IOM, 1995), through trials of prevention of mother-to-child transmission with antiretrovirals, Caesarean sections, and formula feeding, nonvaccine biomedical interventions seemed to hold promise for large-scale control of HIV transmission (International Perinatal HIV Group, 1999; Bulterys et al., 2004).

However, some failures in biomedical trials began to appear by the late-1990s. Notably, only one of six randomized controlled trials (Grosskurth et al., 1995) showed that the control of bacterial sexually transmitted diseases and trichomonas reduced HIV incidence (Grosskurth et al., 1995; Wawer et al., 1999; Gray et al., 2001; Kamali et al., 2003; Kaul et al., 2004; Gregson et al., 2007).

Investigators have continued to pursue a number of new biomedical HIV prevention interventions. Phase 2 and phase 3 trials of several biomedical interventions—including male circumcision, vaginal microbicides, pre-exposure prophylaxis (PrEP), cervical barriers (the latex diaphragm), herpes simplex virus 2 (HSV-2) suppression, and vaccines—have recently been completed or are ongoing (see Table 1-1 and Figure 1-1 for trial specifics and timeline). Recently completed trials have been marked by both successes and disappointments. Male circumcision is the primary success story. Three randomized, controlled trials found that male circumcision reduced the risk of heterosexually acquired HIV infection among men by about 50–60 percent at 18–24 months of follow-up (Auvert et al., 2005;

TABLE 1-1 Ongoing and Recently Completed Phase IIB/III Trials of Biomedical Interventions for HIV Prevention

Product Category and Study Name[a]	Also Known As	Phase	Primary Sponsors and Funders
Microbicides			
Phase 2/2B Safety and Effectiveness Study of Vaginal Microbicides BufferGel and 0.5% PRO2000/5 Gel (P) for the Prevention of HIV Infection in Women	HPTN 035	2/2B	National Institute of Allergy and Infectious Diseases HIV Prevention Trials Network, Indevus, ReProtect
Phase 3 Study of the Efficacy and Safety of the Microbicide Carraguard in Preventing HIV Seroconversion in Women	Carraguard	3	United States Agency for International Development, Bill and Melinda Gates Foundation, Population Council
Phase 3 Randomized Controlled Trial of 6% Cellulose Sulfate Gel and the Effect on Vaginal HIV Transmission (Multisite)	Cellulose sulfate (CONRAD-multisite)	3	United States Agency for International Development, Bill and Melinda Gates Foundation, CONRAD
Phase 3 Randomized Controlled Trial of Cellulose Sulfate Gel and HIV in Nigeria	Cellulose sulfate (Nigeria)	3	United States Agency for International Development, CONRAD
An International Multicentre, Randomised, Double-Blind, Placebo-Controlled Trial to Evaluate the Efficacy and Safety of 0.5% and 2% PRO 2000/5 Gels for the Prevention of Vaginally Acquired HIV Infection	MDP 301	3	Indevus Pharmaceuticals, U.K. Medical Research Council, United Kingdom Department for International Development

Actual or Target Enrollment	Country(ies)	Results
Approx. 3,100 sexually active HIV-uninfected women	Malawi, South Africa, United States, Zambia, Zimbabwe	Expected 2009.
6,202 sexually active HIV-uninfected women	South Africa	The trial failed to demonstrate that Carraguard was effective in preventing HIV infection. There were 134 new infections in the Carraguard group (an incidence of 3.3 infections per 100 woman-years) and 151 new infections in a placebo group (an incidence of 3.7 per 100 woman-years). The difference between the two groups is not statistically significant. The gel was shown to be safe for vaginal use.
1,428 (out of 2,574 targeted) sexually active HIV-uninfected women	Benin, India, South Africa, Uganda, Zimbabwe	In early 2007, the trial was halted because of an apparent increased risk of HIV infection in the CS arm, which was later confirmed in an analysis of the subset of data derived from women who completed the study.
1,644 (out of 2,160 targeted) sexually active HIV-uninfected women	Nigeria	In early 2007, the trial was stopped as a precautionary measure following the closure of the CONRAD CS trial, although there was no indications of increased risk of HIV infection in the Nigeria CS trial.
9,673 sexually active HIV-uninfected women	South Africa, Tanzania, Uganda	Expected 2009.

Continued

TABLE 1-1 Continued

Product Category and Study Name[a]	Also Known As	Phase	Primary Sponsors and Funders
Effectiveness of COL-1492, a Nonoxynol-9 Vaginal Gel, on HIV-1 Transmission in Female Sex Workers	COL-1492 or Nonoxynol-9	2/3	UNAIDS
Randomized Controlled Trial of SAVVY (C31G) Gel for Prevention of HIV infection in Women (Ghana)	Savvy (Ghana)	3	United States Agency for International Development, BIOSYN, Inc.
Phase 3 Randomized Controlled Trial of SAVVY (C31G) Gel for Prevention of HIV infection in Women (Nigeria)	Savvy (Nigeria)	3	United States Agency for International Development, BIOSYN, Inc.
Phase 2B Trial to Assess the Safety and Effectiveness of the Vaginal Microbicide 1% Tenofovir Gel for the Prevention of HIV Infection in Women in South Africa	CAPRISA 004	2B	Centre for the AIDS Programme of Research in South Africa, CONRAD, Family Health International, United States Agency for International Development, LIFElab, Gilead
Cervical Barriers (Diaphragm)			
The Latex Diaphragm to Prevent HIV Acquisition Among Women: A Female-Controlled, Physical Barrier of the Cervix	The MIRA trial	3	Bill & Melinda Gates Foundation
Preexposure Prophlaxis (PrEP)[b]			
Phase 2 Study of Tenofovir Disoproxil Fumarate (TDF) for Prevention of HIV	West Africa Tenofovir study	2	Bill & Melinda Gates Foundation

Actual or Target Enrollment	Country(ies)	Results
892 HIV-uninfected female sex workers	Benin, Côte d'Ivoire, South Africa, Thailand	The trial did not show a protective effect of COL-1492 on HIV-1 transmission in high-risk women. Multiple use of nonoxynol-9 could cause toxic effects enhancing HIV-1 infection. HIV-1 frequency in nonoxynol-9 users was 59 (16%) of 376 compared with 45 (12%) [corrected] of 389 in placebo users (402.5 vs. 435.0 woman-years; hazard ratio adjusted for centre 1.5; 95% CI:1.0–2.2; p = 0.047). 239 (32%) women reported use of a mean of more than 3.5 applicators per working day, and in these women, risk of HIV-1 infection in nonoxynol-9 users was almost twice that in placebo users (hazard ratio 1.8; 95% CI:1.0–3.2). 516 (68%) women used the gel less frequently than 3.5 times a day, and in these, risk did not differ between the two treatments.
2,142 sexually active HIV-uninfected women	Ghana	The number of HIV seroconversion in participants (17 total; 8 in the SAVVY and 9 in the placebo arm) was lower than expected. The study had insufficient power to determine effectiveness of the intervention.
2,152 sexually active HIV-uninfected women	Nigeria	The data monitoring committee determined the trial was unlikely to provide convincing evidence that SAVVY protects against HIV.
980 sexually active HIV-uninfected women	South Africa	Expected 2010.
5,045 sexually active HIV-uninfected women	South Africa, Zimbabwe	No added protective benefit against HIV infection when the diaphragm and lubricant gel were provided in addition to condoms and a comprehensive HIV prevention package.
936 (out of 1,200 targeted) sexually active HIV-uninfected women	Cameroon, Ghana, Nigeria	Daily use of TDF in HIV-uninfected women was not associated with increased adverse events. Effectiveness could not be conclusively evaluated because of premature trial closures in Cameroon and Nigeria which decreased planned person years of follow-up and study power.

Continued

TABLE 1-1 Continued

Product Category and Study Name[a]	Also Known As	Phase	Primary Sponsors and Funders
Study of the Safety and Efficacy of Daily Tenofovir to Prevent HIV Infection Among Injection Drug Users in Bangkok, Thailand	Bangkok Tenofovir study	2/3	Centers for Disease Control
Study of the Safety and Efficacy of Daily Tenofovir Disoproxil Fumarate and Emtricitabine (Truvada) for the Prevention of HIV Infection in Heterosexually Active Young Adults in Botswana	Truvada Botswana study	3	Centers for Disease Control
Chemoprophylaxis for HIV Prevention in Men	Truvada Peru/Ecuador study	3	National Institute of Allergy and Infectious Diseases
Index Partner Treatment with ARV			
A Randomized Trial to Evaluate the Effectiveness of Antiretroviral Therapy Plus HIV Primary Care versus HIV Primary Care Alone to Prevent the Sexual Transmission of HIV-1 in Serodiscordant Couples	HPTN 052	3	National Institute of Allergy and Infectious Diseases
Male Circumcision			
Effect of Safe Male Circumcision on Incidence of Infection by HIV, HSV-2, and of Genital Ulceration	ANRS 1265 (Orange Farm)	3	Agence Nationale de Recherches sur le SIDA (ANRS); National Institute for Communicable Diseases (Johannesburg, SA); Institut National de la Sante et de la Recherche Medicale
RCT of male circumcision for HIV prevention in young men in Kisumu, Kenya	Male Circumcision Trial Kisumu, Kenya	3	National Institute of Allergy and Infectious Diseases, Canadian Institute of Health Research

Actual or Target Enrollment	Country(ies)	Results
2,000 HIV-uninfected IDUs	Thailand	Expected 2008.
1,200 sexually active HIV-uninfected young adults	Botswana	Expected 2009.
3,000 high risk HIV-uninfected MSM	Ecuador, Peru, Other sites TBD	Expected 2010.
1,750 HIV-serodiscordant couples in which the HIV-infected partner is ART naïve and has a CD4+ cell count of 350-550 cells/mm^3	Brazil, India, Malawi, South Africa, Thailand, United States	Expected 2013.
3,274 HIV-uninfected heterosexual men	South Africa	The incidence rate was 0.85 per 100 person years in the intervention group and 2.1 per 100 person years in the control group, corresponding to a RR of 0.40 (95% CI: 0.24–0.68, $p < 0.001$ and a reduction in HIV risk of 60 percent. Average duration of follow-up was 18 months.
2,784 HIV-uninfected heterosexual men	Kenya	The 2-year HIV incidence was 2.1% (95% CI: 1.2–3.0) in the circumcision group and 4.2% (95% CI: 3.0–5.4) in the control group ($p = 0.0065$). Relative risk of HIV infection in circumcised men was 0.47 (95% CI: 0.28–0.78), corresponding to a reduction in risk of acquiring HIV infection by 53 percent. Median length of follow-up was 24 months.

Continued

TABLE 1-1 Continued

Product Category and Study Name[a]	Also Known As	Phase	Primary Sponsors and Funders
RCT of male circumcision for HIV prevention in men in Rakai, Uganda	Male Circumcision Trial Rakai, Uganda	3	NIAID
Trial of male circumcision in HIV positive men, Rakai, Uganda: Safety in HIV positive men and effects on women and the community	Rakai Transmission study	3	Johns Hopkins University, Rakai Health Sciences Project, Bill & Melinda Gates Foundation
HSV-2 Suppression			
Phase III, Randomized, Double-Blind, Placebo-Controlled Trial of Acyclovir for the Reduction of HIV Acquisition Among High Risk HSV-2 Seropositive, HIV-Seronegative Individuals	HPTN 039	3	NIAID
Phase III Randomized Placebo-Controlled Trial of HSV-2 Suppression to Prevent HIV Transmission Among HIV Sero-Discordant Couples	Partners in Prevention	3	Bill & Melinda Gates Foundation
Impact of HSV-2 suppressive therapy on HIV incidence in HSV-2 seropositive women: A randomised controlled trial in Tanzania	Tanzania HSV-2 Suppression	3	Wellcome Trust

[a]Table excludes vaccine and prevention of mother-to-child transmission trials.

[b]Three separate PrEP trials (in Cambodia, Cameroon, Malawi) were stopped before enrollment due to controversy about ethical issues and standard of care and concerns about possible resistance. See http://www.prepwatch.org/pdf/Trials/PrEP_trials_table.pdf.

Actual or Target Enrollment	Country(ies)	Results
4,996 HIV-uninfected heterosexual men	Uganda	HIV incidence over 24 months was 0.66 per 100 person-years and 1.33 per 100 person-years in the control group (estimated efficacy of intervention was 51% (95% CI: 16–72; p = 0.006).
1,015 HIV-seropositive men. Married men (n = 770) were asked to invite their spouses: 556 enrolled of whom 245 were HIV-seronegative.	Uganda	Male circumcision was safe and reduced genitourinary disease in HIV-seropositive men. There were no direct HIV benefits to women, but potentially an increased risk of transmission with early resumption of sex.
3,172 sexually active HIV-uninfected women who have sex with men and men who have sex with men	Peru, South Africa, United States Zambia, Zimbabwe	Acyclovir 400 mg given twice daily (800 mg total) did not reduce the risk of HIV acquisition among high-risk HSV-2 seropositive MSM and women. HIV incidence was 3.9/100 person-years in the acyclovir arm (75 events) and 3.3/100 person-years in the placebo arm (64 events), with an overall hazard ratio of 1.16 (95% CI: 0.83–1.62).
3,300 HIV-discordant couples with HIV-infected partner also HSV-2 coinfected	Botswana, Kenya, Rwanda, South Africa, Tanzania, Uganda, Zambia	Expected 2009.
820 HIV-uninfected, HSV-2 infected sex workers	Tanzania	Acyclovir 400 mg given twice daily did not reduce the risk of HIV acquisition among high-risk HSV-2 seropositive women. The HIV incidence rate was 4.29 per 100 person-years in the acyclovir arm and 4.25 per 100 person-years in the placebo arm. The difference was not statistically significant.

SOURCES: Study protocols, www.clinicaltrials.gov, AVAC HIV Prevention Research: A Comprehensive Timeline, Investigator Presentations to IOM Committee on the Methodological Challenges in HIV Prevention Trials; Publications of trial results.

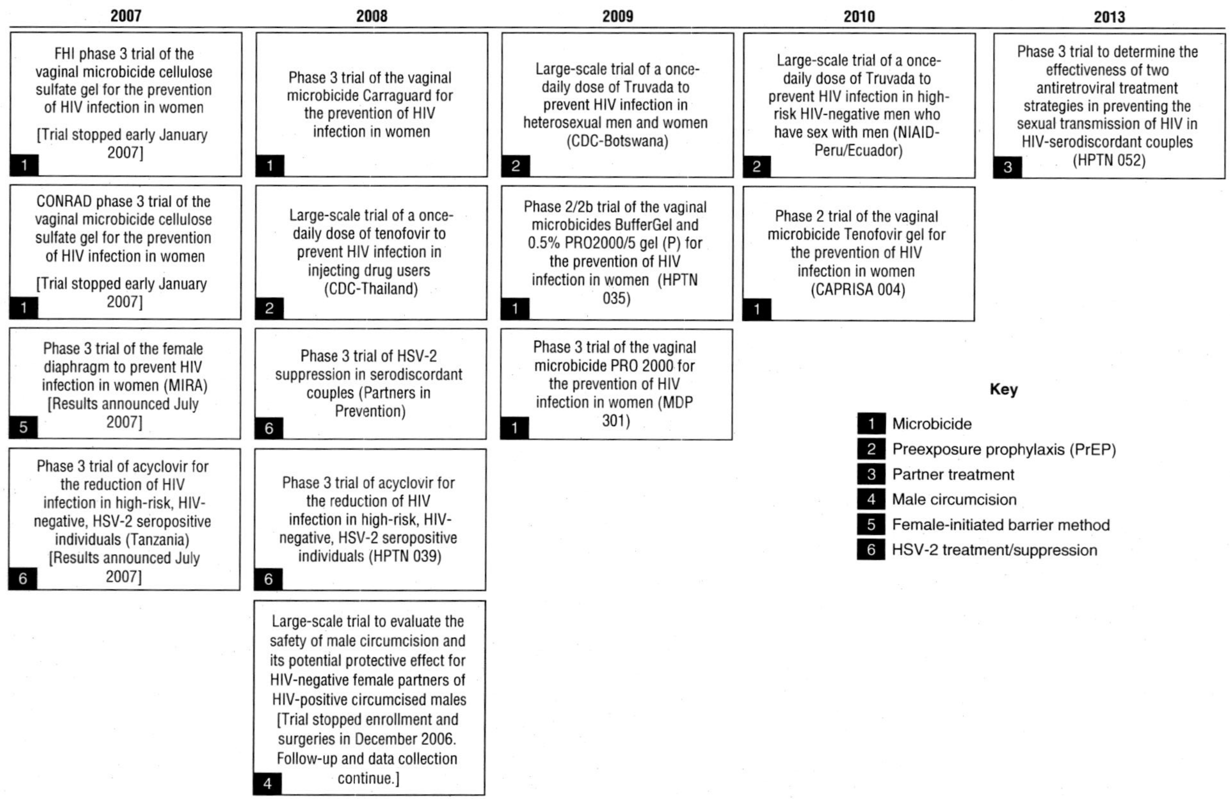

FIGURE 1-1 Timeline for results of non-vaccine biomedical HIV prevention research trials.
SOURCE: Adapted from AIDS Vaccine Advocacy Coalition, 2007, http://www.avac.org/tmeline-website/index.htm.

Bailey et al., 2007; Gray et al., 2007). As a result, an expert consultation convened by the World Health Organization (WHO) and UNAIDS recently recommended increasing the scale-up of male circumcision as an HIV prevention strategy (UNAIDS, 2007).

Other late-stage trials have failed to demonstrate a benefit in reducing HIV infection risk, including a phase 3 trial of the diaphragm and Replens gel (Padian et al., 2007) and two phase 3 trials of HSV-2 suppression with acyclovir (Watson-Jones et al., 2007; Celum et al., 2008). Two vaginal microbicide trials (of N-9 and cellulose sulfate [CS]) were halted because of evidence that they may have a harmful effect (Van Damme et al., 2002; Van Damme, 2007), and a separate trial of CS was stopped as a precautionary measure based on evidence from the other CS trial (Cates, 2007). Several PrEP trials were prematurely closed or canceled because of ethical concerns raised by advocates, governments, and community members (IAS, 2005). One PrEP trial and two microbicide trials (Savvy in Ghana and Nigeria) did not have sufficient power to determine efficacy of the intervention (Peterson et al., 2007a,b). In addition, two trials of an HIV vaccine that were recently stopped based on a lack of evidence of benefit and concerns that they might also increase HIV infection risk.[1]

This chapter begins with an overview of recent late-stage biomedical trials of interventions designed to prevent primary infection of HIV (see Figure 1-2 and Box 1-1 for an overview of clinical trial phases for product development). It then examines the methodological challenges that can undermine trial outcomes, including the design and conduct of such trials, site preparedness, interim monitoring and analysis, and interpretation of results. The chapter concludes with a discussion of how behavior driven by diverse sociocultural and economic factors plays a critical role in the overall effectiveness of most biomedical interventions, as well as in the success of clinical trials themselves.

RECENT LATE-STAGE TRIALS OF NON-VACCINE BIOMEDICAL PREVENTIONS

Topical Microbicides

Microbicides are topical agents designed to reduce or prevent transmission of HIV and/or other sexually transmitted infections (STIs) when

[1]The STEP study was discontinued based on recommendations made by a Data and Safety Monitoring Board, which concluded that the vaccine neither prevented HIV infection nor reduced the amount of virus in those who became infected with HIV (http://www.avac.org/pdf/STEP_data_release.7Nov.pdf), and possibly might have increased the risk of HIV infection. Based on review of the STEP data, the Phambili study in South Africa was also stopped (http://www.hvtn.org/media/pr/PhambiliSAAVIstatement.pdf).

	Discovery/ Preclinical Testing	File IND at FDA	Clinical Trials: Phase I	Clinical Trials: Phase II	Clinical Trials: Phase III	File NDA/BLA at FDA	FDA	Phase IV
Years	6.5		1.5	2	3.5		1.5	
Test Population	Laboratory and animal studies		20 to 100 healthy volunteers	100 to 500 patient volunteers	1,000 to 5,000 patient volunteers		Review process/ approval	Additional post-marketing testing required by FDA
Purpose	Assess safety, biological activity and formulations		Determine safety and dosage	Evaluate effectiveness, look for side effects	Confirm effectiveness, monitor adverse reactions from long-term use			
Success Rate	5,000 compounds evaluated		5 enter trials				1 approved	

FIGURE 1-2 The drug development and approval processin the United States, see also Box 1-1 on the facing page.
SORUCE: Adapted with permission from PhRMA, 2007.

BOX 1-1
The Drug Development and Approval Process in the United States

It takes 10–15 years, on average, for an experimental drug to travel from lab to U.S. patients. Only five in 5,000 compounds that enter preclinical testing make it to human testing. And only one of those five is approved for sale. Once a new compound has been identified in the laboratory, medicines are developed as follows:

Preclinical Testing. A pharmaceutical company conducts laboratory and animal studies to show biological activity of the compound against the targeted disease, and the compound is evaluated for safety.

Investigational New Drug Application (IND). After completing preclinical testing, a company files an IND with the U.S. Food and Drug Administration (FDA) to begin to test the drug in people. The IND becomes effective if FDA does not disapprove it within 30 days. The IND shows results of previous experiments; how, where and by whom the new studies will be conducted; the chemical structure of the compound; how it is thought to work in the body; any toxic effects found in the animal studies; and how the compound is manufactured. All clinical trials must be reviewed and approved by the Institutional Review Board (IRB) where the trials will be conducted. Progress reports on clinical trials must be submitted at least annually to FDA and the IRB.

Clinical Trials, Phase I. These tests typically involve about 20 to 100 normal, healthy volunteers. The tests study a drug's safety profile, including the safe dosage range. The studies also determine how a drug is absorbed, distributed, metabolized, and excreted as well as the duration of its action.

Clinical Trials, Phase II. In this phase, controlled trials of approximately 100 to 500 volunteers assess a drug's effectiveness.

Clinical Trials, Phase III. This phase usually involves 1,000 to 5,000 participants. Physicians monitor patients closely to confirm efficacy and identify adverse events.

New Drug Application (NDA)/Biologic License Application (BLA). Following the completion of all three phases of clinical trials, a company analyzes all of the data and files an NDA or BLA with FDA if the data successfully demonstrate both safety and effectiveness.

Approval. Once FDA approves an NDA or BLA, the new medicine becomes available for physicians to prescribe. A company must continue to submit periodic reports to FDA, including any cases of adverse reactions and appropriate quality-control records. For some medicines, FDA requires additional trials (Phase IV) to evaluate long-term effects.

SOURCE: Adapted with permission from PhRMA, 2007.

applied to genital mucosal surfaces (Alliance for Microbicide Development, ND). Microbicides can be in the form of gel, film, cream, suppository, pre-loaded diaphragm or cervical cap; or vaginal ring that releases the active ingredient over time. Some vaginal microbicides may also have contraceptive effects and help prevent other sexually transmitted infections, such as chlamydia or gonorrhea.

Several vaginal microbicides are in late-stage efficacy testing (Box 1-2). Three candidates have failed to show a protective effect on HIV transmission:

- COL-1492, a Nonoxynol-9–based gel, was the first vaginal microbicide to be tested in a phase 3 trial. The trial—conducted in female sex workers in Benin, Côte d'Ivoire, South Africa, and Thailand—found that the product had no protective benefit against HIV, and that women who were frequent users of the gel appeared to be at increased risk of HIV infection compared with women with similar levels of placebo use (Van Damme et al., 2002).
- Two phase 3 trials of Savvy vaginal microbicide in Ghana and Nigeria were stopped in 2005 and 2006, respectively, because lower-than-expected HIV incidence at the trial sites meant that the study had insufficient power to determine efficacy (Peterson et al., 2007b).
- In early 2007, a phase 3 multicountry trial of the cellulose sulfate (CS) microbicide was halted because of an apparent increased risk of HIV infection in the CS arm, which was later confirmed in an analysis of the subset of data derived from women who completed the study (Van Damme, 2007). A separate, concurrent trial of CS in Nigeria was stopped as a precautionary measure, although there was no apparent increased risk in that trial (Cates, 2007; Van Damme, 2007).

Three candidate microbicides (Carraguard [completed], PRO2000 and Buffer Gel) are now in phase 2B or phase 3 testing. The Carraguard trial results are expected in 2008 while the MDP 301 trial (of different formulations of PRO2000) and the HPTN 035 trial (of PRO2000 and BufferGel) results are expected in 2009. Researchers began enrolling participants in 2007 in CAPRISA 004, a phase 2B trial of a vaginal microbicide containing 1 percent tenofovir gel. The vaginal ring—a coitally independent device for delivering microbicides—and two microbicides (ACIDFORM© and Dapivirine [TMC120]) are slated to begin phase 3 testing in 2008 (Alliance for Microbicide Development, 2008a).

Products designed for vaginal use may or may not be appropriate for rectal use. The rectal lining is more fragile than most of the tissue lining the vagina, and is richer in cells that are particularly vulnerable to HIV infection. These factors further enhance rectal susceptibility to irritation, tearing,

BOX 1-2
Microbicide Candidates

Microbicides can be divided into first- and second-generation candidates. Six candidates in the first generation have advanced to phase 3 efficacy trials. These candidates are nonspecific compounds that work by disrupting the viral envelope, or by electrostatically binding to the virus and preventing it from interacting with its target cells in the vagina (Nuttall et al., 2007). All six candidates are for vaginal use, and require adherence to a coitally dependent dosing strategy.

First-generation products include the following:

- COL-1492 is a Nonoxynol-9–based surfactant that disrupts the cell membranes and protects against pregnancy (Van Damme et al., 2002).
- C31G (Savvy) is a surfactant compound designed to disable HIV by breaking down its outer membrane. C31G may also protect against pregnancy (Global HIV Prevention Work Group, 2007).
- Carbopol 974p (BufferGel) is a vaginal-defense enhancer designed to maintain the vagina's acidity in the presence of semen, to help kill or disable the virus (Global HIV Prevention Work Group, 2007).
- Cellulose sulfate (Ushercell) is an "attachment inhibitor," which prevents HIV from attaching to cells in the vaginal wall. This compound may also prevent pregnancy (Global HIV Prevention Work Group, 2007).
- Naphthalene sulfonate (PRO2000/5) is an "entry/fusion inhibitor," which binds to HIV pathogens to prevent them from entering and infecting healthy human cells (Global HIV Prevention Work Group, 2007).
- PC-515 (Carraguard) is also an entry/fusion inhibitor (Global HIV Prevention Work Group, 2007).

Trials of three of these microbicide candidates (COL-1492, C31G, and cellulose sulfate) failed to show a protective effect on HIV transmission. The efficacy of the remaining three candidates (BufferGel, Carraguard, and PRO2000/5) is also being evaluated (Carraguard, HPTN 035, and MDP 301). The Carraguard trial was recently completed and could show results by the end of 2007; the results of the remaining two trials are expected in 2009.

Second-generation microbicide candidates include those that specifically target HIV or the molecules of the cells it infects, and those that use existing or new classes of antiretroviral compounds (Global HIV Prevention Working Group, 2006). Researchers are now conducting a phase 2B efficacy trial of a vaginal microbicide containing 1 percent tenofovir gel (CAPRISA 004), and two more second-generation vaginal microbicides (ACIDFORM© and Dapivirine [TMC120]) are slated for phase 3 testing in 2008. Researchers are investigating new ways of formulating these microbicides, such as delivering them through a vaginal ring. Early-stage testing of rectal microbicides is also under way. (See Nuttall et al., 2007, for more on these classes.)

and infection during sex (Global Campaign for Microbicides, 2007). One microbicide compound, a topical formulation of the antiretroviral drug UC-781, is in early phase-testing for rectal use (Alliance for Microbicide Development, 2008b).

Pre-Exposure Prophylaxis with Antiretrovirals

Animal studies suggest that antiretroviral drugs used for HIV treatment may also be effective in preventing HIV infection. This approach is known as pre-exposure prophylaxis, or PrEP. Several early PrEP studies were closed to further enrollment or canceled because of ethical concerns raised by advocates, governments, and community members.

- A phase 3 randomized, controlled trial of tenofovir chemoprophylaxis in sex workers in Cambodia was halted in August 2004 in response to statements by the Cambodian prime minister, and after community advocates raised attention to concerns regarding needs among trial participants for medical treatment. An avalanche of commentary regarding the trial highlighted the need for community consultation and review of policies worldwide regarding how HIV prevention trials address antiretroviral treatment and long-term care (potentially associated with trial-related adverse events) for participants.
- In 2004, a phase 2 trial of daily oral tenofovir began in Ghana, Nigeria, and Cameroon in women at high risk for infection. However, research in Cameroon was halted in 2005 after advocates, and later the government and community members, raised similar issues about community involvement in research, and the rights and protections afforded trial participants (IAS, 2005). The Nigerian trial site was closed in 2005 because of an inability to meet protocol requirements. The premature closure of two sites meant that study power was insufficient to assess the efficacy of tenofovir in preventing HIV acquisition among women.
- A planned PrEP trial in Malawi never began because of government concerns that it would foster HIV resistance to tenofovir, which is being used as a treatment for HIV (Prep Watch, 2007).

Three late-stage efficacy trials using two antiretroviral agents—specifically, tenofovir disoproxil fumarate (tenofovir or TDF, brand name Viread®), used alone or in combination with emtricitabine (together TDF/FTC, known by the brand name Truvada®)—are under way. The first trial is testing the efficacy of tenofovir in preventing HIV infection among male and female injecting drug users in Thailand (CDC, 2007). The second trial is testing Truvada® for the prevention of HIV infection in heterosexually active young men and women in Botswana (CDC, 2007). The third trial is testing Truvada® in high-risk men who have sex with men in Peru and Ecuador. Results from the Thai study could be available as early as 2008, with Botswana expected in 2009, and the Peru/Ecuador study expected in 2010.

Planned for 2008, the VOICE Study—Vaginal and Oral Interventions to Control the Epidemic—will compare the safety and efficacy of oral versus topical PrEP in preventing sexual transmission of HIV (Microbicide Trials Network, 2007). VOICE is designed as a five-arm, double-blinded study. Women will first be randomized to receive either gel or oral PrEP. Then, within each group, the women will be randomly assigned to either tenofovir topical gel or placebo gel; or to oral tenofovir, oral Truvada, or oral placebo. The study plans to enroll 4,200 women at 10 sites in sub-Saharan Africa.

In addition to PrEP studies, several observational studies of serodiscordant couples suggest that treating HIV infected persons with ART may reduce the sexual transmission of HIV (Bunnell et al., 2006; Kayitenkore et al., 2006). A randomized control trial (HPTN 052) to determine the effects of antiretroviral drugs on HIV transmission in serodiscordant couples is underway (HPTN, 2007).

Although not addressed in this report, emergency post-exposure (PEP) prophylaxis with antiretroviral drugs is the standard of care for occupational exposures to HIV through infected tissues or fluids, and is increasingly used for nonoccupational exposures (Cohen et al., 2007).

It is well documented that antiretroviral treatment of HIV-infected persons may result in emergent viral resistance, particularly in the setting of monotherapy. For example, use of single dose intrapartum nevirapine results in emergence of resistant HIV in 19–87 percent of mothers (Chaix et al., 2007). However, it is unknown whether the use of antiretroviral agents (either as pre-exposure prophylaxis or as vaginal/rectal microbicides) to prevent HIV acquisition in HIV-uninfected persons will result in infection with resistant viruses or the emergence of resistant virions. In particular, the use of nonnucleoside reverse transcriptase inhibitors as microbicides may be of concern as the genetic barrier for resistance of that class of agents is quite low. Although an assessment of this topic is outside the scope of the report, prevention trials using antiretroviral agents must rigorously address this question, including assessing incident HIV infections for presence of antiretroviral resistance and considering the prevalence of agent-specific resistance.

Male Circumcision

A number of observational and ecological studies, including a systematic review and meta-analysis of studies from sub-Saharan Africa, have suggested that male circumcision may reduce men's risk of becoming HIV infected. The effectiveness of male circumcision was recently confirmed in three randomized, controlled trials conducted in Kenya, Uganda, and South Africa, which found that male circumcision reduced the risk of heterosexually acquired HIV infection among men by about 50–60 percent at 18–24 months of follow-up (Auvert et al., 2005; Bailey et al., 2007; Gray et al., 2007). A recent expert consultation convened by WHO and UNAIDS (UNAIDS, 2007) characterized this evidence as compelling, and recommended that public health officials include male circumcision in a comprehensive HIV prevention package, particularly, expanding it to areas where rates of heterosexually acquired HIV infection among men is high.

A follow-up study was initiated in Rakai, Uganda, to determine whether circumcision among HIV-infected men reduces HIV transmission to female partners (Wawer, 2007). However, after reviewing the data in late 2006, the trial's Data Safety Monitoring Board stopped further enrollment based on futility. The data suggested that transmission of HIV from circumcised, infected men to women may actually rise if they resume sex before the wound is fully healed (Wawer, 2007).

Cervical Barriers

Researchers hypothesized that cervical barriers may help protect women from HIV by covering the cervix and blocking the upper genital track, areas with cells that are more susceptible to certain STIs and HIV infection (Padian et al., 2007). Observational studies have suggested that women using diaphragms have a reduced risk of cervical STIs, pelvic inflammatory disease, and human papillomavirus-associated cervical neoplasia (Padian et al., 2007). In a recent phase 3 trial, researchers evaluated whether the diaphragm, lubricant gel, and condoms/counseling (intervention arm), compared to condoms/counseling alone (control arm) had a protective effect on HIV incidence among women in South Africa and Zimbabwe (Padian et al., 2007). The trial failed to show any additional benefit of a latex diaphragm and lubricant gel (Replens) over standard risk reduction and condom counseling in preventing acquisition of HIV in women, corresponding to a relative hazard of 1.05 (95% confidence interval [CI]: 0.84–1.32). Notably, the proportion of women who reported using condoms was significantly lower in the intervention than in the control group (54 percent versus 85 percent of visits, $p < 0.0001$) (Padian et al., 2007).

Herpes Suppression

Multiple studies have found that individuals with herpes simplex virus-2 (HSV) are at increased risk of HIV infection (Freeman et al., 2006). HIV-infected individuals who are coinfected with HSV-2 are also more likely to transmit HIV to others (Nagot et al., 2006). HSV-2 is one of the most common STIs worldwide. In some parts of Africa, more than 70 percent of adults are infected with HSV-2 (Hogrefe et al., 2002). Several studies have examined whether acyclovir, a widely used drug to suppress HSV-2, can reduce sexual acquisition and transmission of HIV (Global HIV Prevention Work Group, 2007).

Two recently completed trials failed to demonstrate that acyclovir treatment had a protective effect on HIV acquisition. The first was a randomized, placebo controlled trial of acyclovir treatment (400 mg BD) among initially HIV-seronegative, HSV-2 seropositive women in northern Tanzania (Watson-Jones et al., 2007). The trial found no protective effect of acyclovir against HIV acquisition. High rates of pregnancy (resulting in 25 percent of participants being withdrawn from study medication), poor reported participant adherence (50 percent of the women provided with acyclovir failed to achieve the target 90 percent adherence rate), and poor participant retention (60 percent of the women completed the trial) were reported (Watson-Jones et al., 2007).

A second randomized, placebo-controlled trial (HPTN 039) was designed to assess whether HSV-2 suppression twice-daily oral acyclovir of 400 mg (800 mg total) reduced the rate of HIV acquisition among high-risk women in Africa and men who have sex with men in the United States and Peru. The regimen failed to show a protective benefit against HIV. HIV incidence was 3.9/100 person-years in the acyclovir arm (75 events) and 3.3/100 person-years in the placebo arm (64 events), with an overall hazard ratio of 1.16 (95%: CI: 0.83–1.62). There were no significant differences by gender or reported adherence to the drug.

A third phase 3 trial examining the impact of HSV-2 suppression in HIV-infected individuals on transmission of HIV to their partners is underway. Results from this trial (Partners in Prevention study) are due in 2008 (Celum, 2007).

METHODOLOGICAL CHALLENGES IN BIOMEDICAL HIV PREVENTION TRIALS

This report examines methodological challenges in late-stage randomized prevention trials of nonvaccine biomedical interventions, and their impact on study design and conduct, site preparedness, interim monitoring and analysis, and interpretation of results. Key challenges include the lack of a reliable surrogate marker for HIV infection: the difficulty of accurately estimating HIV incidence; the need to provide risk-reduction counseling, which is of uncertain benefit; high rates of pregnancy among trial participants; the difficulty measuring and maintaining adequate levels of product adherence and inadequate participant retention. These challenges are briefly highlighted below. Subsequent chapters contain a more in-depth discussion of these issues. Although the committee's charge did not include examining vaccine, pMTCT trials, and some behavioral risk-reduction trials (outside of their use as a cointervention in biomedical HIV prevention trials), many of the potential responses to these challenges may also have implications for those studies.

Lack of a Surrogate Marker for HIV Infection

HIV infection is, appropriately, by default the primary endpoint in both Phase 2 and 3 HIV randomized prevention trials, because researchers have not identified and validated a surrogate marker of product efficacy. Because HIV infection is a relatively uncommon event even in high-incidence areas, these trials must enroll very large numbers of participants to have the power to detect that a product has a beneficial effect. This requirement increases both the time needed to conduct trials and their cost.

Risk-Reduction Counseling

There is broad agreement among multiple stakeholders that participants in HIV prevention trials should receive behavioral risk-reduction counseling. Trials must therefore show that the biomedical intervention has a benefit in a setting where this counseling also may reduce the HIV incidence rate. That is, if the counseling strategy were effective, it could reduce the study's power to detect a beneficial effect of the biomedical intervention. Yet little is known about the effectiveness of behavioral counseling in many of the settings where biomedical HIV prevention takes place.

Pregnancy

Despite intensive counseling on family planning, and access to contraceptives through referrals to family planning clinics or onsite provision, many women enrolled in HIV prevention trials, particularly in Africa, become pregnant. Trials testing new products and new drug indications typically restrict pregnant women from enrolling and require women to use some form of contraceptive while participating in the trials. Women who become pregnant during a trial are typically taken off the product, either permanently or for the duration of their pregnancy. Time off the product owing to pregnancy has adversely affected study power in trials whose sample size and power calculations do not account for this, or where higher-than-expected pregnancy rates occur.

Discontinuing product use among pregnant women also prevents researchers from learning about the effects of the interventions on pregnant women and on pregnancy outcomes. That presents a problem because once a biomedical intervention is found to be efficacious and approved for use, a recommendation against use during pregnancy is unlikely to be widely followed, particularly when women may use such products throughout childbearing age. This raises ethical questions about how to best collect safety data, and about whether women participating in trials should have the option of remaining on the product if they become pregnant.

Adherence and Reporting of Sexual Behavior

Imperfect adherence to prescribed randomized regimens is common in HIV prevention trials and can obscure the efficacy of a product. If a trial fails to show a protective effect, investigators need to understand whether that failure occurred because the product was not biologically efficacious, or because participants failed to adhere to the product regimen. Each biomedical intervention has its own adherence challenges. For example, coitally dependent products, such as the current generation of microbicides, require women to use the product before or after each sex act. This may pose challenges because sex is not always predictable or controlled by women.

With respect to both adherence and risk behavior, many studies with no or limited objective measures of product adherence rely heavily on self-reported measures of product use and sexual behavior. The accuracy of such data is sometimes questionable, and few objective measures exist to corroborate these reports.

Recruitment and Retention

Effectively recruiting and retaining trial participants is essential for obtaining meaningful study results. A slowly accruing trial can delay the widespread use of an efficacious treatment, or expose participants to an ineffective treatment for longer than necessary. A prolonged trial may also divert resources from newer and more promising approaches.

However, while recruiting participants in a timely manner is important, an emphasis on doing so at all costs can undermine the ability of investigators to retain them. And while enrolling participants from a large region may allow for faster recruitment, the resulting population may be more challenging to retain as access to the clinic and follow-up in the participants' homes would be more difficult.

To ensure confidence in their outcomes, trials must achieve high retention. Lower-than-expected participant recruitment and retention can mean that a trial will be underpowered and its results biased. Yet maintaining adequate retention is a challenge in many of the settings where HIV prevention trials are being conducted.

Estimating HIV Incidence

If a trial is to show that a prevention product is effective, some individuals must become HIV infected during a trial. The sample size and duration of a trial are based on the number of people expected to become infected during the trial's follow-up period. Thus an accurate estimate of the background HIV incidence at the trial site is critical to determining the required sample size and duration. As noted, several trials have been unable to reach definitive conclusions because of a lower-than-expected HIV incidence rate and the resulting insufficient study power.

BEHAVIORAL AND SOCIOCULTURAL INFLUENCES ON BIOMEDICAL TRIALS

Although some of the challenges facing biomedical trials are more technical—including estimating HIV incidence and identifying surrogate markers—other challenges, such as product adherence, condom use, pregnancy, and retention, are profoundly affected by the behavior of trial participants and the macro-level factors (e.g., social, political, economic, environmental) that influence that behavior.

Indeed, the level of product adherence and risk-taking behavior of trial participants has a large impact on the safety and success of clinical trials of biomedical interventions. For example, trial staff members instruct participants to protect themselves from HIV by using condoms, to adhere to study products, to remain in the study, and, in most trials, to avoid pregnancy. However, macro-level factors often work in opposition to these instructions, as the following sections illustrate.

Encouraging Correct and Consistent Condom Use

Biomedical HIV prevention studies counsel participants on the importance of using either male or female condoms to prevent HIV infection. In some cultures, decisions on condom use rest largely with men. For example, in some communities, men use condoms with sex workers and not with their wives or regular sexual partners, and women may be reluctant to ask their partners to use condoms because of their association with sex workers and infidelity (Veldhuijzen et al., 2006). Power dynamics, especially between young women and older sexual partners, may also prevent the former from using condoms and following study instructions regarding the use of HIV prevention products (Kuate-Defo, 2004).

Maintaining High Adherence to Instructions for Using a Product

Suboptimal adherence to the product regimen can obscure the efficacy of a product during trials and reduce its effectiveness in the real world. And adherence may vary depending on the attitudes and practices of individuals within a particular setting. For example, several studies of the acceptability of microbicides have noted that women may not attempt to use a product or may discontinue or reduce the amount they apply, if gel wetness raises concerns among male sexual partners (Bentley et al., 2004; Braunstein and van de Wijgert, 2005).

In some areas of South Africa, cultural norms dictate that women dry their vaginas, and some women may want their vaginas to remain dry to avoid being stigmatized as prostitutes or unfaithful to their partners (Braunstein and van de Wijgert, 2005). In some Rwandan communities, in contrast, vaginal lubrication is the desired norm. The custom is to stimulate vaginal secretions, and women who fail to produce enough during intercourse are sometimes given derogatory names (Veldhuijzen et al., 2006). Thus, sociocultural norms around sexual practices may influence the ability and willingness of individuals and couples to use microbicides (see Box 1-3).

Preventing Pregnancy During a Trial

In most biomedical HIV prevention trials, uncertainties and concerns about the effects of the intervention on pregnancy outcomes prompt investigators to counsel women to avoid pregnancy and to take them off product if they become pregnant. Yet pregnancy is a common and often desired outcome for women of child-bearing age who are likely to use a biomedical intervention after it is introduced into the community.

In some cultures, women are expected to have children, and in some marriages, a lack of children may be grounds for divorce (Yale Law Journal, 1946). Young women may also feel pressure to prove they are fertile, and to increase their chances of getting married by becoming pregnant (Loosli, 2004). In-depth interviews with a subset of women who participated in a PrEP trial in Ghana, Nigeria, and Cameroon revealed the importance of understanding local context when determining how to reduce pregnancies during HIV prevention trials (MacQueen and Karim, 2007).

Maintaining High Recruitment and Retention Rates

Effectively recruiting and retaining trial participants is essential for obtaining meaningful study results. However, while poverty and unemployment may initially encourage participants to enroll to receive financial compensation, these factors can also lead to poor retention. During a site

BOX 1-3
HIV Biomedical Interventions May Enhance Women's Control Over Their Sexual Decision Making But They Are Not a Panacea

Sexual decision making is embedded within complex societal expectations in which both men and women exercise different kinds of control. A female-controlled HIV prevention product that could be used covertly (Morrow and Ruiz, 2007; Morrow et al., 2007) and provide long-lasting protection (Orner et al., 2006) could be a tremendous benefit in reducing women's vulnerability to HIV. Mathematical models have shown that even if a small proportion of women in lower income countries used a 60 percent efficacious microbicide in half of the sexual encounters where condoms are not used, 2.5 million HIV infections could be averted over 3 years (Watts and Vickerman, 2001). Microbicides and other new biomedical interventions such as PrEP may be able to afford women greater control over their sexual decision making. However, the introduction of these new technologies is not a panacea for women's sexual decision making, as illustrated in the examples below.

Many women must still seek partner permission
In Zimbabwe more than 90 percent of the women eligible to participate in a microbicide and diaphragm safety study indicated that they sought permission of their partners to participate in the study and about two-thirds said if they did not do so, they would experience difficulties in their marriage (Montgomery et al., 2006).

Covert use may be difficult
In a simulated vaginal microbicide pilot study done in Massachusetts, more than 86 percent of respondents indicated that their primary sexual partners knew that they were using Replens (Mosack et al., 2005). In an acceptability study of the Carraguard microbicide, only 15 percent of women said they could use the microbicide gel without their male partner's knowledge (Whitehead et al., 2006). Additionally, many women who use microbicides experience vaginal wetness. In some

visit in South Africa, study staff told the committee that some participants had left the study area because of work-related migration or dropped out of a trial once they became employed.

Studies may also fail to enroll participants or lose them to follow-up because of imprisonment or fear of imprisonment, if the study population engages in illegal activities, such as injecting drug use or commercial sex work. For example, in Thailand, the government undertook an aggressive campaign to crackdown on drug use, which resulted in the arrest, incarceration, and sometimes execution of many drug users. In this environment, investigators of a PrEP trial that enrolled injecting drug users were concerned that some of their study participants could be incarcerated. Investi-

cultures, people believe that vaginal wetness must be due to improper hygiene or a sexually transmitted infection, may also limit women's ability to use microbicide products (Bentley et al., 2004; Braunstein and van de Wijgert, 2005).

Fear of violence

Compared to microbicides, women may be able to use oral PrEP more covertly. However, in some instances, women may find it difficult to conceal medication, especially in small households. During the committee's site visits to several African trial sites, some female participants expressed the need to hide pills from their partners for fear of violence stemming from a link between pills and illness. Trial site staff noted that women in the trial are counseled on how to discuss the use of pills for prevention with their partners and families.

Challenging traditional gender norms

Methods that provide women with more control over their sexual lives might challenge traditional gender norms. In some countries, males dominate sexual decision making, and pervasive gender inequities underpin the HIV/AIDS epidemic (Jewkes et al., 2003; Dunkle et al., 2004; Pettifor et al., 2004; Abdool Karim, 2005). Little data exist on what women and men would think of women initiating and controlling sexual decision making and methods of preventing HIV. Moreover, many HIV biomedical interventions will require acknowledgement and discussion of sexuality and sexual practices, issues that policy makers, providers and users can find difficult.

Partially effective products

Microbicides and other biomedical products are likely to be only partially effective and could lead to risk compensation or disinhibition among some people. Thus, new HIV biomedical interventions may be best conceptualized as part of a broader package that should complement traditional HIV prevention strategies, such as condoms, whenever possible. Educating women about a "combination" approach to HIV prevention could also prove challenging.

gators received permission to continue to follow incarcerated participants and give them the study product during incarceration (Smith, 2007).

Another important factor shaping recruitment and retention of participants in HIV prevention trials is the stigma associated with HIV. Participants in HIV-related research may experience stigma regardless of their HIV status. Individuals may therefore choose not to participate in trials because others may believe they are HIV infected or at risk of infection. Indeed, a systematic review of 26 HIV vaccine studies found that social discrimination is one of the leading factors that may limit participation in future HIV prevention research (Mills et al., 2004).

Some people may be wary of participating in a trial because they do not want to know or do not feel it is important to know their HIV status. Participants in HIV prevention trials must undergo routine HIV testing, and be prepared to not only know their status but sometimes discuss it with their partner. The stigma associated with HIV, as well as a lack of access to antiretrovirals, can discourage individuals from being tested (Global HIV Prevention Working Group, 2004). A cross-sectional, population-based study in Botswana found that the key barriers to HIV testing included fear of learning one's status (49 percent), lack of perceived HIV risk (43 percent), and fear of having to change sexual practices after a positive HIV test (33 percent) (Weiser et al., 2006).

Researchers and participants may also differ in their perspectives on what participation in clinical trials can offer individuals and their communities (Benatar, 2002). Divergence between the goals of researchers and the realties of participants often reflects disparities in wealth and health (Benatar, 2004). Many research subjects are among the world's most vulnerable populations. Thus, it is important for investigators to understand the factors that shape individuals' perceptions of research. For example, investigators may need to determine whether participants see research as distinct from health care (Horton, 1995a,b). Investigators may further need to consider the historical and ideological forces that may shape participants' perceptions of research (Loue et al., 1996a,b), how they expect research to benefit them and their society (Benatar and Fleischer, 2005), and whether research will mesh or conflict with community norms and values (Molyneux et al., 2005). Research that takes such concerns into account and incorporates methods to evaluate them is more likely to succeed in addressing health issues that are heavily influenced by complex social and behavioral factors.

Yet many studies of the importance of behavioral change in reducing people's risk of HIV infection have focused on individuals and often ignored the social and cultural context. This thinking has influenced the conduct of biomedical HIV prevention trials, which also target individual risk behavior, such as having multiple sexual partners, engaging in unprotected sex, and sharing needles with other drug users. Increasingly, the emphasis in social science research is on understanding individual behavior within a broader sociocultural and economic context.

The promise of new HIV prevention technologies underscores the need for multidisciplinary teams to be involved in all stages of the trial. Incorporating behavioral and social science research into biomedical research could improve the design, implementation, and analysis of clinical trials, and thus render new technologies more effective. However, despite numerous calls for integrating traditional biomedical and social science research, most biomedical HIV prevention trials have rather limited behavioral and social science research components (IOM and NAS, 1994; Auerbach and

Coates, 2000; Glasgow et al., 2003; Tolley and Severy, 2006). Failure to rectify this shortcoming will frustrate progress in developing effective HIV prevention methods.

REFERENCES

Abdool Karim, Q. 2005. Heterosexual transmission of HIV: The importance of a gendered perspective in HIV prevention. In *HIV/AIDS in South Africa*, edited by S. S. Abdool Karim and Q. Abdool Karim. Cambridge, UK: Cambridge University Press.

AIDS Vaccine Advocacy Coalition. 2007. *AVAC Report 2007: Resetting the Clock*. http://www.avac.org (accessed January 2008).

Alliance for Microbicide Development. ND. http://www.microbicide.org/ (accessed November 1, 2007).

Alliance for Microbicide Development. 2008a. *Microbicide candidates and ancillary devices in planned and funded clinical trials as of February 2008*. http://www.microbicide.org/microbicideinfo/reference/Microbicides.Planned.Funded.Clinical.Trials1Feb08.pdf (accessed February 8, 2008).

Alliance for Microbicide Development. 2008b. *Microbicide candidates in ongoing clinical trials: Summary as of February 2008*. http://www.microbicide.org/microbicideinfo/reference/Microbicide.Ongoing.Clinical.Trials.Summary1Feb08.pdf (accessed February 8, 2008).

Auerbach, J. D., and T. J. Coates. 2000. HIV prevention research: Accomplishments and challenges for the third decade of AIDS. *American Journal of Public Health* 90(7): 1029-1032.

Auvert, B., D. Taljaard, E. Lagarde, J. Sobngwi-Tambekou, R. Sitta, and A. Puren. 2005. Randomized, controlled intervention trial of male circumcision for reduction of HIV infection risk: The ANRS 1265 trial. *PLoS Medicine* 2(11):e298.

Bailey, R. C., S. Moses, C. B. Parker, K. Agot, I. Maclean, J. N. Krieger, C. F. Williams, R. T. Campbell, and J. O. Ndinya-Achola. 2007. Male circumcision for HIV prevention in young men in Kisumu, Kenya: A randomised controlled trial. *Lancet* 369(9562):643-656.

Benatar, S. R. 2002. Reflections and recommendations on research ethics in developing countries. *Social Science and Medicine* 54(7):1131-1141.

Benatar, S. 2004. Rationally defensible standards for research in developing countries. Review of Macklin's "Double standards in medical research in developing countries." *Health and Human Rights* 8(1):197-202.

Benatar, S., and T. Fleischer. 2005. Ethical and policy implications of clinical drug trials conducted in developing countries. *Harvard Health Policy Review* 6(1):9.

Bentley, M. E., A. M. Fullem, E. E. Tolley, C. W. Kelly, N. Jogelkar, N. Srirak, L. Mwafulirwa, G. Khumalo-Sakutukwa, and D. D. Celentano. 2004. Acceptability of a microbicide among women and their partners in a 4-country phase I trial. *American Journal of Public Health* 94(7):1159-1164.

Braunstein, S., and J. van de Wijgert. 2005. Preferences and practices related to vaginal lubrication: Implications for microbicide acceptability and clinical testing. *Journal of Women's Health* (Larchmt) 14(5):424-433.

Bulterys, M., M. G. Fowler, K. K. Van Rompay, and A. P. Kourtis. 2004. Prevention of mother-to-child transmission of HIV-1 through breast-feeding: Past, present, and future. *Journal of Infectious Diseases* 189(12):2149-2153.

Bunnell, R., J. P. Ekwaru, P. Solberg, N. Wamai, W. Bikaako-Kajura, W. Were, A. Coutinho, C. Liechty, E. Madraa, G. Rutherford, and J. Mermin. 2006. Changes in sexual behavior and risk of HIV transmission after antiretroviral therapy and prevention interventions in rural Uganda. *AIDS* 20(1):85-92.

Cates, W. 2007. *Effectiveness of cellulose sulfate gel for prevention of HIV: Results of the phase III trial in Nigeria.* Paper read at the Fourth International AIDS Society Conference on HIV Pathogenesis, Treatment and Prevention, July 25, Sydney, Australia.

CDC (Centers for Disease Control and Prevention). 2007. *CDC trials of pre-exposure prophylaxis for HIV prevention.* http://www.cdc.gov/hiv/resources/factsheets/PDF/prep.pdf (accessed January 15, 2008).

Celum, C. 2007. *Phase III randomized placebo-controlled trial of HSV-2 suppression to prevent HIV transmission among HIV-discordant couples.* Paper read at the second public meeting for the Committee on Methodological Challenges in HIV Prevention Trials, London, UK.

Celum, C., A. Wald, J. Hughes, J. Sanchez, S. Reid, S. Delaney-Moretlwe, F. M. Cowan, J. Fuchs, B. Koblin, L. Corey, and HPTN-039. 2008. *HSV-2 suppressive therapy for prevention of HIV acquisition: Results of HPTN 039.* Paper presented at Conference on Retroviruses and Opportunistic Infections, Boston, Massachusetts.

Chaix, M. L., D. K. Ekouevi, G. Peytavin, F. Rouet, B. Tonwe-Gold, I. Viho, L. Bequet, C. Amani-Bosse, H. Menan, V. Leroy, C. Rouzioux, and F. Dabis. 2007. Impact of nevirapine (NVP) plasma concentration on selection of resistant virus in mothers who received single-dose NVP to prevent perinatal human immunodeficiency virus type 1 transmission and persistence of resistant virus in their infected children. *Antimicrobial Agents and Chemotherapy* 51(3):896-901.

Cohen, M. S., C. Gay, A. D. Kashuba, S. Blower, and L. Paxton. 2007. Narrative review: Antiretroviral therapy to prevent the sexual transmission of HIV-1. *Annals of Internal Medicine* 146(8):591-601.

Dunkle, K. L., R. K. Jewkes, H. C. Brown, G. E. Gray, J. A. McIntryre, and S. D. Harlow. 2004. Transactional sex among women in Soweto, South Africa: Prevalence, risk factors and association with HIV infection. *Social Science and Medicine* 59(8):1581-1592.

Freeman, E. E., H. A. Weiss, J. R. Glynn, P. L. Cross, J. A. Whitworth, and R. J. Hayes. 2006. Herpes simplex virus 2 infection increases HIV acquisition in men and women: Systematic review and meta-analysis of longitudinal studies. *AIDS* 20(1):73-83.

Glasgow, R. E., E. Lichtenstein, and A. C. Marcus. 2003. Why don't we see more translation of health promotion research to practice? Rethinking the efficacy-to-effectiveness transition. *American Journal of Public Health* 93(8):1261-1267.

Global Campaign for Microbicides. 2007. *Rectal microbicides.* http://www.global-campaign.org/rectal.htm (accessed 2007).

Global HIV Prevention Work Group. 2004. *HIV prevention in the era of expanded treatment access.* Prepared for the Bill & Melinda Gates Foundation and Kaiser Family Foundation.

Global HIV Prevention Work Group. 2006. *New approaches to HIV prevention: Accelerating research and ensuring future access.* Prepared for the Bill & Melinda Gates Foundation and Kaiser Family Foundation.

Global HIV Prevention Work Group. 2007. *Bringing HIV prevention to scale.* Prepared for the Bill & Melinda Gates Foundation and the Henry J. Kaiser Family Foundation.

Gray, R. H., F. Wabwire-Mangen, G. Kigozi, N. K. Sewankambo, D. Serwadda, L. H. Moulton, T. C. Quinn, K. L. O'Brien, M. Meehan, C. Abramowsky, M. Robb, and M. J. Wawer. 2001. Randomized trial of presumptive sexually transmitted disease therapy during pregnancy in Rakai, Uganda. *American Journal of Obstetrics and Gynecology* 185(5):1209-1217.

Gray, R. H., G. Kigozi, D. Serwadda, F. Makumbi, S. Watya, F. Nalugoda, N. Kiwanuka, L. H. Moulton, M. A. Chaudhary, M. Z. Chen, N. K. Sewankambo, F. Wabwire-Mangen, M. C. Bacon, C. F. Williams, P. Opendi, S. J. Reynolds, O. Laeyendecker, T. C. Quinn, and M. J. Wawer. 2007. Male circumcision for HIV prevention in men in Rakai, Uganda: A randomised trial. *Lancet* 369(9562):657-666.

Gregson, S., S. Adamson, S. Papaya, J. Mundondo, C. A. Nyamukapa, P. R. Mason, G. P. Garnett, S. K. Chandiwana, G. Foster, and R. M. Anderson. 2007. Impact and process evaluation of integrated community and clinic-based HIV-1 control: A cluster-randomised trial in eastern Zimbabwe. *PLoS Medicine* 4(3):e102.

Grosskurth, H., F. Mosha, J. Todd, E. Mwijarubi, A. Klokke, K. Senkoro, P. Mayaud, J. Changalucha, A. Nicoll, and G. ka-Gina. 1995. Impact of improved treatment of sexually transmitted diseases on HIV infection in rural Tanzania: Randomised controlled trial. *Lancet* 346(8974):530-536.

Hogrefe, W., X. Su, J. Song, R. Ashley, and L. Kong. 2002. Detection of herpes simplex virus type 2-specific immunoglobulin g antibodies in African sera by using recombinant gG2, western blotting, and gG2 inhibition. *Journal of Clinical Microbiology* 40(10):3635-3640.

Horton, E. 1995a. A provider to managed care. *Behavioral Healthcare Tomorrow* 4(6):22, 75.

Horton, R. 1995b. African traditional thought and western science. In *African philosophy*. A. Mosely, ed. Englewood Cliffs, NJ: Prentice Hall.

HPTN (HIV Prevention Trials Network). 2007. http://www.hptn.org/research_studies/hptn052.asp (accessed December 1, 2007).

IAS (International AIDS Society). 2005. *Building collaboration to advance HIV prevention: Global consultation on tenofovir pre-exposure prophylaxis research*. Geneva, Switzerland: International AIDS Society.

International Perinatal HIV Group. 1999. The mode of delivery and the risk of vertical transmission of human immunodeficiency virus type 1—a meta-analysis of 15 prospective cohort studies. *New England Journal of Medicine* 340(13):977-987.

IOM (Institute of Medicine). 1995. *HIV and the blood supply*. Washington, DC: National Academy Press.

IOM and NAS (Institute of Medicine and National Academy of Sciences). 1994. *Assessing the social and behavioral science base for HIV/AIDS prevention and intervention*. Washington, DC: National Academy Press.

Jewkes, R. K., J. B. Levin, and L. A. Penn-Kekana. 2003. Gender inequalities, intimate partner violence and HIV preventive practices: Findings of a South African cross-sectional study. *Social Science and Medicine* 56(1):125-134.

Kamali, A., M. Quigley, J. Nakiyingi, J. Kinsman, J. Kengeya-Kayondo, R. Gopal, A. Ojwiya, P. Hughes, L. M. Carpenter, and J. Whitworth. 2003. Syndromic management of sexually-transmitted infections and behaviour change interventions on transmission of HIV-1 in rural Uganda: A community randomised trial. *Lancet* 361(9358):645-652.

Kaul, R., J. Kimani, N. J. Nagelkerke, K. Fonck, E. N. Ngugi, F. Keli, K. S. MacDonald, I. W. Maclean, J. J. Bwayo, M. Temmerman, A. R. Ronald, and S. Moses. 2004. Monthly antibiotic chemoprophylaxis and incidence of sexually transmitted infections and HIV-1 infection in Kenyan sex workers: A randomized controlled trial. *JAMA* 291(21):2555-2562.

Kayitenkore, K., B. Bekan, J. Rufagari, S. Marion-Landais, E. Karita, S. Allen, and RZHRG. 2006. *The impact of art on HIV transmission among HIV serodiscordant couples*. Paper presented at the XVI International AIDS Conference, Toronto, Canada.

Kuate-Defo, B. 2004. Young people's relationships with sugar daddies and sugar mummies: What do we know and what do we need to know? *African Journal of Reproductive Health* 8(2):13-37.

Loosli, B. C. 2004. *Traditional practices and HIV prevention in sub-Saharan Africa*. Geneva, Switzerland. http://www.gfmer.ch/GFMER_members/pdf/Traditional_HIV_Loosli.pdf (accessed March 25, 2008).

Loue, S., L. Lloyd, and L. Loh. 1996a. HIV prevention in U.S. Asian Pacific Islander communities: An innovative approach. *Journal of Health Care for the Poor and Underserved* 7(4):364-376.

Loue, S., D. Okello, and M. Kawuma. 1996b. Research bioethics in the Ugandan context: A program summary. *Journal of Law, Medicine and Ethics* 24(1):47-53.

MacQueen, K. M., and Q. A. Karim. 2007. Practice brief: Adolescents and HIV clinical trials: Ethics, culture, and context. *Journal of the Association of Nurses in AIDS Care* 18(2):78-82.

Microbicide Trials Network. 2007. http://www.MtnstopsHIV.Org/ (accessed October 25, 2007).

Mills, E., C. Cooper, G. Guyatt, A. Gilchrist, B. Rachlis, C. Sulway, and K. Wilson. 2004. Barriers to participating in an HIV vaccine trial: A systematic review. *AIDS* 18(17):2235-2242.

Molyneux, C. S., D. R. Wassenaar, N. Peshu, and K. Marsh. 2005. "even if they ask you to stand by a tree all day, you will have to do it (laughter) . . . !": Community voices on the notion and practice of informed consent for biomedical research in developing countries. *Social Science and Medicine* 61(2):443-454.

Montgomery, L., S. Napierala, P. Zvivamwe, S. Mtetwa, N. Hammond, T. Chipato, and A. van der Straten. 2006. *Male involvement in a diaphragm and microbicide safety study in Zimbabwe*. Paper read at Microbicides Conference, Cape Town, South Africa.

Morrow, K. M., and M. S. Ruiz. 2007. Assessing microbicide acceptability: A comprehensive and integrated approach. *AIDS and Behavior*. http://www.springerlink.com/content/30u617k8j2203703/fulltext.html (accessed March 25, 2008).

Morrow, K. M. P., J. L. P. Fava, R. K. P. Rosen, S. B. A. Vargas, C. Barroso, A. L. B. A. Christensen, C. P. Woodsong, and L. P. Severy. 2007. Willingness to use microbicides is affected by the importance of product characteristics, use parameters, and protective properties. *Journal of Acquired Immune Deficiency Syndromes* 45(1):93-101.

Mosack, K. E., M. R. Weeks, L. Novick Sylla, and M. Abbott. 2005. High-risk women's willingness to try a simulated vaginal microbicide: Results from a pilot study. *Women & Health* 42(2):71-88.

Nagot, N., A. Ouedraogo, P. Mayaud, I. Konate, L. Vergne, H. Weiss, V. Foulongne, D. Djagbare, M. Segongy, P. Vande Perre, and ANRS 1285 Study Group. 2006. *Effect of HSV-2 suppressive therapy on HIV-1 genital shedding and plasma viral load: A proof-of-concept randomized doubleblind placebo controlled trial (ANRS1285 trial)*. Paper read at 13th Conference on Retroviruses and Opportunistic Infections, Denver, Colorado.

Nuttall, J., J. Romano, K. Douville, C. Galbreath, A. Nel, W. Heyward, M. Mitchnick, S. Walker, and Z. Rosenberg. 2007. The future of HIV prevention: Prospects for an effective anti-HIV microbicide. *Infectious Disease Clinics of North America* 21(1):219-239.

Orner, P., J. Harries, D. Cooper, J. Moodley, M. Hoffman, J. Becker, E. McGrory, R. Dabash, and H. Bracken. 2006. Challenges to microbicide introduction in South Africa. *Social Science and Medicine* 63(4):968-978.

Padian, N., A. van der Straten, G. Ramjee, T. Chipato, G. de Bruyn, K. Blanchard, S. Shiboski, E. Montgomery, H. Fancher, H. Cheng, M. Rosenblum, M. van der Loan, N. Jewell, J. McIntyre, and The MIRA Team. 2007. Diaphragm and lubricant gel for prevention of HIV acquisition in southern African women: A randomised controlled trial. *Lancet* 370:251-261.

Peterson, L., D. Taylor, R. Roddy, G. Belai, P. Phillips, K. Nanda, R. Grant, E. E. K. Clarke, A. S. Doh, R. Ridzon, H. S. Jaffe, and W. Cates. 2007a. Tenofovir disoproxil fumarate for prevention of HIV infection in women: A phase 2, double-blind, randomized, placebo-controlled trial. *PLoS Clinical Trials* 2(5).

Peterson, L., K. Nanda, B. K. Opoku, W. K. Ampofo, M. Owusu-Amoako, A. Y. Boakye, W. Rountree, A. Troxler, R. Dominik, R. Roddy, and L. Dorflinger. 2007b. Savvy(R) (C31g) gel for prevention of HIV infection in women: A phase 3, double-blind, randomized, placebo-controlled trial in Ghana. *PLoS ONE* 2(12):e1312.

Pettifor, A. E., D. M. Measham, H. V. Rees, and N. S. Padian. 2004. Sexual power and HIV risk, South Africa. *Emerging Infectious Diseases* 10(11):1996-2004.

PhRMA. 2007. *PhRMA, HIV/AIDS medicines in development.* Washington, DC: PhRMA. (adapted for use by NAS).

Prep Watch. 2007. Ongoing prep trials as of January 2007. http://prepwatch.org/pdf/Trials/PrEP_trials_table.pdf (accessed November 1, 2007).

Smith, D. 2007. *CDC PrEP trials.* Presentation read at the first public meeting for the Committee on Methodological Challenges in HIV Prevention Trials, Washington, DC.

Tolley, E. E., and L. J. Severy. 2006. Integrating behavioral and social science research into microbicide clinical trials: Challenges and opportunities. *American Journal of Public Health* 96(1):79-83.

UNAIDS. 2007. *New data on male circumcision and HIV prevention: Policy and programme implications*. Geneva, Switzerland: UNAIDS.

Van Damme, L. 2007. *Phase III trial of 6% cellulose sulfate (CS) gel for the prevention of HIV transmission.* Paper read at the Fourth International AIDS Society Conference on HIV Pathogenesis, Treatment and Prevention, Sydney, Australia.

Van Damme, L., G. Ramjee, M. Alary, B. Vuylsteke, V. Chandeying, H. Rees, P. Sirivongrangson, L. Mukenge-Tshibaka, V. Ettiegne-Traore, C. Uaheowitchai, S. S. Karim, B. Masse, J. Perriens, and M. Laga. 2002. Effectiveness of col-1492, a nonoxynol-9 vaginal gel, on HIV-1 transmission in female sex workers: A randomised controlled trial. *Lancet* 360(9338):971-977.

Veldhuijzen, N., J. Nyinawabega, M. Umulisa, B. Kankindi, E. Geubbels, P. Basinga, J. Vyankandondera, and J. Van De Wijgert. 2006. Preparing for microbicide trials in Rwanda: Focus group discussions with Rwandan women and men. *Culture, Health and Sexuality* 8(5):395-406.

Watson-Jones, D., M. Rusizoka, H. Weiss, K. Mugeye, K. Baisley, J. Changalucha, D. Everett, C. Tanton, T. Clayton, D. Ross, and R. Hayes. 2007. *Impact of HSV-2 suppressive therapy on HIV incidence in HSV-2 seropositive women: A randomised controlled trial in Tanzania.* Paper read at the Fourth International AIDS Society Conference on HIV Pathogenesis, Treatment and Prevention, Sydney, Australia.

Watts, C., and P. Vickerman. 2001. The impact of microbicides on HIV and STD transmission: Model projections. *AIDS* 15(Suppl 1):S43-S44.

Wawer, M. 2007. *Lessons learned from STD treatment trials for HIV prevention.* Paper read at Presentation at the second public meeting for the Committee on Methodological Challenges in HIV Prevention Trials, London, UK.

Wawer, M. J., N. K. Sewankambo, D. Serwadda, T. C. Quinn, L. A. Paxton, N. Kiwanuka, F. Wabwire-Mangen, C. Li, T. Lutalo, F. Nalugoda, C. A. Gaydos, L. H. Moulton, M. O. Meehan, S. Ahmed, and R. H. Gray. 1999. Control of sexually transmitted diseases for AIDS prevention in Uganda: A randomised community trial. Rakai Project Study Group. *Lancet* 353(9152):525-535.

Weiser, S. D., M. Heisler, K. Leiter, F. Percy-de Korte, S. Tlou, S. DeMonner, N. Phaladze, D. R. Bangsberg, and V. Iacopino. 2006. Routine HIV testing in Botswana: A population-based study on attitudes, practices, and human rights concerns. *PLoS Medicine* 3(7):e261.

Whitehead, S. J., P. H. Kilmarx, K. Blanchard, C. Manopaiboon, S. Chaikummao, B. Friedland, J. Achalapong, M. Wankrairoj, P. Mock, S. Thanprasertsuk, and J. W. Tappero. 2006. Acceptability of Carraguard vaginal gel use among Thai couples. *AIDS* 20(17):2141-2148.

Yale Law Journal. 1946. Willful refusal to have or bear children as grounds for divorce or annulment. *The Yale Law Journal* 55(3):596-599.

2

Basic Design Features: Size, Duration, and Type of Trials, and Choice of Control Group

When planning a late-stage randomized clinical trial, investigators need to consider a number of design features, including (1) the number of subjects and duration of follow-up; (2) whether the trial will evaluate efficacy or effectiveness; (3) whether to begin with a smaller (phase 2) trial, with the understanding that a larger (phase 3) trial will follow if the results are promising (see Chapter 1, Box 1-1 for a description of clinical trial phases); and (4) how to choose a control group or groups.

A number of factors influence these choices, including the anticipated HIV incidence rate for the control group(s), the rates of product nonadherence and discontinuation owing to pregnancy and other reasons, and the rates of loss to follow-up, as well as the uncertainty surrounding these assumed rates and the resulting effect on the power of the trial. Investigators must also consider how large and long-lasting the effect of the intervention must be to be of scientific interest or public health significance. This chapter discusses these issues in the context of an HIV prevention trial involving a biomedical intervention.

TRIAL SAMPLE SIZE AND DURATION

The power of a clinical trial refers to the probability that it will detect a beneficial effect of a specific magnitude. Investigators commonly measure differences between the study arms as the relative risk, or RR, that someone will become HIV infected. For example, a recently published trial of circumcision (Bailey et al., 2007) compared the probability that participants

TABLE 2-1 Trial Duration as a Function of Accrual Rate and Years of Accrual

Design	Accrual rate (per year)	Years of accrual	Total participants accrued	Trial duration (years)	Expected number of events
1	500	2	1,000	5.43	95
2	300	2	600	8.62	95
3	500	3	1,500	4.42	96
4	300	3	900	6.45	95
5	500	4	2,000	4.18	96
6	300	4	1,200	5.68	96

NOTE: The table assumes a 5 percent type I error, 3 percent annual HIV incidence in the control group, and 90 percent power to detect an RR between intervention and control groups of 0.5.

in the circumcision and control groups would become HIV infected within 2 years of randomization. The results—rates of 2.1 versus 4.2 infections per 100 person years of follow-up for the two groups—yielded an estimated RR of 0.47 for circumcision. Alternatively, investigators could compare the HIV infection rates, or hazards, in the study arms. In that case, researchers would commonly express RR as the ratio of hazards for the two groups.

The power of a trial with a "time-to-event" endpoint, such as HIV infection, is driven by the number of participants who become HIV infected during the trial, not the sample size per se, and by how much investigators expect the number of infections to differ between the intervention and control groups. To illustrate, suppose that a placebo-controlled trial can enroll 500 participants per year, and wishes to have 90 percent power to detect a halving of annual HIV incidence from 3 percent to 1.5 percent, based on a two-sided type I (false positive) error of 5 percent. Table 2-1 illustrates six designs with different combinations of periods for accruing participants and trial durations that will give the desired power.[1]

Phase 3 effectiveness trials typically last for 2 to 4 years. The table assumes that time until infection follows an exponential distribution, that an equal number of participants are randomized to each group, that all participants are followed for the duration of the trial, and that there are no dropouts. An important feature is that despite their differences in sample size and duration, each of the six trial designs has the same type I and II error rates, and each would expect a total of 95–96 participants to become HIV infected during the study, given the assumed difference between treat-

[1]All calculations in this and the following tables and figures were made using EAST software, version 5.1 (Cambridge, MA: Cytel Inc., 2007).

ment groups. However, the designs differ in other important ways. For example, the first design would require only 1,000 participants (500 per arm), but it would require 5.43 years of follow-up from the time of the first randomized subject. In contrast, the fifth design would require twice the number of participants (2,000), but it would be completed more than a year sooner than the first design.

Choosing among such options when designing a trial requires considering several factors. These include the availability of trial participants, the relative costs of enrolling and following subjects, the anticipated number of subjects who become lost to follow-up (which would increase with the duration of follow-up), and the anticipated rates of adherence to the intervention, which could be affected by pregnancy rates, and would vary over time.

Designs with a smaller number of subjects would last longer, and thus provide estimates of cumulative HIV incidence over longer periods of time. Such trials would provide more long-term information on the durability of any intervention effect. However, because smaller studies take more time to complete, they could delay the introduction of an effective intervention into the community.

The above designs suggest that subjects would be enrolled and develop HIV infection at given rates, and therefore that the trials would be completed in the indicated durations of time. However, actual enrollment rates and HIV incidence rates may vary from these assumptions. Thus another approach for implementing these designs is to follow participants until the actual number of events—that is, new HIV infections—equals the expected number. This is sometimes called an "event-driven trial." For example, in design 1, participants would be accrued for 2 years, and the trial would continue until 96 events occurred. If the actual accrual and event rates occurred as assumed during trial planning, the trial would take about 5.43 years to complete.

However, if in fact the accrual rate were only 300 per year (as shown in Table 2-1), and participants were accrued for 2 years, then the trial must last 8.62 years to achieve 96 expected endpoints, and thus the desired power. Although an events-driven approach can compensate for inaccurate assumptions about accrual or incidence rates, investigators and sponsors must also consider the cost of such a trial, the sponsor's willingness to provide longer-term support, and the relevance of the trial result if the time to completion is substantially longer than originally anticipated.

Impact of the Assumed Intervention Effect on Trial Size and Power

One guideline for selecting the magnitude of an intervention effect for the purpose of planning a trial is to use the smallest reduction in HIV incidence that is important from a clinical and public health perspective. For example, investigators might decide that a biomedical intervention would need to reduce the HIV infection rate in a community by at least 50 percent to be practically useful. If so, the trial should ideally be powered to detect an RR between treatment and control of 0.50. Another guideline is to power a study based on the difference investigators expect to see. For example, even though an RR of 0.7 (a 30 percent reduction in risk) might be important from a public health perspective, investigators might expect a new intervention to have a stronger effect, for example, an RR of 0.5, and then power their study to detect this.

All other things being equal, a larger intervention effect requires a smaller or shorter trial. However, if investigators are overly optimistic about the magnitude of this effect, they will end up with a smaller or shorter trial than they need for adequate power.

The power of a trial can drop quickly as the efficacy of an intervention diminishes because of nonadherence, time off of the product, or other factors, so it is important to power a trial against a realistic RR. For example, Figure 2-1 shows how the power of design 5 from Table 2-1 changes when

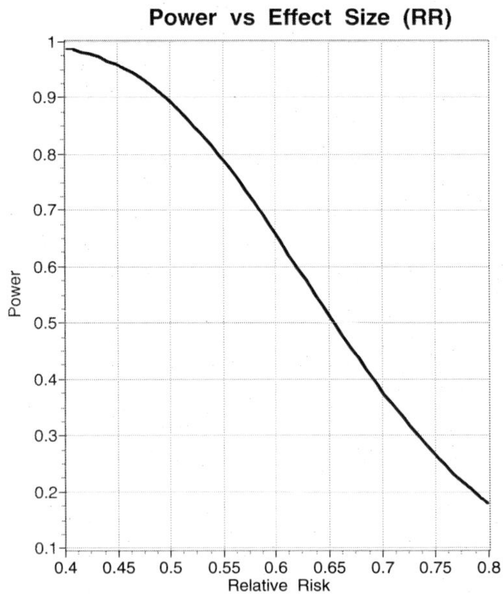

FIGURE 2-1 Power of design 5 as a function of actual product efficacy, as measured by the RR between intervention and control groups.
NOTE: The table assumes a control group incidence rate of 3 percent and a type I error of 5 percent.

the true RR varies from 0.4 to 0.8 with the number of participants held constant. Even with an RR of 0.6, the power drops from the planned 90 percent to 66 percent. Plots such as Figure 2-1 should be part of the planning process, so investigators appreciate how strongly the power of a trial will vary with the assumed RR between intervention and control groups, over ranges of public health significance. Of course, having low power for small intervention effects with no public health importance is not a concern. (See Appendix C for a discussion of the effects of product efficacy on sample size.)

Impact of HIV Incidence on Trial Size and Power

A trial's sample size also depends on the assumed HIV incidence rate in the control group. If investigators overestimate incidence rates when designing a trial, the power to detect an intervention effect could be low. Table 2-2 shows how the power of a study changes as a function of the HIV incidence rate in the control group, assuming a 50 percent reduction in risk in the intervention arm. For example, when the incidence rate in the control group drops from 3 percent to 2 percent in design 5 (2,000 participants, 4.18-year study), the power drops from 0.90 to 0.752. Clearly, when the incidence rate drops, a larger (and sometimes much larger) sample size would be needed to achieve adequate statistical power.

If investigators assume an HIV incidence rate that is too low for an events-driven trial, it may need to last much longer than expected (see Table 2-3).

Because of uncertainty in the expected HIV incidence rate in the control group, use of an events-driven trial can be advantageous to a trial that analyzes results at a prespecified time. However, when actual HIV incidence is substantially lower than investigators originally assume, the extra time

TABLE 2-2 Actual Power of Design 5 When Annual HIV Incidence in the Control Group Differs from the Assumed 3 Percent

Control group incidence rate	Power
5%	.987
4%	.963
3%	.90
2.5%	.84
2%	.752
1%	.464
0.5%	.262

NOTE: The RR between intervention and control is 0.5.

TABLE 2-3 Expected Duration Needed for Design 5 to Achieve 90 Percent Power When Annual HIV Incidence in the Control Group Differs from the Assumed 3 Percent

Control group incidence rate	Expected duration (in years)
4%	3.60
3.5%	3.86
3%	4.18
2.5%	4.62
2%	5.29
1.5%	6.41
1%	8.65

NOTE: The RR between intervention and control is 0.5.

needed to complete a trial with satisfactory power may not be feasible, or the results might be less relevant because of advances in the field. Thus, investigators need to monitor results during a trial to assess whether actual HIV incidence rates are close enough to the assumed rates that the trial remains feasible. (See Chapter 8 for further discussion.)

The Impact of Attrition on Trial Size and Power

In many trials, investigators are not able to follow some participants for HIV infection because they become lost to follow-up (LFU)—that is, leave the study area, refuse further contact participation in the study, or otherwise cannot be reached. If the prognosis for subjects who become LFU at a particular time is the same as that for subjects who remain in the study—called noninformative LFU, a condition that cannot be verified from the data—standard analyses that regard such losses as right-censored observations do not lead to distorted type I (false positive) errors, but the power of the study is diminished because of the resulting loss in person-years of observation for the study endpoint.

To avoid the potential loss of power from this type of LFU, investigators usually adjust the initial sample size to account for the anticipated amount of dropout. For example, if they anticipate that 10 percent of participants will become LFU, they can increase the sample size by 10 percent to yield the same total person-years of observation.

Impact of Product Discontinuation on Trial Size and Power

As described in Chapter 9, subjects that discontinue product use prematurely should continue to be followed for the trial's outcome events, such as HIV infection, and intention-to-treat analyses should be used to compare the intervention groups with respect to these outcomes. Although such an approach avoids biases that can arise from not analyzing outcome events that occur after product discontinuation, the power of the trial to detect an intervention effect on the outcome events can be diminished if the product's effect is lost after it is discontinued, making the observed HIV infection risks for the intervention and placebo groups more alike. As Freedman et al. have shown, the impact on study power can be substantial, depending on the proportion of subjects who discontinue treatment as well as the timing of their discontinuation (Freedman, 1990). (See also Brittain et al., 1989, and Jo, 2002.)

Because of its attenuating effect on the true intervention effect, non-compliance affects sample size more than attrition does (Zelen, 1988; Freedman, 1990). For example, if pregnancies lead to a 10 percent reduction in woman-years of observation, the effect on the power of the trial, if analyzed by intention to treat, is greater than the effect of a 10 percent reduction in sample size. Although this loss of power is typically not addressed by increasing the planned size of the trial, it underscores the need to maximize adherence of study participants.

Recommendation 2-1: Investigators should take steps to develop accurate *a priori* estimates of rates of participant accrual, HIV incidence, product discontinuation, and participant retention, and incorporate those into the sample size calculations. As a guard against inaccurate estimates, investigators should consider using an "events-driven" approach. That is, investigators would analyze study results when the prespecified number of enrolled subjects have become HIV infected, rather than at prespecified calendar times.

Although an events-driven approach can compensate for inaccurate assumptions about participant accrual or HIV incidence rates, investigators and sponsors must consider the cost of such a trial, the sponsor's willingness to provide longer-term support, and the relevance of the trial result if the time to completion is substantially longer than originally anticipated.

EFFICACY VS. EFFECTIVENESS TRIALS

An initial consideration when designing a phase 2 or 3 clinical trial to evaluate a new HIV intervention is whether the objective is to assess efficacy or effectiveness. In this context, efficacy refers to the effect of the intervention in a tightly controlled setting, wherein investigators try to minimize factors such as imperfect adherence to the product regimen, changes in risk behavior, and changes in the risk of exposure to HIV. Effectiveness, on the other hand, refers to how well the intervention would perform in the real world, where these factors and others cannot be rigorously controlled.

The quantitative connection between an intervention's efficacy and effectiveness is discussed in greater detail later in this chapter and in Appendix C. Efficacy trials usually overestimate the real-world effectiveness of an intervention for the outcome in question, and are often undertaken as a "proof of concept" to determine if the intervention, if taken as designed, can lower the risk of becoming infected from an exposure to HIV. Thus, since efficacy does not necessarily imply effectiveness in a real-world setting, a successful efficacy trial would commonly be followed by an effectiveness trial (see, for example, Fleming and Richardson, 2004). If an efficacy trial fails to suggest that an intervention has a positive impact, investigators may abandon further testing.

Efficacy trials can have less practical relevance in situations where adherence to a product is a challenge or includes a strong behavioral component. For example, in recent trials comparing low-carbohydrate and low-fat diets among obese participants (Foster et al., 2003; Samaha et al., 2003), the most important public health question was whether such diets could cause substantial weight loss during the trial period (effectiveness), and not whether the diets would cause weight loss if fully adhered to (efficacy).

Lack of Reliable Surrogate Endpoints

Effectiveness trials have historically measured disease outcomes, such as clinical improvement or survival. In the case of HIV prevention, they have measured time to HIV infection. Efficacy trials can use intermediate, or surrogate, endpoints, if those endpoints are sufficiently predictive of HIV infection or another clinical endpoint, and if the full effect of the interventions on the clinical response is fully explained by the effect on the surrogate (see, for example, Prentice, 1989). Examples of surrogate markers include viral load (of HIV, HCV), tumor response (oncology), bone mineral density (fracture prevention), and serum cholesterol levels (cardiology). In HIV treatment trials, suppression of the HIV virus is such an intermediate outcome. HIV treatment trials using surrogate markers do not require a follow-up trial using a clinical endpoint. In general, studies relying on intermediate endpoints require smaller sample sizes or can be completed in less time.

In some HIV prevention trials that focus on behavioral interventions, investigators have used acute sexually transmitted bacterial diseases, such as gonorrhea, chlamydia, and syphilis, as markers of HIV risk. In biomedical prevention trials, however, these have proven to be less predictive of HIV infection and are not considered reliable proxies.

In studying HIV prevention among injecting drug users, some investigators have used hepatitis B and C as markers of HIV infection (Vlahov and Junge, 1998; Dolan et al., 2003). Some HIV vaccine trials have also used a specific immunogenic effect as a surrogate endpoint. Although investigators know that a vaccine that demonstrates such an effect does not necessarily protect against HIV infection, a lack of immunogenicity may suggest a low protective ability. Investigators also use immunogenicity to prioritize candidate vaccines for further phase 3 testing.

However, surrogate endpoints in HIV prevention trials have in general not reliably predicted clinical efficacy. For example, an HIV adenovirus vaccine produced by Merck had been shown to be immunogenic—that is, capable of inducing a significant HIV-specific cell-mediated immune response. However, the company recently terminated a phase 3 trial because of lack of evidence that the vaccine prevents HIV infection, or that it affects the viral set point of subjects who become infected (NIAID, 2007).

As attractive as the notion of using surrogate markers for trial endpoints is, their use is fraught with many potential difficulties. For instance, a biomarker may be a good surrogate for one type of intervention and useless for another. Surrogates need to be specific for specific interventions and endpoints. Nonetheless, many current trials offer the opportunity to test surrogates against HIV incidence endpoints, and the committee believes that this is a worthwhile secondary goal for appropriate studies. The choice of candidate surrogates must be securely anchored in the knowledge of the pathophysiology of infection and how the surrogate marker relates biologically to the clinical endpoint that it is replacing.

Because no one has yet identified a biological or clinical marker that can reliably serve as a surrogate endpoint for HIV infection in efficacy trials of biomedical interventions, they must rely on HIV infection as the outcome just as effectiveness trials do. This means that efficacy and effectiveness trials will have the same basic design, differing only in the type of study population, duration, and sample size, and perhaps in the steps study staff take to promote product adherence and counsel participants to avoid risky behavior. The next section discusses the attributes of such efficacy and effectiveness trials and their respective sizes.

Attributes of Efficacy and Effectiveness Trials

An efficacy trial would ideally enroll as homogeneous a population as possible, and typically include a blinded control arm and be of short duration—6 months, for example, to attempt to minimize nonadherence and dropout. The shorter duration also serves to get an answer sooner than a trial with longer-term follow-up. An effectiveness trial, in contrast, would typically enroll a more heterogeneous population and last longer, commonly 2 to 4 years. Given the differences in the length of follow-up

TABLE 2-4 Anticipated Attributes of Efficacy and Effectiveness Trials

	Efficacy trial	Effectiveness trial
Duration	Shorter (e.g., 6–9 mos)	Longer (e.g., 2–4 years)
Population	More homogeneous	Less homogeneous
Adherence/behavior education	More	Less
HIV incidence rate in control group	Lower or higher	Lower or higher
Relative efficacy of intervention	Greater	Smaller

between these two types of trials, investigators need to consider the effects of attrition and nonadherence.

Because of potential nonadherence to the product and to condom use in a longer-term study, investigators might expect the magnitude of benefit of an intervention to be lower in an effectiveness trial than in an efficacy trial. Investigators would therefore normally expect the RR of a particular intervention to be as strong or stronger in an efficacy trial than in an effectiveness trial. However, it is not clear which design would have a larger HIV incidence rate in the control group. That is because—by selecting a population felt to be highly adherent to product—an efficacy study might also select individuals more likely to adhere to condom use and other risk-reduction measures. Table 2-4 describes some attributes of efficacy and effectiveness trials using HIV infection as the endpoint.

To see how these factors affect sample size and trial duration, consider an efficacy trial (trial 1) and an effectiveness trial (trial 2), both of which use HIV infection as the endpoint. Suppose that each assigns an equal number of subjects to the intervention and the control group, and the designs differ only in the duration (D) of time each subject is followed for HIV infection, the HIV incidence rate in the control group (I), and the relative risk (RR) of intervention versus control. Let these values for the efficacy and effectiveness trials be denoted (D1, I1, RR1) and (D2, I2, RR2), respectively, and let N1 and N2 denote the corresponding sample sizes for the trials, assuming the same type I and type II errors. Then the relative sample size of the efficacy trial compared with the effectiveness trial can be approximated by

$$\text{Ratio} = N1/N2 = (D2/D1) \times (I2/I1) \times [(1 - RR2)/(1 - RR1)]^2.$$

All other things being equal, the relative size of the efficacy trial will increase with the duration and HIV incidence rate in the effectiveness trial, and decrease with smaller RR in the effectiveness trial. Appendix C shows how nonadherence and efficacy can combine to determine effectiveness.

Shorter-Term vs. Longer-Term Follow-Up

Some investigators and sponsors have suggested that phase 3 trials of HIV prevention agents should be short term, with follow-up lasting only 6 to 9 months (Nunn, 2007). The rationale is that users' adherence to the product regimen may fall with time, perhaps through fatigue. HIV incidence among trial participants could also fall, because of changes in incidence rates unrelated to the trial, or differential dropout of higher-risk individuals.

While short-term trials may demonstrate proof of concept, they may have limited clinical or public health value, especially if the estimated intervention effect size is borderline and adherence to the product regimen is likely to wane over time. Because areas with high HIV incidence have limited resources, those regions may find interventions attractive only if they are clearly effective over a longer period. In that case, investigators would need to pursue a longer-term placebo-controlled trial after a positive efficacy trial. However, such a follow-up trial may pose ethical concerns about maintaining equipoise, because the intervention already would have been shown to be beneficial over the short term.

Information on the longer-term effectiveness of an intervention offers several advantages. For ethical reasons, HIV prevention trials must offer risk-reduction counseling, including on condom use, to participants in both intervention and control arms. If adherence to condoms falls during a longer-term trial, and the HIV infection rate rises, such a trial could be more capable of demonstrating an intervention effect. However, subjects who stop using condoms may also be less adherent to the product. And adherence to some products might actually increase over time as participants and their partners become more familiar with the product.

Moreover, setting up and initiating a trial entails considerable costs and work, and large efficacy trials with short follow-up may cost more than smaller effectiveness trials with a longer follow-up, assuming an equal number of person-years of observation. Thus the value of short-term efficacy trials in the case of HIV prevention is sometimes unclear, given the substantial resource commitment their large sample size would require, and the ethical concerns about undertaking a placebo-controlled effectiveness trial if an intervention turns out to be promising in an efficacy trial.

Two types of modified trial designs can provide information on both efficacy and effectiveness. The first is a way of obtaining some information on longer-term effectiveness in an efficacy trial whose main goal is to assess short-term efficacy, while the second is a way of possibly terminating a longer-term effectiveness trial during an interim analysis if there is insufficient evidence of short-term efficacy. The rationale behind these designs is that a product that has efficacy might not be effective in a real-world setting, and that a product that does not have efficacy would not be expected to be effective in a real-world setting:

- *Efficacy study with extended follow-up:* In this design, an efficacy trial would follow all subjects for HIV infection for a specific time (e.g., 6 months) after the last subject has been enrolled. Thus, for example, if the trial takes 18 months to enroll all subjects, follow-up will range from 6 months for the last enrolled subject to 2 years for the first enrolled subject. Such a trial will have the same power as an efficacy trial comparing the 6-month cumulative HIV infection rates of the intervention and placebo groups and following all subjects for exactly 6 months. However, it will also provide some evidence of cumulative HIV incidence rates through 24 months, and therefore give some measure of the effectiveness of the intervention. This example is based on a passive approach for obtaining more information about longer-term effects in the sense that the maximal follow-up time will be determined by the duration of the accrual period and thus the accrual rate. An alternative is to intentionally control the accrual rate to achieve a desired maximal follow-up time. For example, if follow-up times up to 3 years is desired, then the accrual rate in the example could be chosen to require a total of 2.5 years of accrual, in which case subjects would be followed for up to 3 years. In considering the implementation of such a design, cost and practicality issues would need to be considered.
- *Phase 3 trial with stopping rules for futility:* Similarly, a longer-term effectiveness trial can include an interim analysis that compares the intervention and control groups with respect to cumulative HIV incidence at some early time point, such as 6 months. This trial can terminate owing to futility if the interim data do not show a 6-month benefit of a particular magnitude. We note that power of a study to assess futility will be determined by the number of outcome events (HIV infections) that have occurred by the time point (e.g., 6 months) of interest. The issue of stopping rules is complex, however. In chapter 9, the committee discusses in depth several examples of trials that were stopped for efficacy and for futility, and situations when an unplanned interim analysis might arise.

Phase 2B vs. Phase 3 Trials

Rather than focusing on whether to precede an effectiveness trial with an efficacy trial, investigators may want to pursue a phase 2B trial before undertaking a phase 3 effectiveness trial. Phase 2B trials tend to involve follow-up periods similar to those of phase 3 trials, but to enroll only one-quarter to one-third the number of subjects. Phase 2B trials might also allow for a larger type II (false negative) error, and thus have lower power. Phase 2B trials provide a smaller, and less resource-intensive evaluation of new interventions which—if successful—would typically lead to a larger phase 3 trial.

Fleming and Richardson (2004) provide a detailed discussion of Phase 2B trials and propose that investigators consider using these to evaluate HIV microbicides, based on a four-step rule: (1) if a trial shows that a product has low efficacy, investigators would not study it further; (2) intermediate results would prompt investigators to consider a phase 3 trial; (3) stronger results would spur a confirmatory phase 3 trial; and (4) extremely positive results would enable investigators to submit the product for regulatory approval without further trials.

However, the use of a phase 2B design raises two concerns. First, if a phase 2B trial suggests that a microbicide provides a benefit, but the evidence falls short of that needed for regulatory approval, pursuing a placebo-controlled phase 3 trial would raise ethical concerns, as noted, especially if the trial were conducted in the same region as the phase 2B trial. Second, because of their smaller size, phase 2B trials may lack the power to assess a product's safety and participants' ability to tolerate it over the long term.

As an alternative, a phase 3 effectiveness trial that requires interim analysis could reduce these concerns yet offer some of the efficiencies of a phase 2B trial. Such a design could include guidelines for continuing the trial if early results show that the product has adequate promise of efficacy. The trial design can also include futility criteria, which would prompt investigators to terminate it given adequate evidence that the product is not efficacious.

Identifying reliable surrogate endpoint(s) for assessing the efficacy of biomedical HIV prevention products is a challenging, yet critical scientific goal that requires further research. At present, using an HIV infection endpoint, efficacy and effectiveness trials differ primarily in duration, anticipated HIV incidence rates in the control group, and the relative risks of intervention versus control. Unless an efficacy trial is designed to shed light on longer-term effectiveness, investigators would likely need to follow it with a longer trial, which could raise ethical concerns about equipoise between an intervention and control arm. Similar concerns apply to phase 2B trials.

Recommendation 2-2: Until validated surrogate endpoint(s) for HIV infection or product activity is (are) identified, investigators should use modified trial designs that can provide information on both the short- and long-term benefits of an intervention.

CHOICE OF CONTROL GROUP

Late-stage biomedical HIV prevention trials have relied almost exclusively on a superiority design, which entails comparing a new biomedical intervention to a control arm, and providing counseling and education on condom use and other risk-reduction activities to participants in both arms. Such trials aim to advance the field by assessing whether the new intervention is superior to the control intervention. A natural question arises as to how to select the control intervention for such trials. In many such trials, a placebo-controlled design is highly desirable to help to ensure an unbiased evaluation of the relative effects of the intervention. Although this also would apply to many HIV prevention trials of biomedical interventions, there are circumstances where the use of a blinded control group can be disadvantageous in shedding light on the effectiveness of the intervention if used in the community. The limitations arise from the possibility that people's risk-taking behavior will depend on their knowledge of the intervention they are (or are not) receiving.

In contrast, an unblinded trial comparing the microbicide with no biomedical intervention might provide a more realistic assessment of the impact of a microbicide when used in the community, because women's knowledge of whether they do or do not have access to a microbicide could affect the frequency of their risk-taking behavior, and whether they use a condom.

Consider a randomized trial designed to test a microbicide gel that provides all participants with the same level of counseling on condom use. One issue is whether the control group should receive only counseling on condom use (C), or both counseling and a placebo microbicide (P). That is, if M denotes the microbicide arm, should investigators randomize participants to M versus P, M versus C, or M versus P versus C? The key distinction between the placebo gel arm and the "condom-only" arm is that in the latter, participants know that they are not receiving the microbicide.

To address this question, investigators must consider the goals of the trial as well as the possible impact of a blinded versus unblinded control group on the validity and precision of the study's results and their interpretation and generalizability.

Potential Advantages of Blinding

Blinding treatment arms in a randomized trial is a common practice, and is aimed at preventing biases that could be caused by either the caregiver's or the participant's awareness of which arm he or she is in.

Such awareness can affect the accuracy and uniformity with which the trial's outcome measures are evaluated. For example, knowledge of which treatment a subject is receiving could affect the caregiver's assessment of that subject's health status. This is especially a concern in studies with subjective endpoints, such as trials that evaluate pain or cognition levels, or trials evaluating self-reported risky behavior, such as unprotected sexual intercourse.

Such concerns are substantially lower in studies with objective endpoints, such as HIV infection, which is based entirely on laboratory testing of blood samples. This is especially true if laboratory assessments are blinded to treatment arm (even though participants and caregivers are unblinded). However, self-reported information on other study outcomes, such as sexual risk behavior or adherence to the treatment protocol, could be affected by a subject's knowledge of her or his treatment arm. And investigators cannot easily distinguish differential reporting of such outcomes from differential behavior among study arms.

Blinding can also affect study results in other ways. Specifically, when intervention arms are not blinded, caregivers might offer different levels of support, treatment, and counseling to study participants with otherwise similar risk behavior profiles, and thus affect their primary study outcomes. Failure to account for this might cause investigators to misinterpret study results, if these are based on an assumption that concomitant care is identical in the study arms.

The choice to blind a study or not can also affect study visits and losses to follow-up. For example, participants who know they are not receiving a new intervention might miss more study visits, or drop out of a study at a higher rate, than participants who know they are receiving the intervention. Such differential losses or missing data can reduce the study's power, at a minimum, and more importantly can bias assessments of the relative efficacy of a new intervention.

Thus, for HIV prevention trials, an important concern is the effect of blinding (or not) on the completeness of study visits and retention and comparable counseling. However, numerous unblinded HIV prevention trials have produced excellent and nondifferential retention rates (Guay et al., 1999; Thior et al., 2006).

Potential Disadvantages of Blinding

Blinding through the use of a placebo can also have disadvantages. One would occur if the placebo had a direct effect on the study outcome. For example, a placebo microbicide gel might biologically inhibit the risk of HIV infection, or it might have lubricant properties that reduce vaginal abrasion and thus the risk of becoming infected (Nuttall et al., 2007). Such effects, while beneficial for study participants randomized to a placebo arm, can lead to biased estimates of the benefits of the microbicide gel. (See, for example, Kilmarx and Paxton, 2003.)

Another potential disadvantage of a blinded placebo is that a subject's knowledge of her or his treatment arm could affect behavior, such as the frequency or types of risky behavior, in a way that more accurately reflects the behavior of individuals in the community. If so, the resulting estimates of effectiveness for a placebo control arm in a trial may not reflect the effectiveness if the intervention were implemented (Jones et al., 2003; Padian, 2004).

For example, a recently published unblinded diaphragm trial found that women who were randomized to receive diaphragms did not experience a lower HIV infection rate than those who did not receive diaphragms—yet the former group reported much lower use of condoms (Padian et al., 2007). One view of this trial's results is that it failed because the lack of a placebo diaphragm arm, which presumably would have led to similar condom use as the active diaphragm arm, prevented an assessment of the protective effects of the diaphragm. However, another view is that the trial results reflect what might happen if the diaphragm were introduced into the community: a possible protective effect per sexual act might not translate into a reduced overall risk of HIV infection because of lower condom use.

The next section considers the potential advantages and limitations of three design strategies in the case of a microbicide gel trial.

Design 1: Microbicide (M) vs. Placebo (P)

A potential advantage of this design is that it is more likely to yield study retention rates that are similar between arms compared to design 2. One disadvantage is that investigators will not be able to determine whether the placebo has any direct effect on the risk of becoming HIV infected. Another disadvantage is that the resulting estimates of the benefit of the microbicide are less likely to reflect the actual effectiveness of the microbicide were it introduced into the community, than in design 2, which uses no placebo.

If a trial based on design 1 had high adherence and yielded a positive result, it would establish the biological efficacy of the microbicide gel, though not its effectiveness. If the trial provided convincing evidence of little or no benefit, then investigators might assume that the microbicide would not be effective in a community setting. However, such a result is also consistent with the hypothesis that the placebo was not inert: that is, that both the placebo gel and the microbicide have a biologically inhibitory effect on the risk of HIV infection.

Design 2: Microbicide (M) vs. Condom (C)

A potential advantage of this design is that the trial results would be expected to more closely reflect the true effectiveness of the microbicide if it were introduced into the community than design 1. Another advantage is that the trial would provide information on potentially differential effects of the microbicide and condom arms on reported risky behavior. In Padian et al. (2007), the unblinded trial of diaphragm with lubricant gel and condom provision versus condom provision only, self-reported condom use was significantly higher on the condom-only arm. However, a potential disadvantage of this design is that a subject's knowledge of his or her treatment arm could lead to differential rates of study retention or missed visits.

Suppose that such a trial led to comparable retention rates in the M and C arms. If the trial results were positive, the study would provide more direct evidence than design 1 that the microbicide would be effective if introduced into the community. If trial results were negative, introducing the microbicide into the general study population could not be justified, although this might not rule out evaluation of the microbicide in a different population. For example, if the trial demonstrated disinhibition, also known as risk compensation (Cassell et al., 2006), (that is, that participants will engage in more risky behavior because they believe they are protected by the test intervention) in the M arm, this may have caused the lack of an apparent benefit of the microbicide, and investigators might obtain different results in a different subject population where disinhibition is less likely.

Design 3: Microbicide (M) vs. Placebo (P) vs. Condom (C)

This three-arm design enjoys the advantages of both designs 1 and 2 and also avoids the disadvantages of each, except for the possible differential rates of retention between the M/P and C arms (Fleming and Richardson, 2004).

Comparison of the P and C arms would shed light on the effects on behavior among participants who know they are not receiving a microbicide versus those who know they could be receiving a microbicide and possibly on any direct effects of the placebo. Comparisons of M and P would be expected to reflect the direct effects of the microbicide gel (relative to placebo gel) on susceptibility to HIV infection.

If the P and C groups had similar HIV incidence rates and behaviors during follow-up, future studies in the same population may not require both control groups. A comparison of the relative risks of M:P and M:C would potentially reflect the efficacy versus effectiveness of the intervention.

The ongoing HPTN 035 microbicide trial employs this design (but with two microbicide arms), and will hopefully shed some initial light on these issues. However, the committee cautions that the results of HPTN 035 regarding both the direct efficacy of the product and its impact on behavior would not necessarily generalize to other populations. That is because the impact on behavior of knowing one is not receiving a microbicide versus knowing one might be receiving a microbicide may differ across populations. Thus this trial would not necessarily eliminate the need for other trials with multiple control groups.

Although the M versus P versus C design is more expensive because of the increased sample size and complexity, the benefits of successfully completing one or more such trials could have important potential advantages. As noted, because such a trial could assess the impact of the placebo, the potential benefit of the new intervention would be clearer. Given that so little is understood about the interplay between intervention and risk behavior, and given the strong impact of adherence and risk behavior on the ultimate effectiveness of an intervention, the committee believes that the potential economic disadvantage does not outweigh the substantial potential benefits of a dual-control design.

Recommendation 2-3: Sponsors, investigators, and regulatory agencies should consider using both blinded and unblinded control groups in future trials to more fully understand the effects of the intervention on HIV infection risk and behavior.

REFERENCES

Bailey, R. C., S. Moses, C. B. Parker, K. Agot, I. Maclean, J. N. Krieger, C. F. Williams, R. T. Campbell, and J. O. Ndinya-Achola. 2007. Male circumcision for HIV prevention in young men in Kisumu, Kenya: A randomised controlled trial. *Lancet* 369(9562):643-656.

Brittain, G. P., C. K. Rostron, D. B. Morton, and J. E. Rees. 1989. The use of a biological adhesive to achieve sutureless epikeratophakia. *Eye* 3(Pt 1):56-63.

Cassell, M. M., D. T. Halperin, J. D. Shelton, and D. Stanton. 2006. Risk compensation: The Achilles' heel of innovations in HIV prevention? *British Medical Journal* 332(7541):605-607.

Dolan, K., S. Rutter, and A. D. Wodak. 2003. Prison-based syringe exchange programmes: A review of international research and development. *Addiction* 98(2):153-158.

Fleming, T. R., and B. A. Richardson. 2004. Some design issues in trials of microbicides for the prevention of HIV infection. *Journal of Infectious Diseases* 190(4):666-674.

Foster, G. D., H. R. Wyatt, J. O. Hill, B. G. McGuckin, C. Brill, B. S. Mohammed, P. O. Szapary, D. J. Rader, J. S. Edman, and S. Klein. 2003. A randomized trial of a low-carbohydrate diet for obesity. *New England Journal of Medicine* 348(21):2082-2090.

Freedman, L. S. 1990. The effect of partial noncompliance on the power of a clinical trial. *Controlled Clinical Trials* 11(3):157-168.

Guay, L. A., P. Musoke, T. Fleming, D. Bagenda, M. Allen, C. Nakabiito, J. Sherman, P. Bakaki, C. Ducar, M. Deseyve, L. Emel, M. Mirochnick, M. G. Fowler, L. Mofenson, P. Miotti, K. Dransfield, D. Bray, F. Mmiro, and J. B. Jackson. 1999. Intrapartum and neonatal single-dose nevirapine compared with zidovudine for prevention of mother-to-child transmission of HIV-1 in Kampala, Uganda: HIVNET 012 randomised trial. *Lancet* 354(9181):795-802.

Jo, B. 2002. Statistical power in randomized intervention studies with noncompliance. *Psychological Methods* 7(2):178-193.

Jones, H., J. van de Wijgert, and E. Kelvin. 2003. The need for a "condoms-only" control group in microbicide trials. *Epidemiology* 14(4):505; author reply 505-506.

Kilmarx, P. H., and L. Paxton. 2003. Need for a true placebo for vaginal microbicide efficacy trials. *Lancet* 361(9359):785-786; author reply 786.

NIAID (National Institute of Allergy and Infectious Diseases). 2007. *Statement: Immunizations are discontinued in two HIV vaccine trials.* http://www3.niaid.nih.gov/news/newsreleases/2007/step_statement.htm (accessed December 15, 2007).

Nunn, A. 2007. *Issues in microbicide trial design, monitoring, and analysis.* Paper read at the second public meeting for the Committee on Methodological Challenges in HIV Prevention Trials, April 19, London, UK.

Nuttall, J., J. Romano, K. Douville, C. Galbreath, A. Nel, W. Heyward, M. Mitchnick, S. Walker, and Z. Rosenberg. 2007. The future of HIV prevention: Prospects for an effective anti-HIV microbicide. *Infectious Disease Clinics of North America* 21(1):219-239.

Padian, N., A. van der Straten, G. Ramjee, T. Chipato, G. de Bruyn, K. Blanchard, S. Shiboski, E. Montgomery, H. Fancher, H. Cheng, M. Rosenblum, M. van der Loan, N. Jewell, J. McIntyre, and the MIRA Team. 2007. Diaphragm and lubricant gel for prevention of HIV acquisition in southern African women: A randomised controlled trial. *Lancet* 370:251-261.

Padian, N. S. 2004. Evidence-based prevention: Increasing the efficiency of HIV intervention trials. *Journal of Infectious Diseases* 190(4):663-665.

Prentice, R. L. 1989. Surrogate endpoints in clinical trials: Definition and operational criteria. *Statistics in Medicine* 8(4):431-440.

Samaha, F. F., N. Iqbal, P. Seshadri, K. L. Chicano, D. A. Daily, J. McGrory, T. Williams, M. Williams, E. J. Gracely, and L. Stern. 2003. A low-carbohydrate as compared with a low-fat diet in severe obesity. *New England Journal of Medicine* 348(21):2074-2081.

Thior, I., S. Lockman, L. M. Smeaton, R. L. Shapiro, C. Wester, S. J. Heymann, P. B. Gilbert, L. Stevens, T. Peter, S. Kim, E. van Widenfelt, C. Moffat, P. Ndase, P. Arimi, P. Kebaabetswe, P. Mazonde, J. Makhema, K. McIntosh, V. Novitsky, T. H. Lee, R. Marlink, S. Lagakos, and M. Essex. 2006. Breastfeeding plus infant zidovudine prophylaxis for 6 months vs. formula feeding plus infant zidovudine for 1 month to reduce mother-to-child HIV transmission in Botswana: A randomized trial. The Mashi Study. *Journal of the American Medical Association* 296(7):794-805.

Vlahov, D., and B. Junge. 1998. The role of needle exchange programs in HIV prevention. *Public Health Reports* 113(Suppl 1):75-80.

Zelen, M. 1988. Statistical issues in the planning of prevention studies. *Cancer Investigation* 6(5):615-620.

3

Design Considerations: Risk-Reduction Counseling

Numerous stakeholders have reached a consensus that investigators who work with at-risk, uninfected populations have an ethical obligation to provide behavioral risk-reduction counseling to participants in HIV prevention trials (UNAIDS, 2000, 2007). Yet determining the appropriate level or "standard" of risk-reduction intervention in biomedical HIV prevention trials has been difficult. Two main reasons are the uncertainties about the effectiveness of specific behavioral interventions in reducing HIV infection risk in areas where many HIV prevention trials are conducted, and the uncertainties associated with adapting behavioral interventions that have been shown to reduce risky behaviors or specific sexually transmitted infections (STIs) from one geographical or cultural setting to another. In addition, determining the appropriate standard risk-reduction intervention requires stakeholders to consider the sustainability and costs of the risk-reduction intervention.

To help investigators address these dilemmas, this chapter first highlights the ethical arguments for providing risk-reduction counseling to participants in an HIV prevention trial of a biomedical intervention. The next section then reviews findings from randomized, comparative studies of behavioral risk-reduction interventions in the United States and other countries, efforts to adapt these findings to different regions and cultural settings, and the need to evaluate the effectiveness of such adapted strategies in new settings. The final section argues for the incorporation of randomized comparisons of behavioral intervention strategies in late-stage biomedical intervention trial, highlights several ethical considerations that need to be addressed about the standard of behavioral risk-reduction interventions in future HIV prevention trials, and makes recommendations for practice and research.

ETHICAL REASONS FOR RISK-REDUCTION COUNSELING

In discussions over the past decade about the ethics of vaccine trials, researchers, community representatives, human rights advocates, and ethicists reached broad agreement—based on several ethical principles, including beneficence, autonomy, and justice—that participants in clinical trials of HIV prevention interventions should receive risk-reduction counseling, and access to condoms and other means to reduce their risk of becoming infected with HIV (UNAIDS, 2000, p. 522).

Ethicists have advanced three reasons for this obligation. As discussed by Lie et al. (2006): "The ethical requirements to provide counselling and condoms as part of HIV preventive trials . . . are based on the general requirements (1) to provide relevant information to participants in clinical trials, (2) not to impede or place any barriers on access to known preventive methods, and (3) to actively promote the use of known preventive methods" (p. 522).

Ethicists have put forth several other considerations to justify provision of known prevention methods to participants. First, they argue that investigators must attempt to counterbalance any increased risk that participants will become HIV infected owing to disinhibition: that is, that they may engage in more risky behavior if they erroneously believe they are protected by the test intervention. Thus the duty to minimize risks in clinical trials dictates that investigators provide counseling on methods to prevent HIV infection (Lie et al., 2006).[1]

Second, some ethicists have suggested that providing such counseling to trial participants is a form of "justice as reciprocity." That is, because participants contribute to the social good, they are owed recompense in the form of HIV prevention counseling and access to information and technologies prevention methods that can reduce their risk of HIV infection (Lie et al., 2006).

Finally, some ethicists have argued that participants should receive risk-reduction counseling prevention methods because of the "fundamental ethical requirement for any person to do what they can to help others in need" (Lie et al., 2006, p. 523). This Good Samaritan proposition imposes special duties on those who conduct clinical trials (Lie et al., 2006).

However, despite widespread agreement that participants in clinical

[1]Lie et al. (2006) discuss these principles in their examination of the ethical obligation of researchers to provide male circumcision as part of the prevention standard for HIV prevention trials, but these arguments also apply to risk-reduction counseling and condom promotion.

trials should receive risk-reduction interventions, considerable uncertainty remains about what the nature and intensity of such interventions should be. Some ethicists have called for "high-quality counseling" (Wolf and Lo, 2001). UNAIDS and the World Health Organization (WHO) recommend a more comprehensive standard, suggesting that investigators should provide "appropriate counseling and access to all state of the art HIV risk-reduction methods . . . to participants throughout the duration of the biomedical HIV prevention trial" (UNAIDS, 2007, p. 47). UNAIDS and WHO also call for adding new HIV risk-reduction methods "based on consultation among all research stakeholders including the community, as they are scientifically validated or as they are approved by the relevant authorities" (UNAIDS, 2007, p. 47).

Uncertainty about the appropriate standard of care in biomedical HIV prevention trials stems in part from ethical considerations. For example, should the standard risk-reduction intervention be the one shown to be most effective, regardless of cost or sustainability? The ethical uncertainties are compounded by the lack of definitive findings on the effectiveness of behavioral risk-reduction interventions in many of the resource-poor settings where biomedical HIV prevention trials are conducted. Investigators have conducted only a limited number of studies of the efficacy of behavioral risk-reduction interventions in these settings. Indeed, a significant amount of the research evaluating the efficacy of behavioral risk-reduction interventions has occurred in the United States. This limitation is compounded by the difficulty of extrapolating behavioral risk-reduction interventions shown to be efficacious in one setting and population to different settings with different populations, risk behaviors, and cultural norms. In particular, behavioral risk-reduction interventions that have been shown to be efficacious in developed countries may not always be easily transferable to settings and populations in developing countries. Finally, there is uncertainty about the effectiveness of behavioral intervention strategies in reducing the risk of HIV infection.

The next section reviews the evidence on the effectiveness of behavioral risk-reduction interventions in reducing risk behaviors, with an emphasis on sexual behaviors, the incidence of STIs, and incidence of HIV infection.

EFFECTIVENESS OF BEHAVIORAL RISK-REDUCTION INTERVENTIONS

Voluntary Counseling and Testing (VCT Programs)

Voluntary counseling and testing (VCT) is widely used throughout the world to prevent HIV acquisition and transmission, and to identify individuals for treatment or monitoring. A number of nonrandomized studies have assessed the impact of VCT on risky behavior, but results from randomized trials are limited.

Perhaps the most definitive study of the effectiveness of VCT on reported risk behavior was that of the Voluntary HIV-1 Counseling and Testing Efficacy Study Group (2000), which conducted a trial of 3,120 individuals and 586 couples in Kenya, Tanzania, and Trinidad. Participants were randomized to receive VCT versus basic health information. The primary efficacy endpoint was self-reported unprotected intercourse with a nonprimary partner by the time of the 6-month study visit.

The study showed that individuals assigned to VCT reported a significantly greater reduction in unprotected intercourse with a nonprimary partner than individuals assigned to basic health information (overall odds ratio [OR] = 0.68, 95% confidence interval [CI]: 0.56–0.82). In other analyses, the study showed that couples randomized to VCT reported significantly greater reductions in unprotected intercourse with each another than did couples randomized to basic health information. The study found no significant differences in reported unprotected intercourse between participants and unenrolled partners (OR = 1.09, 95% CI: 0.92–1.29). The trial also did not detect a beneficial impact from VCT on the incidence of STIs (OR = 0.80, 95% CI: 0.53–1.20), although the study was not designed for that endpoint.

Although there is limited evidence of the effectiveness of VCT in reducing some sexual risk behaviors, overall the findings are mixed. This sentiment is echoed in a recent meta-analysis of VCT of behavioral risk-reduction interventions in developing countries based on papers published between 1990 and 2005, which included the VCT Study Group (2000) study and 6 nonrandomized studies (Allen et al., 1992; Muller et al., 1995; Wang et al., 2002; Farquhar et al., 2004; Kawichai et al., 2004; Matovu et al., 2005). Denison and colleagues (2007) found that the combined data from these showed a moderate effect of VCT on unprotected sex (OR = 1.69; 95% CI: 1.25–2.31) but VCT showed no significant effect on number of sex partners (OR = 1.22; 95% CI: 0.89–1.67).

Randomized studies comparing the effect of different types of VCT on HIV incidence are very limited. Corbett et al. (2007) assessed the relative efficacy of two forms of VCT in Zimbabwe. The investigators found no evidence that more intensive VCT (rapid testing and counseling provided onsite) reduced HIV infection rates compared with standard VCT (providing participants with prepaid vouchers for use with an external provider).

Studies Evaluating Behavioral Risk-Reduction Interventions

Numerous studies and meta-analyses have compared different behavioral risk-reduction interventions that aim to reduce the risk of HIV infection or transmission. These studies have involved different populations, including injecting drug users, men who have sex with men (MSM), heterosexuals, adolescents, ethnic and racial minorities, and HIV-infected individuals. Most studies have used a behavioral endpoint, such as self-reported unprotected sex, but some have examined biological endpoints, including the acquisition of non-HIV STIs, and a few have used HIV infection. Meta-analyses of the behavioral risk-reduction interventions for these different populations have been reported by Copenhaver et al. (2006) for injecting drug users, Johnson et al. (2002) and Herbst et al. (2005) for MSM, Neumann et al. (2002) for heterosexuals, Mullen et al. (2002) for adolescents, Crepaz et al. (2007) for ethnic and racial minorities, and Johnson et al. (2005) for persons living with HIV.

One of the earliest and most important trials of behavioral risk-reduction interventions was Project RESPECT, a randomized, controlled trial conducted at five public STI clinics in the United States. This study compared the efficacy of two personalized ("client-centered") HIV/STI counseling interventions in increasing rates of condom use and reducing STIs among heterosexual clients (Kamb et al., 1998). The two test interventions were (1) enhanced counseling, involving four visits and a total of 200 minutes of counseling; and (2) brief counseling, involving two visits and a total of 40 minutes of counseling. The study compared these interventions with a control arm given didactic prevention messages.

The study found that self-reported condom use was significantly higher in subjects randomized to each of the counseling arms than in subjects randomized to the didactic message arm ($P < 0.05$ for each comparison). This was the first randomized trial to show that client-centered counseling could reduce the number of new STIs. After 6 months, 30 percent fewer subjects in the counseling arms than in the didactic arm had acquired new STIs ($P < 0.01$ for each comparison). The study found no significant differences between the more intense and less intense risk-reduction counseling, so the investigators suggested that clinics provide the short counseling intervention.

Lyles and colleagues (2007) recently conducted a systematic review of randomized and nonrandomized U.S.-based research from 2000 to 2004 on behavioral risk-reduction interventions, to identify those with the best evidence of efficacy in reducing HIV risk behaviors. Their review focused on behavioral risk-reduction interventions delivered to the individual or small group, and evaluated them in three domains: study design, implementation and analysis, and strength of evidence.

To meet the strength-of-evidence criterion, a study had to have shown a statistically significant ($P \leq 0.05$) positive effect for at least one outcome measure at least three months post-intervention, and no significant negative evidence for reducing HIV risk. A study also had to have a retention rate of

70 percent, base its results on at least 50 participants per arm, and avoid any limitations considered a fatal flaw.

One hundred behavioral intervention studies met the criteria for eligibility for review. Of those, 18 met the criteria for demonstrating a positive intervention effect, and were thus identified as "best evidence." Fourteen of the studies targeted uninfected populations at risk for HIV. These were conducted among drug users (four studies), heterosexual adults (six studies), MSM (two studies), and adolescents (two studies).

All "best-evidence" behavioral risk-reduction interventions applied at least one theory or model on behavioral change. These included social cognitive theory, social learning theory, the AIDS risk-reduction model, the information-motivational-behavior model, and the theory of gender and power. Interventions were typically conducted in research sites (eight studies), community or public areas (five studies), health care clinics (four studies), HIV or STI clinics (three studies), or community-based agencies (three studies). Although the content of these interventions differed, most entailed building technical (such as condom use), personal, or interpersonal skills.

The majority of the significant intervention effects were based on the endpoint of self-reported reduction of unprotected sexual intercourse (12 studies). Studies of the five interventions targeting injecting drug users also measured the effect on self-reported injection-related risk behaviors, such as frequency of injection or needle sharing with three of the five finding a reduction.

Lyles and colleagues (2007) identified four randomized interventions that demonstrated a significant reduction in incident STIs: Baker and colleagues (2003) compared the effect of two 16-session group interventions that provided skills training versus health education in 287 heterosexual women in Washington state. The endpoint was the development of an STI, including gonorrhea, mucopurulent cervicitis (including chlamydia), pelvic inflammatory disease, syphilis, HIV, or herpes simplex virus 2 (HSV-2). During follow-up, 18 of 104 women in the control group developed an STI, compared with 9 of 105 women in the skills-training group ($P = 0.05$), with mucopurulent cervicitis (14 cases) and HSV-2 (7 cases) the main STIs. No women in either arm became HIV infected.

In the second study, DiClemente et al. (2004) conducted a randomized comparison of an intervention emphasizing ethnic and gender pride, HIV knowledge, communication, condom skills, and healthy relationships with a control emphasizing exercise and nutrition in 522 sexually experienced African American girls aged 14 to 18 in the U.S. South. STI infection (chlamydia, trichomonas, gonorrhea) at the study's 6-month or 12-month assessment was a secondary endpoint. The authors reported a significantly lower risk of chlamydia in the experimental arm compared with the control arm ($OR = 0.17$, 95% CI: 0.03–0.92, $P = 0.04$).

Third, Wingood and colleagues (2004) reported on a randomized trial of 366 women living with HIV in Alabama and Georgia. That study compared an intervention emphasizing gender pride, participants' personal networks, knowledge of HIV transmission, communication and condom skills, and healthy relationships with a control arm receiving health promotion. A secondary endpoint of the trial was the occurrence of chlamydia or gonorrhea during the 12-month follow-up period. The intervention group experienced a significantly lower rate of chlamydia and gonorrhea than the control group (OR = 0.20, 95% CI: 0.1–0.6, P = 0.006).

Finally, Shain and colleagues (2004) reported on a two-year randomized trial comparing standard and enhanced gender- and culture-specific counseling offered in small groups (to 209 and 232 women, respectively) with interactive STI counseling (249 women) in minority women from Texas. The primary endpoint—acquisition of chlamydia or gonorrhea—occurred significantly less often in the intervention groups (15.4 percent versus 39.8 percent, P = 0.004) during the entire follow-up period.

Only a few randomized trials of behavioral interventions have evaluated HIV infection as the study endpoint. Lyles et al. (2007) reviewed one U.S.-based study that used HIV infection as the study endpoint: Project EXPLORE (HIVNET 015) compared the efficacy of an intense behavioral intervention to that of standard risk-reduction counseling among U.S. MSM (EXPLORE Study Team, 2004), with HIV infection as primary endpoint and behavioral outcomes, including unprotected anal intercourse and unprotected anal intercourse with a serodiscordant partner, as secondary endpoints. (The control group received the "brief" counseling intervention recommended by the Project RESPECT trial noted above.) The study found that the rates of unprotected receptive anal intercourse with HIV-positive and unknown-status partners was 20.5 percent lower in the intervention arm than in the control arm (OR = 0.80, 95% CI: 0.71–0.89). The observed rate of HIV infection was 18.2 percent lower in the intervention group than in the standard group, but the difference was not statistically significant (95% CI for difference: –5% to +36%).

Several behavioral intervention HIV prevention trials done outside the United States were designed and powered to assess HIV infection as an endpoint. Kamali et al. (2003) undertook a large community-level randomized trial comparing the efficacy of a behavioral intervention alone, and a behavioral intervention plus STI control, with routine care in preventing HIV infection in 18 communities in Uganda. The study enrolled more than 40,000 subjects, of whom more than 300 became HIV infected. However, the study found no significant difference in HIV incidence between the behavioral counseling arm (incidence rate ratio = 0.94, 95% CI: 0.60–1.45, P = 0.72) or the behavioral-plus-STI arm (incidence rate ratio = 1.00,

95% CI: 0.63–1.58, P = 0.98) and the control arm, although both interventions reduced the rate of specific non-HIV STIs.

Ross and colleagues (2007) conducted a community-randomized trial in Tanzania that compared a specially designed program of behavioral and educational interventions with standard activities in school-aged youth, with HIV incidence as a primary endpoint. Few (5) seroconversions occurred among the young men, so the study could not adequately compare groups. Among young women, the study found no significant difference in HIV incidence between the intervention and control groups (Relative risk [RR] = 0.75, 95% CI: 0.34–1.66). Nor did it find significant differences between the interventions in either gender with respect to HSV-2 infection, the second primary endpoint.

Gregson and colleagues (2007) reported the results of a cluster-randomized trial in eastern Zimbabwe. The intervention group received targeted and population-level strategies to promote safer sexual behavior and to improve treatment of STIs that facilitate HIV. Both the intervention and control groups received standard government services plus social marketing of condoms. There was no evidence that the intervention communities had a lower risk of HIV infection, other STIs, or high-risk behaviors than the control communities (incidence rate ratio = 1.27, 95% CI: 0.92–1.75).

Two additional behavioral risk-reduction trials using HIV endpoints are underway. First, the National Institute of Mental Health (NIMH) Collaborative HIV/STD Prevention Trial is a community-level HIV prevention intervention study conducted in international settings, using behavioral outcomes and HIV infection as the primary study endpoints. The trial is evaluating the effectiveness of an intervention using a community popular opinion leader to convey HIV prevention messages to the community. The study phases consist of an ethnographic study, pilot studies, an epidemiological study, and a community-randomized trial. Results are not yet available.

The second study, Project Accept (HPTN 043), is a community-randomized HIV prevention trial involving 34 communities in South Africa, Tanzania, and Zimbabwe, and 14 communities in Thailand (Morin et al., 2006). These communities are being randomized to receive either a community-based HIV voluntary counseling and testing (CBVCT) intervention plus standard clinic-based VCT (SVCT), or SVCT alone. The CBVCT intervention aims to make VCT more available in community settings, to engage communities through outreach, and to provide posttest support. These strategies are designed to change community norms and reduce the risk of HIV infection among all members of a community, whether or not they participate directly in the intervention. This is the first international randomized, controlled phase 3 trial to determine the efficacy of a behavioral or social science intervention with HIV incidence as an endpoint.

In sum, behavioral risk reduction interventions have lowered the incidence of specific self-reported sexual risk behaviors and specific non-HIV STIs. However, none of these strategies has yet shown a beneficial effect in reducing the incidence of HIV infection.

ADAPTING EFFICACIOUS BEHAVIORAL RISK-REDUCTION INTERVENTIONS

If an intervention has been shown to be effective in one setting, it is important to adapt it for use by a diverse array of providers of HIV prevention services (NIH, 2007; Wingood and DiClemente, 2008). This often requires providers to enhance the acceptability of the intervention among a new target population. This is particularly true if an organization in a developing country would like to use an intervention designed in the United States or other developed countries. If providers do not pay attention to the cultural context and HIV-related risks of the new target population, the intervention may remain faithful to the underlying theoretical framework and core elements but lack relevance, sustainability, and acceptability.

Researchers have recently developed several frameworks to guide the adaptation of a HIV behavioral intervention to a different setting. For example, the Centers for Disease Control and Prevention (CDC) has articulated the Map of Adaptation Process (MAP) (McKleroy et al., 2006). This approach includes an assessment phase, in which an organization evaluates the target population's HIV risk, the appropriateness of the behavioral risk-reduction intervention, and the organization's capacity to implement it. The assessment phase is followed by a preparation phase, in which the organization adapts the evidence-based intervention: then comes the implementation phase, in which the organization pilots the adapted intervention. Other adaptation models take a more stringent approach, and encourage evaluating the adapted behavioral risk-reduction intervention as part of a phase 2B trial (Wingood and DiClemente, 2008).

A number of studies have adapted behavioral HIV risk-reduction interventions shown to be efficacious in developed countries to developing country settings. For example, Kalichman and colleagues (2005) relied on collaborative interdisciplinary workshops to adapt a brief theory-based HIV risk-reduction counseling intervention developed in the United States for use in an STI clinic in South Africa. Wingood and DiClemente (2008) used a process known as theatre testing to adapt an efficacious behavioral risk-reduction intervention developed in the United States. for young Zulu-speaking women in KwaZulu-Natal, South Africa. In theatre testing, facilitators implement the core elements of an intervention while integrating new materials and activities to enhance its cultural relevance and efficacy for the target population.

However, behavioral risk reduction interventions that have been shown to be efficacious in one setting may not necessarily be efficacious in another. Thus, when adapting an HIV intervention to a new setting and population, investigators should evaluate its effectiveness in the new target population, and identify potential ways to enhance it.

EVALUATING BEHAVIORAL RISK-REDUCTION INTERVENTIONS IN THE CONTEXT OF A BIOMEDICAL INTERVENTION TRIAL

If definitive evidence on the effectiveness of behavioral risk-reduction interventions in settings where biomedical HIV prevention trials are planned were to become available, investigators would face questions on the cost and sustainability of integrating behavioral risk-reduction interventions into such trials. Unfortunately, as noted, researchers face considerable uncertainty about which behavioral risk-reduction interventions are most effective in many settings where biomedical HIV prevention trials occur. In the face of such uncertainty, it becomes critical to undertake research that may provide evidence on this question. Such studies are necessary because behavioral risk-reduction interventions will remain an important component of the overall HIV prevention effort regardless of the efficacy of biological approaches. The committee believes strongly that integrating that research into a biomedical intervention trial provides an excellent opportunity to move forward on both fronts.

Given such uncertainty, however, communities must participate in decisions regarding the conduct of trials, including the choice of behavioral interventions. UNAIDS and WHO have advocated that the "technique, frequency, and message content of counseling should be agreed upon by the community–government–investigator–sponsor partnership" (UNAIDS, 2007, p. 49).

Chapter 6 explores specific study designs, such as factorial designs, for late-stage effectiveness trials of biomedical prevention interventions that also allow a comparative evaluation of two or more behavioral risk-reduction interventions. As noted, the choice of such strategies should reflect current knowledge about which strategies have been shown to be effective and can be adapted to the setting of the biomedical prevention trial, and which strategies the community, donors, researchers, and other relevant stakeholders consider feasible and sustainable. When two or more behavioral strategies are implemented during a biomedical intervention trial, they must satisfy principles of research ethics, just as the biomedical interventions must.

The committee recognizes that the incorporation of a behavioral intervention comparison into a biomedical intervention trial will increase the trial's logistical complexity. For example, if an individual and group behavioral intervention were provided by a site, it would create additional scheduling, training, and manpower responsibilities for the site. On the other hand, if some sites were randomized to evaluate one behavioral intervention while the rest were randomized to evaluate another, using the ideas of cluster randomization (Chapter 10), the additional logistical complexity to a site would be far less. For either scenario, careful site preparation should be adequate to allow the incorporation of an evaluation of behavioral interventions, and the potential gains from finding improved behavioral interventions would provide lasting benefits to the community.

In addition to the need for clinical equipoise among these behavioral strategies, other critical ethical questions about the standard of care, costs and sustainability, and obligations of researchers must be answered. Although it is outside the scope of the committee's review to address these issues, we highlight some of the critical questions below.

Standard of Care

- What is the minimal or standard behavioral intervention that the trial can ethically use as a control group?
- Because most uninfected populations in developing countries do not receive individualized HIV behavioral counseling outside the context of a research study, what defines the "community standard" for risk-reduction counseling?
- Can the trial ethically limit the counseling in a control group to the level already (nominally) provided in a particular community, when more intensive behavioral interventions have not been shown to be effective in reducing HIV infection risk in that context?

Costs and Sustainability

- What is the next course of action if an expensive behavioral risk-reduction intervention is shown to be highly efficacious in developed countries, but is not sustainable in developing countries?

Obligations of Researchers

- What is the duty for those studying biomedical investigations to undertake concurrent investigations of behavioral risk-reduction interventions?
- Should risk-reduction counseling that occurs during a biomedical HIV prevention trial be provided through an organization that is independent of the investigators? If the risk-reduction interventions were fully effective, none of the participants in the trial would become infected, and

there could be no evaluation of the efficacy of the biomedical intervention. To address any possible conflict between the desires of researchers to provide counseling and their wish to demonstrate benefits from the biomedical intervention, UNAIDS and WHO suggest investigators consider having an independent organization counsel participants as one way to minimize such conflicts (UNAIDS, 2000).

There are no simple solutions to such complex challenges. The answers to these questions will in general vary with different intervention trials and over time. It is important, however, that in decisions about these issues be determined through a fair and transparent process. Daniels and Sabin have proposed a framework for setting priorities in resource allocation (Daniels and Sabin, 1997) which has also been applied to roll-out of ARVs (Daniels, 2005) and has bearing on the resolution of these questions. According to this framework, a fair process would dictate the following:

- Decisions should be based on evidence, and reasons for those decisions should be contextually relevant. This requires that all stakeholders who will be affected by the priority-setting process have some say, so the effort to make decisions and set priorities takes into account a variety of values.
- The rationale for decisions and disagreements must be publicly accessible.
- Appeals must be allowed, so decisions can be reconsidered in light of new evidence or arguments.

Such a priority-setting process could be useful in clinical research in determining whether specific interventions meet the needs of a community in a particular setting.

SUMMARY

In late-stage HIV prevention trials of biomedical interventions, investigators and donors also have an excellent and unique opportunity to evaluate and compare different behavioral risk-reduction interventions as part of the trial's research objectives (see Chapter 10 for specific study designs). The identification of improved behavioral interventions will benefit at-risk populations even if the biomedical intervention being studied has no efficacy, and will potentiate its effectiveness if it does have efficacy.

Recommendation 3-1: Given the lack of evidence on the effectiveness of behavioral risk-reduction interventions in settings where many HIV biomedical trials are planned, investigators planning such trials should

incorporate randomized comparisons of behavioral risk-reduction interventions into their designs whenever possible.

Recommendation 3-2: Donors and investigators should involve behavioral and social scientists in the early planning stages of a trial, to identify the most appropriate behavioral risk reduction interventions, and to efficiently plan their implementation during the trial.

Recommendation 3-3: Investigators planning to test behavioral risk-reduction interventions as part of a late-stage biomedical HIV prevention trial should consult with the community, governments, donors, and other stakeholders about the cost and sustainability of those interventions in the community.

Recommendation 3-4: If a trial will adapt specific behavioral interventions shown to be effective in other settings, investigators should field-test the strategies during the planning of the trial, to ensure that they can be implemented as envisioned.

REFERENCES

Allen, S., J. Tice, P. Van de Perre, A. Serufilira, E. Hudes, F. Nsengumuremyi, J. Bogaerts, C. Lindan, and S. Hulley. 1992. Effect of serotesting with counselling on condom use and seroconversion among HIV discordant couples in Africa. *British Medical Journal* 304(6842):1605-1609.

Baker, S. A., B. Beadnell, S. Stoner, D. M. Morrison, J. Gordon, C. Collier, K. Knox, L. Wickizer, and S. Stielstra. 2003. Skills training versus health education to prevent STDs/HIV in heterosexual women: A randomized controlled trial utilizing biological outcomes. *AIDS Education and Prevention* 15(1):1-14.

Copenhaver, M. M., B. T. Johnson, I. C. Lee, J. J. Harman, and M. P. Carey. 2006. Behavioral HIV risk reduction among people who inject drugs: Meta-analytic evidence of efficacy. *Journal of Substance Abuse Treatment* 31(2):163-171.

Corbett, E. L., B. Makamure, Y. B. Cheung, E. Dauya, R. Matambo, T. Bandason, S. S. Munyati, P. R. Mason, A. E. Butterworth, and R. J. Hayes. 2007. HIV incidence during a cluster-randomized trial of two strategies providing voluntary counselling and testing at the workplace, Zimbabwe. *AIDS* 21(4):483-489.

Crepaz, N., A. K. Horn, S. M. Rama, T. Griffin, J. B. Deluca, M. M. Mullins, and S. O. Aral. 2007. The efficacy of behavioral interventions in reducing HIV risk sex behaviors and incident sexually transmitted disease in black and Hispanic sexually transmitted disease clinic patients in the United States: A meta-analytic review. *Sexually Transmitted Diseases* 34(6):319-332.

Daniels, N. 2005. Fair process in patient selection for antiretroviral treatment in WHO's goal of 3 by 5. *Lancet* 366(9480):169-171.

Daniels, N., and J. Sabin. 1997. Limits to health care: Fair procedures, democratic deliberation, and the legitimacy problem for insurers. *Philosophy & Public Affairs* 26(4):303-350.

Denison, J. A., K. R. O'Reilly, G. P. Schmid, C. E. Kennedy, and M. D. Sweat. 2007. HIV voluntary counseling and testing and behavioral risk reduction in developing countries: A meta-analysis, 1990–2005. *AIDS and Behavior*.

DiClemente, R. J., G. M. Wingood, K. F. Harrington, D. L. Lang, S. L. Davies, E. W. Hook, 3rd, M. K. Oh, R. A. Crosby, V. S. Hertzberg, A. B. Gordon, J. W. Hardin, S. Parker, and A. Robillard. 2004. Efficacy of an HIV prevention intervention for African American adolescent girls: A randomized controlled trial. *Journal of the American Medical Association* 292(2):171-179.

EXPLORE Study Team. 2004. Effects of a behavioural intervention to reduce acquisition of HIV infection among men who have sex with men: The EXPLORE randomised controlled study. *Lancet* 364(9428):41-50.

Farquhar, C., J. N. Kiarie, B. A. Richardson, M. N. Kabura, F. N. John, R. W. Nduati, D. A. Mbori-Ngacha, and G. C. John-Stewart. 2004. Antenatal couple counseling increases uptake of interventions to prevent HIV-1 transmission. *Journal of Acquired Immune Deficiency Syndromes* 37(5):1620-1626.

Gregson, S., S. Adamson, S. Papaya, J. Mundondo, C. A. Nyamukapa, P. R. Mason, G. P. Garnett, S. K. Chandiwana, G. Foster, and R. M. Anderson. 2007. Impact and process evaluation of integrated community and clinic-based HIV-1 control: A cluster-randomised trial in eastern Zimbabwe. *PLoS Medicine* 4(3):e102.

Herbst, J. H., R. T. Sherba, N. Crepaz, J. B. Deluca, L. Zohrabyan, R. D. Stall, and C. M. Lyles. 2005. A meta-analytic review of HIV behavioral interventions for reducing sexual risk behavior of men who have sex with men. *Journal of Acquired Immune Deficiency Syndromes* 39(2):228-241.

Johnson, W. D., L. V. Hedges, G. Ramirez, S. Semaan, L. R. Norman, E. Sogolow, M. D. Sweat, and R. M. Diaz. 2002. HIV prevention research for men who have sex with men: A systematic review and meta-analysis. *Journal of Acquired Immune Deficiency Syndromes* 30(Suppl 1):S118-S129.

Johnson, W. D., D. R. Holtgrave, W. M. McClellan, W. D. Flanders, A. N. Hill, and M. Goodman. 2005. HIV intervention research for men who have sex with men: A 7-year update. *AIDS Education and Prevention* 17(6):568-589.

Kalichman, S. C., D. Cain, L. Weinhardt, E. Benotsch, K. Presser, A. Zweben, B. Bjodstrup, and G. R. Swain. 2005. Experimental components analysis of brief theory-based HIV/AIDS risk-reduction counseling for sexually transmitted infection patients. *Health Psychology* 24(2):198-208.

Kamali, A., M. Quigley, J. Nakiyingi, J. Kinsman, J. Kengeya-Kayondo, R. Gopal, A. Ojwiya, P. Hughes, L. M. Carpenter, and J. Whitworth. 2003. Syndromic management of sexually-transmitted infections and behaviour change interventions on transmission of HIV-1 in rural Uganda: A community randomised trial. *Lancet* 361(9358):645-652.

Kamb, M. L., M. Fishbein, J. M. Douglas, Jr., F. Rhodes, J. Rogers, G. Bolan, J. Zenilman, T. Hoxworth, C. K. Malotte, M. Iatesta, C. Kent, A. Lentz, S. Graziano, R. H. Byers, and T. A. Peterman. 1998. Efficacy of risk-reduction counseling to prevent human immunodeficiency virus and sexually transmitted diseases: A randomized controlled trial. Project Respect Study Group. *Journal of the American Medical Association* 280(13):1161-1167.

Kawichai, S., C. Beyrer, C. Khamboonruang, D. D. Celentano, C. Natpratan, K. Rungruengthanakit, and K. E. Nelson. 2004. HIV incidence and risk behaviours after voluntary HIV counselling and testing (VCT) among adults aged 19–35 years living in peri-urban communities around Chiang Mai city in northern Thailand, 1999. *AIDS Care* 16(1):21-35.

Lie, R. K., E. J. Emanuel, and C. Grady. 2006. Circumcision and HIV prevention research: An ethical analysis. *Lancet* 368(9534):522-525.

Lyles, C. M., L. S. Kay, N. Crepaz, J. H. Herbst, W. F. Passin, A. S. Kim, S. M. Rama, S. Thadiparthi, J. B. DeLuca, and M. M. Mullins. 2007. Best-evidence interventions: Findings from a systematic review of HIV behavioral interventions for U.S. populations at high risk, 2000–2004. *American Journal of Public Health* 97(1):133-143.

Matovu, J. K., R. H. Gray, F. Makumbi, M. J. Wawer, D. Serwadda, G. Kigozi, N. K. Sewankambo, and F. Nalugoda. 2005. Voluntary HIV counseling and testing acceptance, sexual risk behavior and HIV incidence in Rakai, Uganda. *AIDS* 19(5):503-511.

McKleroy, V. S., J. S. Galbraith, B. Cummings, P. Jones, C. Harshbarger, C. Collins, D. Gelaude, J. W. Carey, and A. Team. 2006. Adapting evidence-based behavioral interventions for new settings and target populations. *AIDS Education and Prevention* 18(4 Suppl A):59-73.

Morin, S. F., G. Khumalo-Sakutukwa, E. D. Charlebois, J. Routh, K. Fritz, T. Lane, T. Vaki, A. Fiamma, and T. J. Coates. 2006. Removing barriers to knowing HIV status: Same-day mobile HIV testing in Zimbabwe. *Journal of Acquired Immune Deficiency Syndromes* 41(2):218-224.

Mullen, P. D., G. Ramirez, D. Strouse, L. V. Hedges, and E. Sogolow. 2002. Meta-analysis of the effects of behavioral HIV prevention interventions on the sexual risk behavior of sexually experienced adolescents in controlled studies in the United States. *Journal of Acquired Immune Deficiency Syndromes* 30(Suppl 1):S94-S105.

Muller, O., S. Sarangbin, K. Ruxrungtham, W. Sittitrai, and P. Phanuphak. 1995. Sexual risk behaviour reduction associated with voluntary HIV counselling and testing in HIV infected patients in Thailand. *AIDS Care* 7(5):567-572.

Neumann, M. S., W. D. Johnson, S. Semaan, S. A. Flores, G. Peersman, L. V. Hedges, and E. Sogolow. 2002. Review and meta-analysis of HIV prevention intervention research for heterosexual adult populations in the United States. *Journal of Acquired Immune Deficiency Syndromes* 30(Suppl 1):S106-S117.

NIH (National Institutes of Health). 2007. *Conference on building the science of dissemination and implementation in the service of public health*. Bethesda, MD.

Ross, D. A., J. Changalucha, A. I. Obasi, J. Todd, M. L. Plummer, B. Cleophas-Mazige, A. Anemona, D. Everett, H. A. Weiss, D. C. Mabey, H. Grosskurth, and R. J. Hayes. 2007. Biological and behavioural impact of an adolescent sexual health intervention in Tanzania: A community-randomized trial. *AIDS* 21(14):1943-1955.

Shain, R. N., J. M. Piper, A. E. Holden, J. D. Champion, S. T. Perdue, J. E. Korte, and F. A. Guerra. 2004. Prevention of gonorrhea and chlamydia through behavioral intervention: Results of a two-year controlled randomized trial in minority women. *Sexually Transmitted Diseases* 31(7):401-408.

UNAIDS. 2000. *Ethical considerations in HIV preventive vaccine research*. Geneva, Switzerland: UNAIDS.

UNAIDS. 2007. *Ethical considerations in biomedical HIV prevention trials*. Geneva, Switzerland: UNAIDS.

Voluntary HIV-1 Counseling and Testing Efficacy Study Group. 2000. Efficacy of voluntary HIV-1 counselling and testing in individuals and couples in Kenya, Tanzania, and Trinidad: A randomised trial. The Voluntary HIV-1 Counseling and Testing Efficacy Study Group. *Lancet* 356(9224):103-112.

Wang, X., J. Ma, Z. Xu, H. Liu, Y. Zhang, and C. Han. 2002. Effectiveness of post-exposure prophylaxis using live attenuated hepatitis alpha vaccine (h(2) strain) among schoolchildren. *Zhonghua Yi Xue Za Zhi* 82(14):955-957.

Wingood, G., and R. DiClemente. 2008. The ADAPT-ITT model: A novel method of adapting evidence-based HIV interventions. *Journal of Acquired Immune Deficiency Syndromes* 47(Suppl 1):S40-S46.

Wingood, G. M., R. J. DiClemente, I. Mikhail, D. L. Lang, D. H. McCree, S. L. Davies, J. W. Hardin, E. W. Hook, 3rd, and M. Saag. 2004. A randomized controlled trial to reduce HIV transmission risk behaviors and sexually transmitted diseases among women living with HIV: The WILLOW program. *Journal of Acquired Immune Deficiency Syndromes* 37(Suppl 2):S58-S67.

Wolf, L., and B. Lo. 2001. *Ethical dimensions of HIV/AIDS.* http://hivinsite.ucsf.edu/InSite?page=kb-08-01-05#S2X (accessed December 12, 2007).

4

Design Considerations: Pregnancy

Many late-stage biomedical HIV prevention trials are conducted among sexually active women of reproductive age in areas with high fertility rates. Despite intensive counseling on family planning, and provision of or access to contraceptives, a large percentage of women enrolled in biomedical HIV prevention trials become pregnant. Trials testing new products and devices (or new indications of existing drugs) restrict pregnant women from enrolling, and typically take women who become pregnant during the trial off the product, either permanently or for the duration of their pregnancy. High pregnancy rates and the product use implications for women who become pregnant have important implications for the design, conduct, and generalizability of biomedical HIV prevention trials, including loss in trial power when the occurrence of pregnancies has not been adequately accounted for when planning the size and duration of the trial, and potential interpretational problems when women who become pregnant are taken off product. Beyond the loss of study power and generalizability of results that the occurrence and handling of pregnancies can produce, removal of product in trial participants that become pregnant raises questions about the real-world use of approved products during pregnancy, because safety and efficacy data for pregnant women will not be available. That concern challenges the assumption that pregnant women should always be taken off the study product. The committee therefore considers variations on trial designs that may allow some pregnant women to remain on certain products to enable investigators to collect valuable information on their safety and efficacy.

WHEN PREGNANCY OCCURS DURING TRIALS

Women involved in clinical trials of any kind where the potential teratogenicity—or likelihood of birth defects—of the agent is unknown are usually counseled to employ at least two birth control methods to prevent pregnancy. As noted, studies of biomedical HIV interventions promote condoms and provide them to participants, primarily to protect them from HIV infection, but also to prevent pregnancy while they are exposed to an investigational drug or device whose risks to the fetus are unknown. Biomedical HIV prevention trials involving sexually active women of childbearing age also usually make other forms of contraception available, such as hormonal patches or injections, oral contraceptives, and to a lesser extent, intrauterine devices, through onsite provision of contraception or referrals to local family planning clinics.

However, women are often unable to negotiate condom use with their sexual partners, and adherence to other contraceptive methods is less than universal (Raymond et al., 2007). Thus a significant number of women may become pregnant during a trial. Microbicide trials in West Africa observed pregnancy rates ranging from 32 to 76 per 100-person-years at sites in Ghana and Nigeria (Macqueen et al., 2007). Because most trials conduct frequent pregnancy testing with highly sensitive tests, these rates may overestimate true pregnancy rates because they detect chemical pregnancies that never result in clinical pregnancies. Clinical pregnancy rates are nevertheless extremely high among participants in HIV prevention trials, even when reported condom use or oral contraceptive use is high (Raymond et al., 2007). Condoms are generally insufficient as the only contraceptive method for sexually active women with a high frequency of coital acts to result in a low pregnancy rate (Raymond et al., 2007). For example, Skoler et al. (2006) estimate that the 12-month cumulative probability that a woman engaging in 20 coital acts per month will become pregnant—given a 90 percent rate of condom use and no other contraceptive—is 51 percent.

High pregnancy rates among participants in such trials reflect high background pregnancy rates in populations to which these products will ultimately be targeted. That is, pregnancy is not an incidental occurrence in HIV prevention trials, but rather a predictably common event. Because an approved prevention product will, on introduction into a community, be used by many women even after they become pregnant, it is important that trials obtain information on the safety and efficacy of a product when used during pregnancy. When an efficacy trial does not obtain such information, it is important that additional studies do so.

Regulatory agencies and sponsors have required that women who become pregnant during trials of new products, including drugs and devices, without established benefit in humans discontinue the study product. Some trials allow women to go back on the product once they are no longer pregnant, provided they are not breast-feeding, while other trials require that pregnant women permanently discontinue use of the product. However, the occurrence of pregnancy during a trial, and the requirement that women discontinue use of a study product upon pregnancy diagnosis, have major statistical and ethical implications for the trial.

STATISTICAL IMPLICATIONS OF PREGNANCIES OCCURRING DURING TRIALS

As discussed in Chapter 9, study results can be seriously biased if women in a trial who become pregnant are no longer followed for HIV infection. Thus, it is important that investigators continue to follow women who may discontinue their product owing to pregnancy, or any other reason, and use this information in analyzing trial results.

As Chapter 9 also notes, discontinuing product use among pregnant women can diminish a study's power to detect a beneficial product by attenuating the intervention effect.[1] However, when investigators can estimate the pregnancy rate before the trial begins, they can increase the sample size or duration of follow-up of participants to compensate for this loss (see Chapter 2 on sample size). Data monitoring committees (discussed in Chapter 9) can also monitor actual pregnancy rates during a trial, and adjust its sample size and duration if these exceed expectations. Of course, this strategy may come at a significant cost in time (for events-driven trials) and money.

Discontinuing product use among pregnant women also complicates the interpretation of trial results because agents that are proven efficacious will be used by women who will become pregnant. Thus, if the relative efficacy of the product in pregnant women differs from that in women who are not pregnant, or if the product affects the fetus, the results of the trial would not be representative of the impact if the product were introduced into the community. This concern makes it imperative that investigators gather information regarding product safety and efficacy as soon as possible. If they cannot do this during the registrational trial for licensing a product, then the product development plan devised before the trial should specify how investigators can reliably obtain such information after the trial.

[1] More frequent testing reduces the amount of time that a woman takes a product after she becomes pregnant. Yet very early and very frequent pregnancy testing using a highly sensitive method may detect many "chemical" pregnancies—those that will not progress. Although women are required to terminate product use, many can resume product use shortly thereafter because of the short duration of chemical pregnancies.

Recommendation 4-1: Investigators should take several steps to minimize the loss of study power and potential biases in results that can occur when women become pregnant during a trial:

- **Before the start of the trial, investigators should attempt to accurately estimate the rate of pregnancy that will occur during participant follow-up, and use these estimates in calculating sample size and trial duration.**
- **Data Monitoring Committees should monitor actual pregnancy rates during the trial, and recommend appropriate adjustments to sample size and trial duration if these rates exceed expectations.**
- **Investigators should continue to follow all women who become pregnant for HIV infection, regardless of whether they discontinue the study product.**

COLLECTING INFORMATION ON BENEFITS AND RISKS

Ultimately, from a public health perspective, the goal is to develop products that people at high risk of HIV acquisition can use. And in most countries, women of childbearing age, with high background rates of pregnancy, are one of the populations at highest risk. As noted, many women who become pregnant are likely to use a product with demonstrated efficacy in preventing HIV infection, regardless of recommendations on the product label. Therefore, investigators and sponsors are obligated to collect as much information, as early as possible, about potential risks and benefits of the product to pregnant women and their fetuses.

As discussed later, relying only on posttrial pregnancy registries to collect information about the safety of a product in pregnant women is insufficient, and perhaps unethical, in a case where a high proportion of likely users will become pregnant, and where the epidemiologic infrastructure is inadequate to support such registries. This raises important questions about the best ways to collect safety information, and whether there are circumstances under which it would be ethical to allow women who become pregnant to continue receiving the study product.

Historical Context

In evaluating whether there are circumstances when women who become pregnant during a trial should have the option of remaining on product, it is important to understand the historical context, legal transformations, and ethical considerations that have shaped current policy and practice. (See Box 4-1 for more detail.)

Some groups and ethicists have suggested allowing pregnant women

BOX 4-1
Historical Perspectives on Including Pregnant Women in Clinical Trials

Because many developing countries do not have the regulatory capacity to process applications for new drugs, product approval in these countries is heavily influenced by approval of the FDA or regulatory agencies in other developed countries.

Historically, two competing concerns drove the FDA's policies regarding the inclusion of women in clinical trials: "(1) the need to protect research participants, and (2) the 'rights' of participants to gain access to clinical studies" (IOM, 1994, p. 36).

Early FDA guidelines reflected a protectionist orientation. In 1977, the FDA issued guidelines that specified the conditions under which women of childbearing potential could participate in trials (FDA, 1977). However, in practice, such trials almost universally barred premenopausal women. These standards reflected a move toward greater protection for vulnerable populations in response to research abuses, and, most notably, the fetal injuries that occurred during the thalidomide disaster.

Moreover, until the 1990s, developers of biomedical products rarely relied on animal studies to identify potential reproductive risks to women and the effects on their offspring until phase 3 clinical trials revealed a product's efficacy. Because the potential reproductive toxicity of a drug was usually unknown before a trial began, women of childbearing potential were considered ineligible to participate, because they could not make a valid risk-benefit assessment during the consent process. The result of these exclusionary standards was that women were systematically underrepresented in U.S. federally funded research (IOM, 1994).

During the 1990s, AIDS activists and women's health groups called on the FDA to revise its protectionist regulations. Rather than excluding all fertile women from trials, they urged a standard of informed consent.

In response, the Institute of Medicine convened the Committee on the Ethical and Legal Issues Relating to the Inclusion of Women in Clinical Studies, which issued *Women and Health Research: Ethical and Legal Issues of Including Women in Clinical Studies* (IOM, 1994). The committee's conclusions and recommendations represented a profound challenge to prevailing practice. Based on the urgent need to include women in trials, and the impor-tance of respecting their reproductive rights and autonomy, the committee concluded that the potential for becoming pregnant during a trial should not be used to exclude or limit a woman's participation.[a]

---

[a]The IOM concluded that "investigators and IRBs not exclude persons of reproductive age from participation in clinical studies. In the case of women of reproductive age, the potential or prospect of becoming pregnant during the study may not be used as a justification for precluding or limiting participation. Risks to the reproductive system should be considered in the same manner as risks to other organ systems. Risks to possible offspring of both men and women who are not pregnant or lactating should not be considered in the risk-benefit calculation. It is the responsibility of the investigators and IRBs to assure that the informed consent process includes an adequate discussion of risks to reproduction and potential

BOX 4-1 Continued

More significantly, the committee called for allowing pregnant women to participate in trials based on informed consent. In the face of uncertainty about potential fetal risks, the IOM committee concluded that the pregnant woman should be able continue to participate. The committee also concluded that only when a clinical investigation had no direct clinical benefit to the woman herself and "a risk of significant harm to potential offspring is known or can be plausibly inferred" was it permissible to exclude women from trials. These proposed policy changes would have dramatically increased the burden of proof required to exclude pregnant women.

Some of the IOM committee's conclusions mirrored those of the FDA itself, which had abandoned its earlier position of excluding women of childbearing potential from trials in 1993. FDA guidelines recommended screening women for pregnancy before enrollment, and counseling them about the use of contraception. The guidelines also recommended that investigators complete reproductive toxicity studies before phase 2 or phase 3 trials, and the informed-consent process was to include all available information about potential reproductive toxicities. In contrast to the IOM committee's position, however, FDA guidelines said that the potential risk to the fetus took precedence over the choice of the woman who had become pregnant in trials before efficacy had been established.

During this time trials in pregnant women showed that antiretroviral therapy was effective in interrupting mother-to-child transmission of HIV. This was a somewhat different case, since the trials were designed to benefit newborns. Still, sponsors continued to prohibit HIV treatment trials from enrolling pregnant women and to require investigators to discontinue study drugs when pregnancy occurred until after phase 3 trials had demonstrated both safety and efficacy. The FDA also recommended the establishment of pregnancy registries to record the outcomes in women exposed to antiretroviral product during pregnancy, as phase 4 clinical trials in pregnant women were usually not conducted.

In 2001, the U.S. Department of Health and Human Services modified its regulations and abandoned the universal exclusion of pregnant women, in part because "information on maternal safety and efficacy and fetal safety can be collected in well-designed research settings" (Uhl et al., 2004). However, these regulations have important caveats that limit the circumstances in which pregnant women can participate in research. Specifically, "pregnant women or fetuses may be involved in research only if a trial meets all the following conditions:

• Where scientifically appropriate, preclinical studies, including studies on pregnant animals, and clinical studies, including studies on nonpregnant women,

---

offspring, including, where appropriate, an adequate discussion of relevant considerations of birth control. The committee recommends that the participant be permitted to select voluntarily the contraceptive method of his or her choice where there are no relevant study-dependent, scientific reasons for excluding certain contraceptives (e.g., drug interaction). The committee recommends that pregnancy termination options be discussed as part of the consent process in clinical studies that pose unknown or foreseeable risks to potential offspring" (IOM, 1994, p. 15).

continued

BOX 4-1 Continued

have been conducted and provide data for assessing potential risks to pregnant women and fetuses;

- The risk to the fetus is caused solely by interventions or procedures that hold out the prospect of direct benefit to the woman or the fetus: or, if there is no such prospect of benefit, the risk to the fetus is not greater than minimal and the purpose of the research is the development of important biological knowledge that cannot be obtained by any other means;
- Any risk is the least possible for achieving the objectives of the research;
- If the research holds out the prospect of direct benefit to the pregnant woman, the pros-pect of a direct benefit both to the pregnant woman and the fetus, or no prospect of benefit for the women nor the fetus when risk to the fetus is not greater than minimal and the purpose of the research is the development of important biomedical knowledge that cannot be obtained by any other means, her consent is obtained in accord with the informed consent provisions of subpart A of this part (45 CFR 46.204)."[b]

More recently, several groups have recommended that women who become pregnant be given the option to remain in the trial based on an informed consent standard. A recent report by UNAIDS and the World Health Organization, Ethical Considerations in Biomedical HIV Prevention Trials, recommends a more inclusionary approach (2007, p. 37):

> Although the enrollment of pregnant or breast-feeding women complicates the analysis of risks and benefits, because both the woman and the fetus or infant could be benefited or harmed, such women should be viewed as autonomous decision makers, capable of making an informed choice for themselves and for their fetus or child. In order for women to be able to make an informed choice for their fetus/breast-fed infant, they should be duly informed about any potential for teratogenesis and other known or unknown risks to the fetus and/or the breast-fed infant.

Similarly, the Council for International Organizations of Medical Sciences' International Ethical Guidelines for Biomedical Research Involving Human Subjects (CIOMS, 2002) states that:

> The justification of research involving pregnant women is complicated by the fact that it may present risks and potential benefits to two beings—the woman and the fetus—as well as to the person the fetus is destined to become. . . . Even when evidence concerning risks is unknown or ambiguous, the decision about acceptability of risk to the fetus should be made by the woman as part of the informed consent process.

---

[b]A description of this section of the Common Rule can be found at http://www.bioethics.gov/reports/reproductionandresponsibility/chapter5.html. The regulation itself is found at http://a257.g.akamaitech.net/7/257/2422/13nov20061500/edocket.access.gpo.gov/cfr_2006/octqtr/pdf/45cfr46.203.pdf.

to enter trials, or allowing women who become pregnant during a trial to continue to receive a product by disclosing possible reproductive risks during the informed-consent process (IOM, 1994; CIOMS, 2002; UNAIDS, 2007). However, historically regulators and sponsors have tended to adopt a more protectionist view (FDA, 1977; IOM, 1994). This approach involves removing pregnant women from exposure to an experimental drug or device unless earlier research has established some potential benefit to study subjects. In the absence of knowledge about such benefit, the prevailing understanding of research ethics dictates that a woman's right to autonomy should not take precedence over the potential hazard to the fetus. According to this perspective, the principle of justice also dictates that the vulnerable fetus be protected from unfair risks.

If the benefits of the product to women are clearer, the balance between maternal rights and fetal concern shifts, on the grounds of both autonomy and justice. In practice, however, investigators do not know the potential efficacy, benefits, and harm of a product for the mother and fetus with certainty, making it more difficult to weigh risks and benefits.

Several sources can provide information on the potential benefits and risks of an HIV prevention product or device. These include preclinical studies in animals, experience with a product in other clinical trials or applications, follow-up of women who are exposed to the product and become pregnant during the trial, and research and monitoring during the posttrial phase.

Preclinical Studies

Several types of preclinical tests performed on animals are particularly important in assessing the potential risks of a new product to women and their fetuses (see Box 4-2). Reproductive toxicity studies assess the product's effects on conception, gonadal function, birth defects, and offspring development. Pharmacokinetic studies, which evaluate absorption, distribution, excretion, and metabolism of a product, look for evidence of carcinogenicity and systemic toxicity. These studies are important even in the case of topically applied agents (such as vaginal microbicides), where the degree of systemic exposure must be established.

Preclinical reproductive toxicity studies can help researchers and policy makers establish the potential risks against which to weigh the potential benefits to pregnant women who participate in clinical trials, although they cannot absolutely rule out the risk of harm. These studies, conducted in more than one mammalian species, can screen for potential human teratogenicity—or birth defects—although they are imperfect predictors of teratogenicity in humans (Ward, 2001; Kennedy et al., 2004). For example, aspirin is teratogenic in mice but not in humans (Corby, 1978). And while

BOX 4-2
Preclinical Testing of HIV Prevention Compounds

Before human dosing of HIV prevention compounds begins, preclinical studies are conducted in animals to identify a safe starting dose in humans, and to identify the types of expected toxicity for which human trials will require meticulous monitoring. In 1997, the International Conference on Harmonisation (ICH) issued guideline M3, which was adopted by the United States, European Union (EU), and Japanese drug regulatory authorities, on the type and extent of preclinical safety studies needed for the conduct of clinical trials of investigational pharmaceuticals in humans (ICH, 2000). This document provides guidance on the timing of multiple types of preclinical studies (including safety pharmacology, toxicokinetic and pharmacokinetic, single dose toxicity, repeated dose toxicity, local tolerance, genotoxicity, carcinogenicity, reproductive toxicity studies and supplementary studies) with respect to clinical testing. The guidelines also identify areas that are not harmonized among the three regions.

As noted, two types of studies are particularly important to understanding the effects of investigational drugs on pregnant women and their fetuses: toxicokinetic and pharmacokinetic studies and reproductive toxicity studies. Toxicokinetic and pharmacokinetic studies consist of animal pharmacology studies, and absorption, metabolism, distribution and excretion studies (ADME) and systemic absorption studies. These are usually completed prior to phase 1 clinical trials of an investigational drug (ICH, 2000).

Reproductive toxicity tests examine three "segments" of mammalian reproduction. Segment I (fertility and general reproductive studies) examines fertility and reproductive function in male and female animals, which reveals the drug's effects on an animal's ability to get pregnant. Segment II studies (developmental studies) examine developmental toxicity and malformation, to reveal the effects of the drug on fetal development in animals. Segment III studies (late-gestation and lactation studies) examine fertility, growth, and development to examine the drug's postnatal and perinatal toxicity, to determine its effects during gestation, and on newborn animals during birth or breast-feeding (Ponce and Faustman, 1998).

The type and timing of reproductive toxicity studies depends on many factors, including the toxicity profile of the drug and the reproductive potential of the population in clinical trials (see ICH Guideline S5A/B). There are regional differences in the timing of reproductive toxicity tests, particularly with respect to drugs being tested in women of childbearing potential on highly effective birth control (ICH, 2000). The guidelines also recommend that all female reproductive toxicity studies and the standard battery of genotoxicity studies be completed prior to inclusion in any clinical trial for women of childbearing potential who are not using highly effective birth control or whose pregnancy status is unknown and for women who are pregnant. Prior to inclusion of pregnant women in trials, safety data from previous human exposure are also generally needed (ICH, 2000).

thalidomide is a potent human teratogen, studies in mice and rats did not observe limb malformations (McBride, 1961). Animal studies with positive findings (for example, an agent tests positive as a developmental toxin) tend to be more predictive of human effects than animal studies showing negative effects (Rogers and Kavlock, 1998). Concordance between animal and human effects is strongest when there are positive findings in multiple animal test species, although certain effects do not extrapolate well across species (Rogers and Kavlock, 1998).

Absorption, distribution, metabolism, and excretion (ADME) studies can provide information on the potential of a compound to produce systemic toxicity. Compounds that show systemic toxicity in animal tests—that is, drugs with hepatic, gastrointestinal, hematological, pulmonary, neurological, or cardiac toxicity—would create concern if intended for widespread use as HIV prevention interventions. Any compounds showing systemic toxicity would be poor candidates for use during pregnancy, as such effects would be unwelcome in both mother and fetus.

If a topical compound is designed to be nonabsorbable, systemic absorption studies in animals can provide information on whether, in fact, the compound is absorbed through the skin or vaginal mucosa into the bloodstream, and how long it persists. Products with systemic absorption carry a higher risk of systemic drug-related toxicity for both mother and fetus during pregnancy, and potentially for the infant while breast-feeding. Topical agents with no systemic absorption may have less capacity to produce teratogenic effects during pregnancy.

Although ADME studies must be completed before phase 1 testing in humans, reproductive toxicity tests for new products, particularly those without commercial sponsors, are sometimes not completed until the products are approved for licensure. This is a problem when the ultimate target population for these products has a high rate of pregnancy. Although there is no mandate to complete all segments of reproductive toxicity studies at any specific time, the International Conference on Harmonization (ICH) has issued guidelines on the timing of such studies. The guidelines on timing of reproductive toxicity studies vary by region, particularly with respect to trial populations of women of childbearing potential on highly effective birth control (ICH, 2000). For women of childbearing potential who are not on highly effective birth control or whose pregnancy status is unknown, and for women who are pregnant, ICH guidance recommends that all female reproductive toxicology studies be completed before enrolling these populations in any clinical trial (ICH, 2000). (See Box 4-2.) Guidance issued by FDA for topical microbicides indicates that all reproductive toxicity studies should be completed prior to Phase 2/3 trials (FDA, 2005).

The first trial of a candidate microbicide in pregnant women (MTN 002) is expected to start in early 2008. This study, involving 16 pregnant women, seeks to understand the extent of drug absorption during pregnancy, and the degree to which the gel's active ingredient may be transferred to the fetus. A single dose of tenofovir topical gel, an antiretroviral-based candidate microbicide, will be given prior to caesarean delivery (Microbicide Trials Network, 2007).

Prior Experience with a Product

Some agents that are now being tested for efficacy in preventing HIV infection are already licensed for other indications, and their use has shed light on their effects in pregnant women and fetuses. For instance, there is considerable evidence regarding the safety of tenofovir, an approved antiretroviral drug for treating HIV-infected persons, and growing experience with the use of tenofovir during pregnancy. Oral tenofovir is now being tested as a preexposure prophylaxis agent to prevent HIV acquisition, and tenofovir-based microbicides are also in phase 2 testing. Other antiretroviral agents (such as zidovudine or nevirapine) have been extensively studied in pregnant women, and have been found to be effective and safe when used during pregnancy to prevent mother-to-child transmission of HIV (Guay et al., 1999; Dorenbaum et al., 2002; Mofenson, 2002; Moodley et al., 2003; Dabis et al., 2005). For serodiscordant couples trying to conceive naturally, researchers have also suggested giving PrEP to the uninfected woman, to reduce her susceptibility to HIV infection while trying to get pregnant (Barreiro et al., 2006a,b; Vernazza et al., 2006). No data have yet been published to demonstrate the efficacy of this approach.

Information Collected During a Trial

Given high pregnancy rates during clinical trials of HIV interventions, some late-stage efficacy trials will accrue significant experience with product exposure early in the first trimester, one of the most vulnerable times for teratogenicity, even when the trial is designed to discontinue product upon detection of pregnancy. The length of exposure will depend on the frequency of pregnancy testing, which typically occurs monthly or every two months. Information on birth outcomes from women in clinical trials exposed to a product during pregnancy can thus provide information on possible adverse effects on the fetus.

To assess such information, investigators can compare pregnancy outcomes in the control and intervention groups, and also examine these outcomes as a function of the duration of exposure to the product during pregnancy within the intervention group. For example, if a two-arm placebo-controlled microbicide trial of 2,000 women experienced a 50 percent pregnancy rate, investigators could obtain information on pregnancy outcomes on as many as 500 women in each of the placebo and microbicide groups. If pregnancy testing occurred monthly, women participating in the trial who became pregnant would be exposed to the product for up to one month after conception. Such a trial could thus provide valuable information about the effects of the product on birth outcomes. Indeed, investigators could obtain useful information about the safety of the product while the trial is continuing. In that case, the risk-benefit ratio could change enough to justify use of the product during pregnancy.

Posttrial Phase

Many developed countries use pregnancy registries to collect information on birth outcomes of children born to women who were exposed to a product during pregnancy. For example, drug companies that produce antiretrovirals support a pregnancy registry that is intended to provide early signals of birth defects associated with prenatal exposure. Health care professionals may register pregnant women who have used the drugs, so information on pregnancy outcomes can be recorded. Registration of exposed women is entirely voluntary. However, it is not clear how effective such registries would be in detecting signals of teratogenicity from agents used to prevent HIV acquisition. Establishing new registries is also not likely to be feasible in developing countries that lack the needed epidemiological infrastructure and health care reporting. Regulators and others should therefore not rely on pregnancy registries as a major source of postmarket information.

If a trial is likely to support market approval, then the "rollover" period between the availability of the findings and product approval provides another opportune time to collect information on experiences during pregnancy. For example, because sponsors typically take 6 months to prepare an application for regulatory approval, and the U.S. Food and Drug Administration (FDA) and other agencies take at least 6 months to complete a review, trial participants who are still in follow-up might be allowed to remain on the product if they become pregnant during this period and no contravening safety issues arise. Alternatively, women from both the original intervention and control groups who have not yet developed HIV or become pregnant could be randomized to discontinue or not discontinue the study product upon pregnancy during this period. In both cases, the resulting data could provide useful insights into the efficacy and safety of the product during pregnancy. Investigators would therefore do well to prepare a protocol for studying women who become pregnant and consent to use a biomedical intervention during this time. Such a study could continue past regulatory approval, to accrue more data on experiences with the product during pregnancy.

Overall, the committee believes that the current "one-size-fits-all" policy requiring women to discontinue product use upon pregnancy is unnecessary and potentially counterproductive. No single approach to product use during pregnancy should apply to all biomedical HIV prevention trials, partly because of the diversity of such interventions themselves.

Recommendation 4-2: Although the current policy of excluding pregnant women from biomedical HIV prevention and other trials stems from an historically protectionist orientation adopted by regulators, the principles of research ethics neither mandate nor preclude use of the product by pregnant women. Because any approved product subsequently would likely be used by many woman who become pregnant, sponsors and investigators of a biomedical intervention should specify in advance of any late-stage trial how they will establish its safety and efficacy for pregnant women and their fetuses, based on information collected both during and after clinical trials. At a minimum, investigators should take the following steps to collect such information.

- **Investigators should conduct appropriate preclinical tests in animals, including reproductive toxicity and pharmacokinetic studies, to allow a more informed decision on whether to continue product use in pregnant women participating in late-stage trials. These tests would ideally be completed before the product or device enters phase 2 testing, but should be completed no later than phase 3 testing.**
- **Investigators should routinely collect and analyze information about birth outcomes from women who become pregnant during a trial, regardless of whether a product is discontinued upon detection of pregnancy.**
- **In trials that discontinue the use of a product by women who become pregnant, investigators should allow women who are no longer pregnant to have the choice of resuming the study medication.**
- **Investigators should conduct observational or randomized studies in pregnant women in the postapproval, premarketing, and posttrial periods, to provide additional information on the safety and efficacy of biomedical HIV prevention interventions for pregnant women.**

Recommendation 4-3: Regulators, sponsors, and investigators should evaluate the strength of the evidence on the beneficial and harmful effects to both a pregnant woman and her fetus on a product-by-product basis, and evaluate whether there are circumstances in which women who become pregnant can continue to receive the study product, based on what is known about its benefits and risks.

Recommendation 4-4: Trials using products with favorable risk-benefit profiles, but which are nonetheless discontinued upon pregnancy, should monitor pregnancy outcomes during the interim analysis of trial results, as this information might alter the risk-benefit profile to allow continuation of the product during pregnancy. Such trials might be modified to thereafter allow women who become pregnant to remain on product or offer them the opportunity to be randomized to remain on product versus to discontinue product.

Recommendation 4-5: Regulatory agencies and institutional review boards (IRBs) should receive periodic safety updates during a trial that include experience with the product during pregnancy. When interim analyses provide evidence of fetal safety and potential benefit to women, regulators and IRBs should consider allowing women to stay on product while pregnant.

REFERENCES

Barreiro, P., J. del Romero, M. Leal, V. Hernando, R. Asencio, C. de Mendoza, P. Labarga, M. Nunez, J. T. Ramos, J. Gonzalez-Lahoz, and V. Soriano. 2006a. Natural pregnancies in HIV-serodiscordant couples receiving successful antiretroviral therapy. *Journal of Acquired Immune Deficiency Syndromes* 43(3):324-326.

Barreiro, P., A. Duerr, K. Beckerman, and V. Soriano. 2006b. Reproductive options for HIV-serodiscordant couples. *AIDS Reviews* 8(3):158-170.

CIOMS (Council for International Organizations of Medical Sciences). 2002. *International ethical guidelines for biomedical research involving human subjects.* Geneva, Switzerland.

Corby, D. G. 1978. Aspirin in pregnancy: Maternal and fetal effects. *Pediatrics* 62(5 Pt 2 Suppl):930-937.

Dabis, F., L. Bequet, D. K. Ekouevi, I. Viho, F. Rouet, A. Horo, C. Sakarovitch, R. Becquet, P. Fassinou, L. Dequae-Merchadou, C. Welffens-Ekra, C. Rouzioux, and V. Leroy. 2005. Field efficacy of zidovudine, lamivudine and single-dose nevirapine to prevent peripartum HIV transmission. *AIDS* 19(3):309-318.

Dorenbaum, A., C. K. Cunningham, R. D. Gelber, M. Culnane, L. Mofenson, P. Britto, C. Rekacewicz, M. L. Newell, J. F. Delfraissy, B. Cunningham-Schrader, M. Mirochnick, and J. L. Sullivan. 2002. Two-dose intrapartum/newborn nevirapine and standard antiretroviral therapy to reduce perinatal HIV transmission: A randomized trial. *Journal of the American Medical Association* 288(2):189-198.

FDA (Food and Drug Administration). 1977. *General consideration for the clinical evaluation of drugs.* Rockville, MD: FDA.

FDA. 2005. *Points to consider in the nonclinical pharmacology/toxicology development of topical drugs intended to prevent the transmission of sexually transmitted diseases (STD) and/or for the development of drugs intended to act as vaginal contraceptives.* http://www.fda.gov/cder/guidance/ptcnonclinical.htm (accessed October 2007).

Guay, L. A., P. Musoke, T. Fleming, D. Bagenda, M. Allen, C. Nakabiito, J. Sherman, P. Bakaki, C. Ducar, M. Deseyve, L. Emel, M. Mirochnick, M. G. Fowler, L. Mofenson, P. Miotti, K. Dransfield, D. Bray, F. Mmiro, and J. B. Jackson. 1999. Intrapartum and neonatal single-dose nevirapine compared with zidovudine for prevention of mother-to-child transmission of HIV-1 in Kampala, Uganda: HIVnet 012 randomised trial. *Lancet* 354(9181):795-802.

ICH (International Conference on Harmonisation). November 9, 2000. *Guideline M3 (Step 4 version): Non-clinical safety studies for the conduct of human clinical trials for pharmaceuticals.* http://www.ich.org/LOB/media/MEDIA506.pdf (accessed February 4, 2007).

IOM (Institute of Medicine). 1994. *Women and health research: Ethical and legal issues of including women in clinical studies, Volume 1.* Washington, DC: National Academy Press.

Kennedy, D. L., K. Uhl, and S. L. Kweder. 2004. Pregnancy exposure registries. *Drug Safety* 27(4):215-228.

Macqueen, K. M., L. Johnson, P. Alleman, B. Akumatey, T. Lawoyin, and T. Nyiama. 2007. Pregnancy prevention practices among women with multiple partners in an HIV prevention trial. *Journal of Acquired Immune Deficiency Syndromes* 46(1):32-38.

McBride, W. B. 1961. Thalidomide and congenital abnormalities. *Lancet* 1358(2).

Microbicide Trials Network. 2007. *MTN-002: Phase I study of the maternal single-dose pharmacokinetics and placental transfer of tenofovir 1% vaginal gel among healthy term gravidas.* http://www.mtnstopshiv.org/files/attachments/MTN%20002%20Final%20Version%201%200%20082907%20(2).pdf (accessed March 25, 2008).

Mofenson, L. M. 2002. U.S. Public Health Service task force recommendations for use of antiretroviral drugs in pregnant HIV-1-infected women for maternal health and interventions to reduce perinatal HIV-1 transmission in the United States. *MMWR Recommendations and Reports* 51(RR-18):1-38; quiz CE31-34.

Moodley, D., J. Moodley, H. Coovadia, G. Gray, J. McIntyre, J. Hofmyer, C. Nikodem, D. Hall, M. Gigliotti, P. Robinson, L. Boshoff, and J. L. Sullivan. 2003. A multicenter randomized controlled trial of nevirapine versus a combination of zidovudine and lamivudine to reduce intrapartum and early postpartum mother-to-child transmission of human immunodeficiency virus type 1. *Journal of Infectious Diseases* 187(5):725-735.

Ponce, R., and E. Faustman. 1998. Reproductive and developmental toxicity of metals: issues for consideration in human health risk assessment. In *Reproductive and developmental toxicology*, edited by K. S. Korach. New York: Marcel Dekker, Inc. Pp. 449-474.

Raymond, E. G., D. Taylor, W. Cates, Jr., E. E. Tolley, D. Borasky, A. Cancel, B. Masse, E. A. Bukusi, and B. R. Johnson. 2007. Pregnancy in effectiveness trials of HIV prevention agents. *Sexually Transmitted Diseases* 34(12):1035-1039.

Rogers, J. M., and R. J. Kavlock. 1998. Developmental toxicology. In *Reproductive and developmental toxicology,* C. D. Klaassen, ed. New York: Marcel Dekker, Inc. Pp. 47-72.

Skoler, S., L. Peterson, and W. Cates, Jr. 2006. Our current microbicide trials: Lessons learned and to be learned. *Microbicide Quarterly* 4(1):6.

Uhl, K., M. A. Miller, and D. L. Kennedy. 2004. Complex clinical, legal, and ethical issues of pregnant and postpartum women as subjects in clinical trials. *Journal of Womens Health (Larchmt)* 13(6):743-744.

UNAIDS. 2007. *Ethical considerations in biomedical HIV prevention trials.* Geneva, Switzerland.

Vernazza, P. L., L. Hollander, A. E. Semprini, D. J. Anderson, and A. Duerr. 2006. HIV-discordant couples and parenthood: How are we dealing with the risk of transmission? *AIDS* 20(4):635-636.

Ward, R. M. 2001. Difficulties in the study of adverse fetal and neonatal effects of drug therapy during pregnancy. *Seminars in Perinatology* 25(3):191-195.

5

Design Considerations: Adherence

For a new biological HIV prevention product to be effective, users must adhere to the prescribed regimen. During a clinical trial, imperfect adherence reduces the product's effectiveness, and also makes it difficult for investigators to assess efficacy. If a trial shows that a product provides an overall benefit, relating the level of protection to the level of adherence is valuable for interpreting the results. Understanding who was protected during the trial and under what circumstances also has important implications for predicting how effective the product will be in various real-world settings.

To properly interpret the results of a clinical trial that failed to show a protective effect, investigators need to distinguish the extent to which the product was not biologically efficacious, participants did not use it as directed, or they engaged in more risky behavior because they thought the product was protecting them. Regardless of whether a trial demonstrates an effect, understanding when and why participants did not adhere to the product regimen can provide valuable insights into the design and delivery of future HIV prevention interventions.

While interventions given once or a very few times, such as vaccines or circumcision, usually do not entail adherence challenges, other existing and new biomedical HIV interventions such as condoms, PrEP, and microbicides require longer-term administration. Adherence is more than "simply remembering medications, but rather, a complex issue involving social, cultural, economic, and personal factors" (Chesney, 2006). In the antiretroviral treatment (ART) field, there has been insufficient progress in understanding the correlates of adherence and strategies to increase adherence (Sankar et al., 2006). Adherence to biomedical HIV prevention interventions is even less well understood. This underscores the importance of understanding the context and factors that affect individuals' adherence and risk behavior. Researchers should not assume that definitions or models of adherence (or risk reduction) developed in one sociocultural context are equally as valid in another (Ware et al., 2006). They should be evaluated and adapted to new settings as appropriate (see Ware et al., 2006, for one such adaptation model). Studies that disregard the sociocultural context of adherence, or that rely on models of adherence that are not appropriate to the cultural context, are more likely to find their efforts to understand and improve adherence ineffective or irrelevant (Sankar et al., 2006; Ware et al., 2006). Although underutilized in the HIV field, qualitative research methods can be particularly useful to understanding the multiple factors that influence adherence and risk behavior patterns and developing suitable adherence measurements and improvement strategies (Friedland, 2006; Sankar et al., 2006).

This chapter examines four important aspects of adherence: defining it, measuring it, improving it, and analyzing data on it. The committee makes recommendations for future practice and research in each area. The chapter also highlights the need for multidisciplinary teams to collaborate in addressing challenges to adherence in trials of HIV prevention interventions.

DEFINING ADHERENCE

Although researchers agree on the importance of product adherence in both research and real-world settings, there is less agreement on how to define it. Despite the complexity of adherence, clinical trials often report it as a simple number, such as the percentage of coital acts in which participants use a gel, or the percentage of pills they take over a given time period (Chesney, 2006). The use of a single number to define adherence may mask crucial insights into adherence problems, product acceptability, and potential areas for intervention (Kerr et al., 2005; Berg and Arnsten, 2006). This number can also reflect variability stemming from adherence behaviors that the measure is not intended to address ("construct-irrelevant variance") (Kerr et al., 2005).

Consider a trial to investigate whether suppression of HSV-2, the herpes simplex virus, prevents HIV infection. The perfectly adherent patient would take one dose in the morning and one in the evening at the same times each day (Vrijens et al., 2006). Suppose the study identifies four participants with imperfect adherence who take 79 percent of prescribed doses during an observation interval. That simple percentage can mask highly disparate adherence patterns (see Figure 5-1): The first patient was

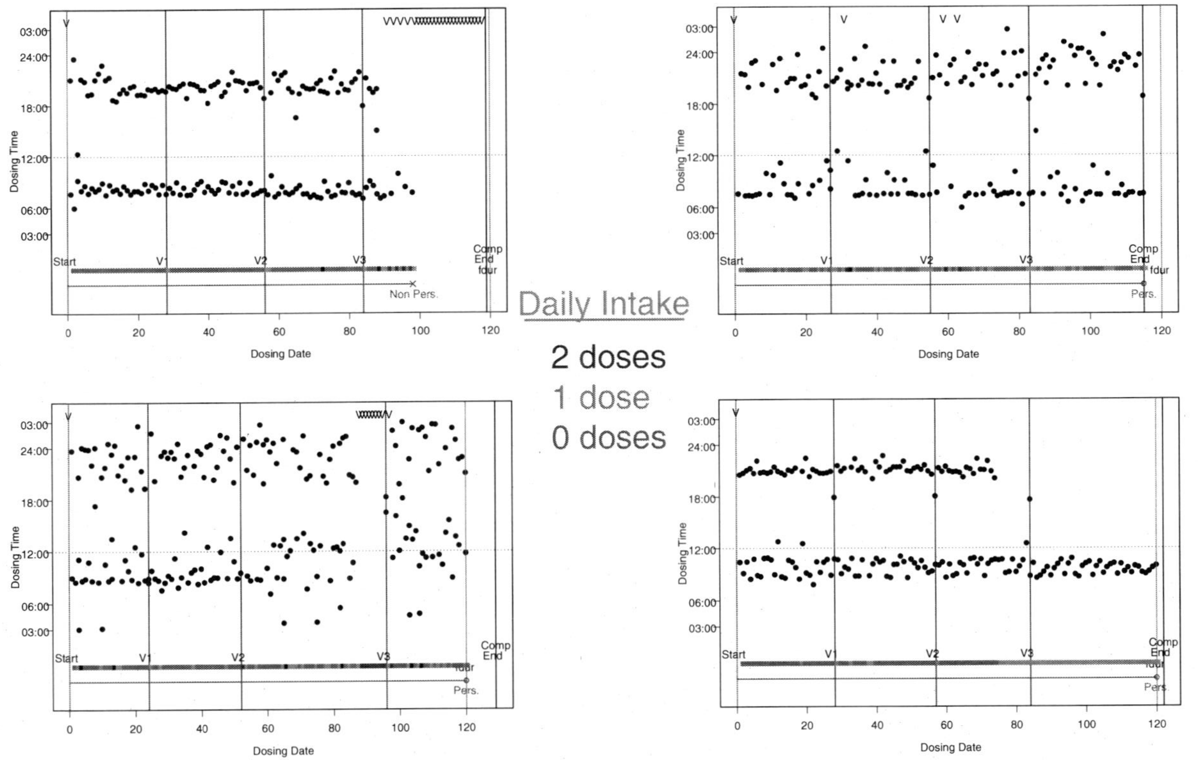

FIGURE 5-1 Differing patterns of product use among four patients—all of whom are 79 percent adherent.
SOURCE: Vrijens, 2007.

adherent but discontinued the prescribed regimen early. The second patient took the morning doses consistently but missed several evening doses. The third patient took the dosages erratically and stopped altogether for a period of time. The fourth patient decided to take only the morning dose and stopped taking the evening dose. Even though each patient was "79 percent adherent," the clinical consequences of those four patterns could be very different, and the actions needed to improve adherence would differ for the four participants.

As Figure 5-1 shows, product adherence is a complex concept. It involves three major components: acceptance of the prescribed regimen, execution of the regimen, and discontinuation of the regimen (Vrijens and Urquhart, 2005; Friedland, 2006) While acceptance and discontinuation tend to happen at a single point in time, quality of execution varies over time.

Two aspects of adherence are particularly important in analyzing the results of a clinical trial: persistence, and quality of execution—commonly called compliance. Persistence is the amount of time between when a patient first uses a product and when she or he discontinues it. Quality of execution is the correspondence between the prescribed regimen and the patient's actual application history during the period of persistence (Vrijens and Urquhart, 2005). That is, quality of execution measures whether a patient has complied with instructions for using a product.

Figure 5-2 illustrates these concepts in 20,000 patients who were prescribed regular doses of drugs for various diseases, aggregated across multiple clinical trials (Vrijens, 2007). The horizontal line at the top of the graph represents perfect adherence. The persistence curve reflects the proportion of patients who continued product use during the first year. While persistence varied across disease and trials, these data indicate that 40 percent of participants discontinued the prescribed intervention in the first 12 months. The adherence/compliance curve reflects on a daily basis the proportion of trial participants who executed product use according to the ideal regimen. About half of the participants did so.

Describing and analyzing persistence separately from quality of execution provides insights into whether a product is acceptable at both the individual and population levels, and suggests different modes of action. A trial population consisting of 50 percent nonpersisters who are otherwise perfect executers would have very different implications than if all subjects skip every other application. In the first instance, the product would work very well for a select subgroup. The second situation would require more complex analysis and intervention.

Recommendation 5-1: Because simple measures of adherence can mask substantially different underlying adherence problems, investigators

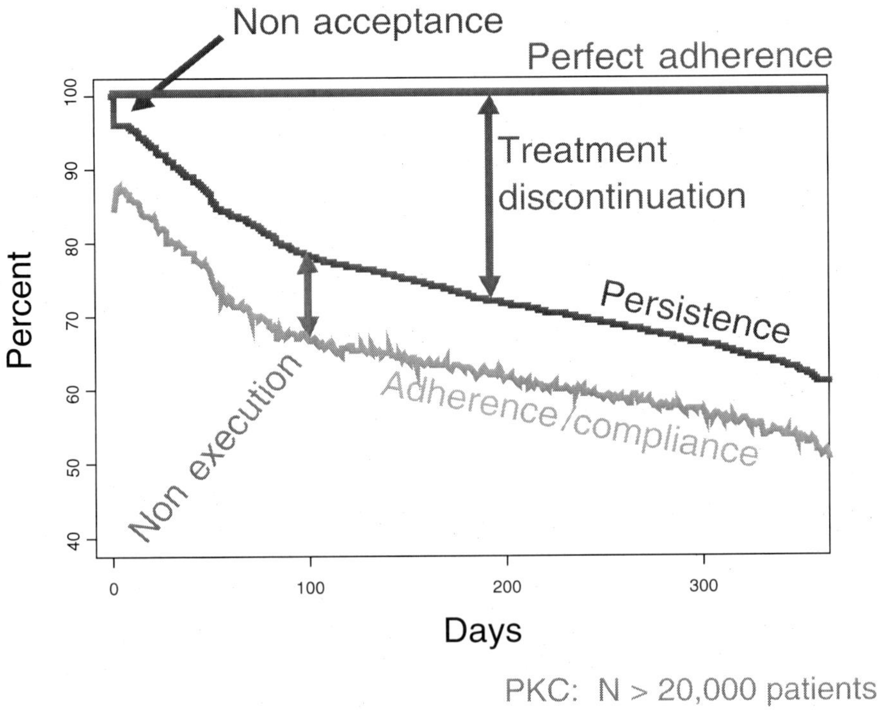

FIGURE 5-2 Different aspects of adherence among 20,000 patients in multiple clinical trials.
SOURCE: Vrijens, 2007.

should develop and use adherence measures that can capture different adherence patterns over time.

MEASURING ADHERENCE, SEXUAL BEHAVIOR, AND CONDOM USE

Investigators can gather information on product adherence and risk behavior through a variety of indirect and direct measures. Adherence and risk behavior are commonly measured by self-report through self-administered questionnaires, audio computer-assisted self-interviewing (ACASI), face-to-face interviews with participants, and participant diaries. Other indirect measures include pill counts, electronic product monitoring, pharmacy refills, and biomarkers of product exposure and risk behavior, such as applicator staining for vaginal insertion, or presence of semen indicating unprotected sex. Direct measures of product adherence include pharmacokinetic studies (which measure drug levels or metabolites in subjects' blood or bodily fluids), and directly observed therapy. These measures can vary substantially in expense, the effort required of participants and their partners, their perceived invasiveness, and their accuracy and reliability (Berg and Arnsten, 2006). Complicating matters is the lack of a "gold standard" for measuring adherence.

Most research on measuring adherence in HIV studies has examined HIV-infected individuals' adherence to ART. Measuring individuals' risk behavior is also critical to knowing whether a product worked. Given the limited published empirical evidence on adherence measures for nonvaccine biomedical HIV prevention interventions, the committee draws heavily on the fields of ART adherence and sexual risk behavior assessment in making its assessment and recommendations.

Indirect Measurement Methods

Self-Reports of Product Adherence and Risk Behavior

Self-report of product adherence and risk behavior is widely used in research and clinical settings because it is relatively inexpensive, easy to administer, allows for probing about nonadherence, and has low participant burden (Berg and Arnsten, 2006). However, the accuracy of self-reports is controversial and has been the focus of substantial research.

Reliability and validity are the two most important psychometric aspects of self-report measurements. Reliability refers to whether the instrument is free of random error and validity refers to whether the instrument is measuring what it intends to measure (Pequegnat et al., 2000). Self-reports can be incorrect because a person fails to respond truthfully or does not accurately recall their behavior (Pequegnat et al., 2000). Participants may respond untruthfully to questions about their adherence and risk behavior because they want the interviewer, study staff, or other participants to view them more favorably—a phenomenon known as "social desirability" bias (Pequegnat et al., 2000; Schroder et al., 2003b; Simoni et al., 2006b). Even with truthful responses, the accuracy of self-reports can be affected by the length of the recall period (for retrospective reports), the question format, appropriateness of the assessment mode, and individual factors (e.g., such as the frequency of behaviors, educational level, age, or use of alcohol and drugs) (Pequegnat et al., 2000; Schroder et al., 2003a,b, 2007).[1]

[1] See Pequegnat et al., 2000; Simoni et al., 2006b; and Schroder et al., 2003a,b, 2007, for a detailed discussion of psychometric factors related to adherence and risk behavior assessment and associated references.

Studies have found that self-reports of adherence tend to be positively skewed, producing higher estimates of adherence compared to more objective measures (e.g., electronic drug monitoring) (Berg and Arnsten, 2006; Simoni et al., 2006b). In contrast, studies comparing self-reports of sexual behavior with biomarkers of semen exposure indicate that individuals may underreport sensitive or stigmatized risk behavior (see, for example, Gallo et al., 2007).

Researchers have identified several methods to help mitigate these problems. First, investigators can enhance the validity and reliability of self-reports by stressing the importance of truthful responses, ensuring anonymity or confidentiality of responses, and allowing for privacy in answering questions (Pequegnat et al., 2000). Guidelines for minimizing social desirability bias in ART adherence assessment include using self-administered measures with either open-ended or forced choices, acknowledging the difficulty of perfect adherence to the participant ("normalizing" imperfect adherence), querying reasons for nonadherence, focusing on recent behavior, clearly specifying a time frame, using recall aids and anchoring reports to salient events, and conducting reliability checks (Simoni et al., 2006b).

Investigators can also use methods of collecting self-reported information that are more likely to promote reliable and valid self-reports. Face-to-face interviews can be prone to overreporting of adherence and underreporting of sensitive risk behaviors (Jadack et al., 2001; Rogers et al., 2005). Use of interviewers who are independent of the study staff can help create a neutral climate (UNAIDS, 2007). Self-administered questionnaires may also decrease the likelihood of social desirability bias. While written self-administered questionnaires are inappropriate in areas with low literacy rates, the use of ACASI can address some of the problems with face-to-face interviews.

A number of studies have suggested that participants are more likely to report sensitive behaviors, such as sexual behavior or drug use, if investigators rely on ACASI rather than in face-to-face interviews. ACASI can also help researchers check the consistency of participants' answers and reduce the number of missing data fields, or "don't know" responses. Several studies have shown that this technique is feasible and acceptable in a variety of international settings among different at-risk populations with varying literacy rates and computer skills (Van De Wijgert et al., 2001; Simoes et al., 2006a,b; NIMH Collaborative HIV/STD Prevention Trial Group, 2007).

Contraception trials have used prospective methods, such as coital diaries, extensively to collect self-reported information, and to validate retrospective self-reports of sexual behavior (Schroder et al., 2003a). The first phase 3 trial of a microbicide (Nonoxynol-9, or N9) initially used diaries in the form of pictorial log charts (Van Damme et al., 2002). However, after finding that women sometimes filled in their diaries while waiting at the clinic, the trial abandoned the diaries in favor of interviews (Van Damme et al., 2002). The Microbicide Development Program's phase 3 trial of the PRO2000 microbicide is now using coital diaries in a subset of women to capture information on sexual behaviors and product use. In a feasibility study prior to the start of the phase 3 trial, investigators found that women tended to report sexual behaviors more frequently in diaries than in face-to-face interviews (Allen et al., 2007).

Electronic diaries such as personal digital assistants (Bartley et al., 2004), mobile phones (Hays et al., 2001), pagers (Shrier et al., 2005), and Web applications (Baer et al., 2002) have also been tested, and could offer important advantages over paper diaries. Electronic diaries can allow internal checks on the validity of the data, and could record time and date information (Raymond and Ross, 2000). Electronic diaries also eliminate the need to transcribe and code data, allowing more detailed and timely analysis (Bartley et al., 2004). Studies have shown that subjects are willing to use electronic diaries, and that they may actually do so more often than paper diaries (Hufford, 2002).

Despite extensive work, several psychometric aspects of self-report measurements remain unresolved. A key problem is the lack of standardization in adherence and risk behavior measurement instruments across research and clinical settings (Schroder et al., 2003b; Berg and Arnsten, 2006). These measures vary in terms of length of recall period, the type of measure (qualitative versus quantitative measures), the question format, among other factors. There is poor agreement between various self-report measures and the variation makes it difficult to compare results across studies (Berg and Arnsten, 2006). Recent review papers suggest that cognitive interviewing, which examines how target audiences interpret questions, process information, and form responses to survey questions, and additional empirical evaluations of self-reported adherence questions can further improve the validity and reliability of self-reports (Berg and Arnsten, 2006).

Pill and Applicator Counts

Many clinical trials rely on less specific but possibly more objective measures of product adherence, such as pill counts. Asking participants to return unused pills and product applicators during routine visits is a relatively inexpensive measure. However, such measures can be time consuming and subject to bias if participants "dump" unused products prior to a visit (Berg and Arnsten, 2006). To address these concerns, some studies have found that unannounced pill counts at participants' homes can provide a reliable measure of ART adherence (Bangsberg et al., 2000, 2001). This approach reduces the problems with asking participants to return unused product at scheduled visits, reduces their opportunity to empty pill containers, and does not require them to bring all their medications to the clinic (Bangsberg et al., 2001).

Yet unannounced pill counts at participants' homes can be expensive and logistically difficult, and some participants may prefer not to have home visits (Kalichman et al., 2007). In a recent study of 77 HIV infected individuals in Atlanta, Kalichman and colleagues (2007) found that unannounced telephone-based pill counts were a logistically feasible and economical method for monitoring adherence to ART medication.

Pharmacy Refills

Maintaining pharmacy refill records is another method for indirectly measuring product adherence. If patients do not receive timely refills from the pharmacy, the investigator can assume that the patient is either missing doses or not taking the medication at all. "Medication gaps" or the period that the patient's supply of product is assumed to be exhausted is determined by a comparison of the actual refill dates with the expected refill dates (Berg and Arnsten, 2006).

This method of measuring adherence relies on two major assumptions. Participants who do not receive timely refills are not obtaining product from other sources, and participants who do receive timely refills use the product as prescribed.

In the clinical setting, a patient may have multiple opportunities to access medication, such as through family members and friends or other pharmacies. However, in the trial setting, access to the product usually is limited to the study pharmacy and study population, though product sharing among trial participants has been raised as a concern in some studies. Given that distribution of the study product is more tightly controlled, the use of pharmacy refill records may have greater applicability for measuring adherence in the trial setting than in the clinical setting.

Similar to pill counts, pharmacy refill records are not immune to bias, as participants may "dump" or share unused products. Timely refills do not guarantee that the participant took the product as instructed. Despite this limitation, several HIV treatment studies have shown a significant correlation between pharmacy refill adherence and HIV viral load (Maher et al., 1999; Low-Beer et al., 2002; Grossberg et al., 2004; Fairley et al., 2005) all studies can be found in Berg and Arnsten (2006).

Electronic Medication Monitoring

A commonly used approach to measuring adherence to ART is the "medication event monitoring" system (MEMs). MEMs uses microcircuitry in pharmaceutical packages to detect, time-stamp, analyze, and store information on when users remove a dose, and communicates that information to investigators (Urquhart, 1997). MEMs provides an "objective" and time-specific measure of adherence, and thus is often considered more valid than other types of measures, such as self-reports (Berg and Arnsten, 2006).

Yet MEMs has several important limitations. It requires participants to store all medications in the MEMs container, to remove only the correct number of pills at each dosing, to open the container only during dosing, and to close the monitor after dosing (Bangsberg et al., 2001). Several studies have documented "pocket dosing," in which participants remove multiple doses from the container at one time, which can lead to underestimates of adherence (Bova et al., 2005). Other studies have identified "curiosity checks," in which participants open the containers to test them, or to see how many tablets they have left, which may lead to overestimates of adherence (Bangsberg et al., 2001; Bova et al., 2005; Berg and Arnsten, 2006).

MEMs may be valuable in assessing adherence to medication-based approaches such as PrEP or HSV-2 suppression therapy. Researchers have also tested modifications of MEMs-type monitors for topical medications and found them feasible (Tusa et al., 2006). Investigators may find it useful to adapt MEMs to microbicide applicators. Other approaches being developed is the "smart" vaginal microbicide applicator, called Xigo, that stores information about product use (Rosenberg, 2007) and the "sexometer"—an intravaginal ring called Paragon that attempts to capture the time and date of sexual intercourse based on motion indicators (Rosenberg, 2007).

Biomarkers of Product Use and Sexual Activity

Researchers have developed biomarkers of product use and sexual activity that have potential for validating self-reported information in trial settings. To assess microbicide product use, researchers developed an assay that assesses lactobacillus growth on returned used applicators to determine exposure to the vagina (Wallace et al., 2004; Hogarty et al., 2007). This method was used in the Carraguard microbicide trial to distinguish applicators that had been inserted vaginally versus those that were not inserted (Skoler, 2007). The assay cannot reveal when the gel was used, which is important information for coitally dependent microbicides, or whether it was used by the participant or someone else. Nor can it determine whether the product was used each time it should have been. It can, however, reveal the absolute level of exposure to a product. A subsequent study of this approach in a 14-day microbicide trial of 0.5% PRO 2000 and placebo gel returned applicators found that there was high concordance between self-report and applicator staining (Hogarty et al., 2007).

Although incidence of sexually transmitted infections (STIs) has been suggested as a potential biomarker for unprotected sexual behavior, transmission of STIs also depends on individual susceptibility, sexual partners, and the characteristics of the infection (Pequegnat et al., 2000). Researchers have recently examined biomarkers of semen exposure as potential tools for validating self-reports of condom use and recent sexual activity. These candidate biomarkers can be classified into two categories: those that detect seminal plasma, and those that detect spermatozoa and other cells present in semen (see Mauck and Doncel, 2007 for a review of methods).

The seminal plasma biomarker with the most extensive testing in clinical trials is the prostate specific antigen (PSA) (Lawson et al., 1998; Macaluso et al., 1999). Because PSA begins to clear from the vagina immediately after it is exposed to semen, PSA detection likely underestimates exposure (Gallo et al., 2007). Another biomarker for semen exposure is the Y-chromosome (Yc) DNA. Researchers developed a Yc polymerase chain reaction (PCR) assay (Jadack et al., 2001; Zenilman et al., 2005). Yc-DNA may offer advantages over PSA because it can be detected several weeks post-coitus (Mauck and Doncel, 2007).

Such biomarkers have been used primarily to evaluate the effectiveness of contraceptives, but they may have a role in validating self-reports of sexual activity in HIV/STI prevention trials (Mauck and Doncel, 2007). For example, a recent study used PSA to assess the validity of self-reported condom use among female sex workers in Kenya, and found that 11 percent of samples from women who reported no unprotected sex in the prior 48 hours tested positive for PSA (Gallo et al., 2007). A follow-up study to the phase 3 MIRA diaphragm trial also used PSA to assess the validity of self-reported sexual behavior (Mauck and Doncel, 2007). Upon completion of the trial, investigators randomized a subset of women to an additional session using either ACASI or face-to-face interview. They then conducted a PSA analysis on women who reported no intercourse in the previous 48 hours, to assess whether misreporting differed by interviewing technique. The investigators have not yet reported the results of this analysis.

These or future assays may help validate self-reports of sexual behavior, and possibly help investigators assess the safety and efficacy of microbicides (Mauck and Doncel, 2007). However, the use of vaginal products, vaginal washing, menses, and infection may affect the sensitivity of the assays, so the ultimate value of the approach requires further research (Zenilman et al., 2005; Mauck and Doncel, 2007).

Direct Measurement Methods

Drug Monitoring

Biological assays of active drug, metabolite, or other markers in blood, urine, or other specimens can provide information on individuals' exposure to drug products. The value of examining drug levels depends on the half-life of the product (Osterberg and Blaschke, 2005). Such tests are thus most valuable for products with longer half-lives. Studies suggest that when exposure is measured during scheduled clinical visits, "white-coat compliance" can occur: that is, heightened awareness may spur participants to have better-than-normal adherence to treatment prior to their scheduled visit (Cramer et al., 1990). Measurements at those intervals may not be an accurate reflection of overall adherence.

Directly Observed Therapy

Directly observed therapy (DOT)—in which members of the study staff administer all doses of a product regimen to individuals, or observe their intake—is most commonly used as an intervention to increase adherence. It is also the only approach that provides near-perfect information on individuals' adherence and exposure to an HIV prevention product.

DOT is quite feasible in some settings and populations. For example, DOT and modified DOT (in which only a portion of the product regimen is taken under supervision) have been used extensively with ART (Goggin et al., 2007), including in resource-poor settings (Pearson et al., 2007). One late-stage biomedical HIV prevention trial now using DOT is the CDC-sponsored phase 2/3 PrEP trial in injecting drug users in Thailand. Participants were given the option of daily DOT or monthly follow-up. Approximately 85 percent of participants opted for daily DOT of their PrEP dose of Truvada, along with their daily methadone treatment (Smith, 2007). Researchers are also considering using DOT for other products that require application once a day, such as a microbicide gel, or once a month or less often, such as the vaginal ring (Rosenberg, 2007).

More widespread use of DOT is often limited by cost and logistical constraints, and by the fact that it cannot be used for coitally dependent products such as the first generation of microbicides. Nevertheless, DOT and modified DOT could be very useful in efficacy or proof-of-concept trials to minimize interpretation problems that result from nonadherence. However, the committee has concerns about using DOT in effectiveness trials of biomedical HIV interventions, if that approach cannot be sustained in real-world practice because the trial results may be poor predictors of the effectiveness of the interventions.

Since no adherence measurement tool is perfect, several studies have found that using multiple measures to "triangulate" adherence levels and risk behaviors is helpful in reducing the error introduced by any particular method (Liu et al., 2001; Pool et al., 2006). However, investigators relying on that approach must directly address inconsistencies in the results from different measures, rather than simply identifying them (Pool et al., 2006).

And any adherence measures that rely on recall must entail short recall periods.

Recommendation 5-2: In light of the uncertainty about the accuracy of various methods for collecting data on adherence and risk behavior, investigators of biomedical HIV prevention trials should strive to use multiple types of measures to triangulate adherence estimates. Rather than collecting detailed information on all participants, investigators could collect more detailed information on a well-chosen random sample, and collect less detailed information on all participants.

Recommendation 5-3: Although directly observed therapy or modified DOT could be very useful in proof-of-concept trials, investigators should not use these methods in effectiveness trials if that approach will not be used in real-world practice, because the trial results may then be poor predictors of the effectiveness of the interventions.

STRATEGIES TO IMPROVE ADHERENCE

High levels of adherence to a product regimen by participants in a clinical trial are critical to determining that product's efficacy—and ultimately its public health impact. However, little empirical evidence exists on the effectiveness of strategies to improve adherence to nonvaccine biomedical HIV prevention interventions.

The committee was unable to identify any publications specifically evaluating adherence strategies for such interventions. However, evidence on the effectiveness of methods to improve the adherence of HIV-infected patients to ART may inform efforts to enhance adherence in biomedical HIV prevention trials. Studies of ART adherence interventions may have particular relevance for medication-based HIV prevention strategies, such as PrEP or acyclovir for HSV-2 suppression.

Although some aspects of adherence undoubtedly differ between the two arenas, they have important similarities: biomedical HIV prevention trials target products to uninfected individuals, and HIV-infected individuals often start ART while they are still asymptomatic. In addition, both treatment and prevention interventions may require patients to follow daily regimens indefinitely.

This section reviews the effectiveness of strategies to improve adherence to ART, examines the lessons learned and knowledge gaps, and makes recommendations for applying such strategies in biomedical HIV prevention trials.

Effectiveness of Strategies to Improve Adherence to ART

Given the advent of combination antiretroviral therapy in the 1990s, the field of improving adherence to HIV treatment is still relatively young (Simoni et al., 2006a). However, a number of literature reviews on strategies to increase adherence to ART have been completed. Early qualitative reviews found that most studies of adherence strategies lacked sufficient methodological rigor, such as inadequate sample size, lack of randomization or control conditions, and failure to use intent-to-treat analyses, among others (Simoni et al., 2003).

Amico and colleagues (2006) conducted the first quantitative review of randomized and uncontrolled studies of strategies to improve adherence to ART published between 1996 and 2004 (24 studies). They found that these strategies had a significant ($P < 0.05$) aggregated effect on adherence to ART, but that the magnitude of the effect varied greatly across studies.

For example, Amico and colleagues found that strategies targeting participants with poor pretest adherence had greater effects than strategies targeting groups with a variety of pretest adherence levels. The analysts conclude that to design effective strategies, investigators must carefully delineate the target population. Amico and colleagues found no evidence that the effects of adherence strategies decayed over time, but few of the studies included extended follow-up periods. Like earlier qualitative reviews, they found that many of the studies were generally underpowered and would not have been able to detect a small to moderate sized effects.

In an update and extension of this work, Simoni and colleagues (2006b) conducted a meta-analysis of 19 randomized, controlled trials of strategies to improve ART adherence, measuring their impact on reported adherence and participants' HIV-1 RNA viral load. They found that participants receiving adherence strategies were about 1.5 times as likely (95% CI: 1.16–1.94) to report at least 95 percent adherence as participants in comparison conditions, and about 1.25 times as likely (95% CI: 0.99–1.59) to achieve an undetectable viral load. However, some strategies did not improve adherence, and most of those that did had only modest and short-term effects.

A Cochrane Collaboration review examined 57 randomized, controlled trials of interventions to improve adherence to medication across a variety of medical conditions, and found similar limitations. The reviewers concluded that "almost all of the interventions that were effective for long-term care were complex," and that "even the most effective interventions did not lead to large improvements in adherence and treatment outcomes" (Haynes et al., 2005, p. 1).

While the two meta-analyses of strategies to improve ART adherence suggest that they can be somewhat effective, the reviews offer few guidelines on which strategies are most effective (Simoni et al., 2007). Despite these limitations, several interventions to improve adherence to ART have shown promise, and could be worth further exploring in biomedical HIV prevention trials. These include cognitive-behavioral strategies (e.g., Pradier et al., 2003; Mannheimer et al., 2006; Petersen et al., 2007; Rueda et al., 2007), social support interventions (Remien et al., 2005; Williams et al., 2006), and directly observed therapy or modified directly observed treatment (e.g., Goggin et al., 2007; Pearson et al., 2007), and contingency management (Haug and Sorenson, 2006; Rosen et al., 2007).[2]

Applying ART Adherence Improvement Strategies to HIV Prevention

The findings from studies and meta-analyses of strategies to improve ART use suggest ways to improve adherence to biomedical HIV prevention interventions. However, important knowledge gaps remain:

- As noted in a recent meta-analysis (Amico et al., 2006) and several qualitative reviews (Haddad et al., 2000; Fogarty et al., 2002; Simoni et al., 2003), many studies of adherence strategies for ART lacked sufficient methodological rigor, were underpowered, and lacked theoretic underpinnings.
- Publications on trials of strategies to improve adherence often do not describe in enough detail the nature, content, and intensity of the strategies. Yet this information is important in evaluating the adherence intervention, and comparing outcomes across studies (Amico et al., 2006). In reviewing the protocols for non-vaccine biomedical HIV prevention trials, the committee generally found a similar paucity of information on the types and frequency of planned adherence improvement strategies, and the factors that might trigger changes in those strategies.
- Most studies evaluating ART adherence strategies have focused on individuals, even though substantial research indicates that factors at the provider, clinic, and sociocultural level can affect adherence to HIV interventions (Gordon, 2006).
- Because most trials evaluating ART adherence strategies were conducted in high-income countries, their applicability to resource-poor areas is uncertain (Gordon, 2006).
- A key unknown is the extent to which strategies that improve adherence to HIV treatment apply to uninfected individuals who must take

[2]Contingency management (CM) typically involves a voucher- or monetary-based reinforcement technique in which individuals are rewarded for sustaining positive behavior. CM has been used successfully in substance abuse treatment settings to reinforce treatment goals such as drug abstinence or completion of certain activities. CM may also help promote adherence in the HIV field (Haug and Sorensen, 2006).

an experimental HIV prevention agent over a long period of time. While the consequences of imperfect adherence for HIV-infected individuals are tangible, those for uninfected individuals are less so.

- Different subgroups within a given population may need different adherence strategies. Such strategies may also exert different effects across subgroups (Chesney, 2006; Simoni et al., 2006a).

Studies of strategies for improving adherence to HIV prevention interventions are lacking but essential. Evidence is especially needed in the context where adherence matters most, and where it may well be most challenging: for coitally dependent microbicides, and for interventions that individuals must use indefinitely, such as PrEP, microbicides, and HSV-2 suppression.

Successful research on strategies to improve product adherence requires collaboration among behavioral, social, and quantitative scientists, despite the barriers to such collaboration. It is critical for multidisciplinary teams to study adherence challenges in a given setting, and to develop socially and culturally relevant strategies for improving adherence. Such teams also need to pursue research on how best to translate strategies that are effective in one setting to settings with different personal, economic, and sociocultural influences on adherence and risk behaviors (Chesney, 2006).

Investigators designing clinical trials of biomedical HIV prevention interventions may need to adapt and combine various strategies to maximize adherence (Haynes et al., 2005). As discussed in Chapter 10, factorial study designs, and dynamic designs, can allow such investigators to empirically evaluate alternative adherence strategies. Investigators of HIV prevention trials also need to consider using adherence strategies that target couples, groups, and communities as well as individuals (Gordon, 2006).

Recommendation 5-4: Donors should fund and investigators should undertake empirical evaluations of strategies to increase adherence to biomedical HIV prevention products during and after a clinical trial. These evaluations should be adequately powered, methodologically rigorous, socially and culturally relevant, grounded in behavioral and social science theories, and conducted in the regions where the strategies will be utilized.

Recommendation 5-5: Investigators should specify in the study protocol detailed plans for monitoring, measuring, and analyzing adherence data, and steps they will take to improve adherence if it is poorer than anticipated.

ANALYZING ADHERENCE

Exposure to a product, adherence to instructions for using it, and behavior related to that use are key factors on the causal path from preventive intervention to HIV infection. Figure 5-1 illustrates how randomization of participants in a clinical trial has a direct effect on their product exposure, but is not itself influenced by their baseline characteristics, including pre-randomization sexual behavior. It is this particular feature that enables investigators to estimate the causal effect of study arm assignment in the traditional intention-to-treat analysis, which compares groups "as randomized" (that is, based on the intended intervention). However, baseline characteristics of participants may influence how much product exposure they ultimately experience, and both factors can influence changes in behavior. In Figure 5-3, arrows emanating from each of these features point to a direct impact on HIV incidence. Additional variables, observed or unobserved, may also enter the picture.

Analyzing patterns of exposure to the product, adherence to the product regimen, and accompanying behavior—including vaginal, anal, and oral sex, with or without various forms of protection (condom and/or product)—can yield important information about the study population. Such analyses also yield information on the acceptability and feasibility of the intervention, and the extent to which the trial results will apply to the target population.

Analyzing the association between exposure or adherence patterns and HIV incidence can help investigators estimate the causal effect of different interventions and reveal whether the primary intention-to-treat analysis is estimating efficacy or some particular form of effectiveness, given the observed dosing schedule. However, "measurement error," (less-than-perfect information on adherence and behavior, due to inaccurate reporting or measuring of adherence) will limit investigators' ability to interpret intention-to-treat analyses, and to recognize and monitor adherence problems, distinguish nonresponders from nonadherers, and provide adherence-specific estimates of the effects of the product, which can guide further development.

This section examines the major sources of variation in adherence patterns within a trial. In each case, the committee discusses how random and systematic measurement error introduced by subjective adherence measures can affect the results and their interpretation. Table 5-1 summarizes this analysis. The committee also suggests adherence analyses that can reveal subject-specific baseline variables (sometimes called moderator variables) and variations in behavioral responses (sometimes called mediator variables)—both of which can shed light on the potential impact of an intervention (Mackinnon and Dwyer, 1993).

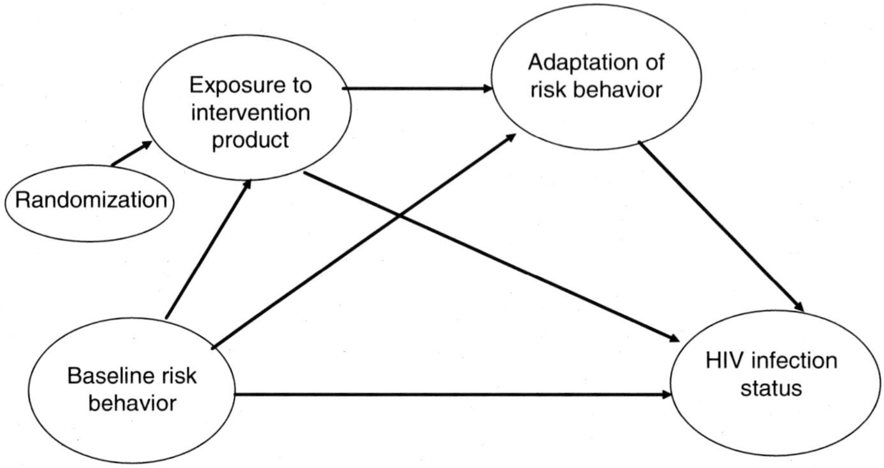

FIGURE 5-3 A causal diagram: some key variables and their potential direct effects (the arrows).

Investigators of trials with low levels of adherence will have difficulty assessing a product's efficacy. Such levels may also indicate that the product will be unacceptable or infeasible for wider use in the community.

Effect of Measurement Error

Because measurements of adherence usually overestimate true adherence, low reported levels of adherence can usually safely be assumed to reflect low actual adherence. However, even if reported adherence levels in a trial are high, doubt may remain about true adherence levels, and thus about the product's efficacy and value in the community.

Comparing Adherence Between Study Arms

Differences in adherence between the intervention and control arms in a randomized trial imply that different products have different side-effect profiles, or otherwise affect participants differently. These differences may emerge early in a trial or become apparent over time. If the latter occurs, blinding has not necessarily failed. A small increase in a mild side effect in the intervention arm could lead to lower adherence even if participants are not aware of which arm they are in. Such an outcome may produce a higher dropout rate in the intervention arm, and hence lower adherence. On the

TABLE 5-1 What Adherence Analyses Can Reveal

Analysis	Possible Results	Interpretation
Analyze level of product adherence in each study arm.	The measured levels indicate how much participants deviate from the prescribed dose timing, and possibly the method of using the product.	Efficacy trial: This shows to what extent the measured effect should indeed be seen as a measure of efficacy. Effectiveness trial: This may reveal problems with the feasibility and acceptability of the intervention in the study population within the trial setting.
Analyze differences in product exposure, adherence, and risk behavior between study arms.[a]	The measured levels of product adherence and sexual behavior differ between study arms.	This might indicate that the active product versus placebo produce different side effects, prompting subjects to comply differently with the assignment.[b]
Analyze differences in product exposure, adherence, and risk behavior between subjects within randomized arms.	People within study arms differ greatly in how they use the product, and possibly also in their risk-taking behavior.	Some subpopulations might be better suited to another type of protection than the one under study.
Analyze changes over time in product exposure, adherence, and risk behavior among subjects within randomized arms.	People within randomized arms differ greatly in how they use the product over time.	If rates of adherence among individual subjects drop dramatically over time, this might indicate that the intervention is not sustainable. That, in turn, may indicate that side effects emerge after cumulative use, or the need for supportive measures to improve adherence. If long-term use of the intervention is envisaged, suggestions that sustainability is limited would require investigators to further examine the appropriateness of the intervention. If adherence rates increase over time, subjects may be getting better at adhering to the intervention.

continued

TABLE 5-1 Continued

Analysis	Possible Results	Interpretation
Analyze how levels of risky behavior differ from those that can be expected outside the trial.	Subjects appear to be highly sexually active, or they engage in more risky behavior than expected outside the trial context.	This could reflect disinhibition, or that subjects want to become pregnant within the healthy study setting. Such behavior could lead to sexual acts against which the product is not designed to protect, and may put subjects at higher risk of HIV infection.
Analyze how levels of risky behavior differ between study arms.	Subjects differ between arms in the amount of risky behavior they pursue against which the product is not designed to protect (such as anal sex).	This could distort the intention-to-treat effect. That, in turn, could give a distorted view of the direct impact of the product under real-world conditions.

[a]Any interpretation of observed differences in adherence between arms will need to account for differential dropout rates over time. Such differences in dropout rates could occur, for instance, if a product is protective, and HIV incidence differs between arms. The least-protected people will tend to drop out first owing to HIV infection.

[b]This does not mean that blinding has failed. A small increase in a mild side effect in the study arm could lead to lower product adherence without participant awareness. These differences may emerge early in the trial or become apparent with accumulated product use over time.

other hand, if a product is protective and HIV incidence differs between arms, the least-protected participants would tend to drop out sooner.

Effect of Measurement Error

Investigators would have no reason to expect measurement error to differ between study arms in a blinded randomized trial. They can therefore expect significant differences in adherence between arms to reflect true differences.

The interpretation of reported adherence differences between arms in an unblinded trial is usually less clear. For example, in the MIRA diaphragm/Replens trial, observed rates of condom use were much higher in the "condom-only" control arm than in the intervention arm (Padian et al., 2007). One explanation is that subjects in the condom-only arm adhered to guidelines on condom use more than did subjects in the condom-plus-diaphragm arm, because they felt that this was their only form of protection against

HIV infection. However, a different explanation is that they over-reported condom use because they could not report diaphragm use and wished to appear compliant.

Comparing Adherence Patterns Within Randomized Arms

Large variations in reported adherence between subjects within a study arm may indicate that some subpopulations are better suited for another type of protection. For example, if participants in one arm used a product for 80 percent of sexual acts, it matters whether all subjects failed to use the product for 20 percent of the acts, versus whether 20 percent of subjects did not use the product at all and 80 percent used it every time. In the latter case, investigators would hope to recognize the 20 percent of nontakers early on and offer them a different intervention option. If most people use the product only 80 percent of the time, the intervention may be impractical. Investigators need to address these differences in their analyses, rather than reporting only the percentage of people who comply with the regimen in each arm.

Effect of Measurement Error

If subjects within a study arm differ significantly in their reported exposure to the product, adherence to the product regimen, and sexual behavior, investigators will need to consider whether the differences reflect true differences, errors in measurement, or a combination of both.

Adherence patterns for individuals may change over time. If compliance rates for individuals drop dramatically during a trial, investigators should determine whether side effects are emerging. If adherence declines are common across subjects within an arm, investigators should consider providing additional support or other interventions, especially if the product is intended for long-term use. If measurement errors remain stable, such differences probably reveal actual trends.

When Behavior Differs from That Expected Outside the Trial

Participants in a clinical trial might pursue higher rates of sexual activity or other risky behavior because of disinhibition, or because they are trying to become pregnant in the healthy environment of the trial. Such behavior would put them at higher risk of HIV transmission, especially if they pursue more risky behavior against which the product is not designed to protect, such as anal sex. In such cases, the results of the trial's intention-to-treat analysis could give a distorted view of the impact of product use outside the study.

Effect of Measurement Error

This aspect of the adherence analysis is quite sensitive to measurement error, although systematic errors are again likely to reflect underreporting among trial participants.

Association Analyses: Linking Adherence Patterns to HIV Incidence

Investigators can attempt to analyze information on reported sexual activity, adherence, and HIV exposure to assess their association with HIV infection. Such analyses may allow them to interpret and explain the observed intention-to-treat effect, judge whether to explore different ways of administering a product, and estimate the effect the product will have in other populations.

The observed association between reported product use and HIV incidence is prone to confounding, and does not necessarily reflect a real (causal) effect even if reported use is correct. For microbicides, for instance, higher sexual activity tends to increase the risk of HIV transmission as well as the number of gel applications. Investigators would therefore expect to find a positive association between the product use (such as applications per day) in the experimental arm and HIV incidence, even in the absence of any causal effect of the product.

Nevertheless, information on variations in product use can help investigators interpret the effect revealed by an intention-to-treat analysis, and help them estimate the product's effectiveness in future populations. As in the N-9 trial, higher HIV incidence rates may occur at high levels of product use in the intervention arm than at corresponding levels of product use in the placebo arm (Van Damme et al., 2002), and this might reflect an increased risk of HIV infection with use of the intervention.

However, investigators need to consider and exclude other explanations before regarding such an effect as causal. The main reason is that a measured compliance level—such as use of gel in at least 80 percent of sexual acts—is a post-randomization category that may itself be influenced by the product, and need not be influenced in the same way among study arms. (In technical investigations of causality, this phenomenon is known as a lack of "exchangeability.") For instance, if a product is associated with more sexually transmitted diseases, some women may start to use it less often, and hence different subpopulations may have similar use levels in both trial arms. However, when the study arms are blinded and investigators observe similar distributions of adherence between them, they can be more confident in the exchangeability of subpopulations with similar compliance levels among study arms.

Errors in reported adherence will further complicate the interpretation of data. Such errors may depend on the actual level of adherence, as more bias may be expected when true adherence is low, and on the study endpoint, as participants may be more reluctant to admit to imperfect adherence after high-risk behavior or an HIV diagnosis, for example. If these biases are at play equally in both study arms, an adherence-adjusted comparison of study arms would tend to convey the correct signal, at least qualitatively. However, assessments of safe adherence levels would tend to be overestimates. In unblinded trials, such as the MIRA diaphragm trial, subjects in the unblinded arm may be under higher pressure to comply with condom use, and may therefore overreport adherence to a larger extent. An adherence-adjusted analysis would then tend to compare HIV incidence rates between somewhat different subpopulations.

Statisticians have developed sophisticated causal models that attempt to address questions such as: "What would have occurred if exposure had been different?" One such model links potential responses to different levels of treatment and risk behavior, and allows estimation of the model's parameters based on the randomization used to assign patients to study arms. The corresponding statistical tests are approximately valid under the null hypothesis of no causal effect, even if the assumed form for the causal model is incorrect (Robins and Tsiatis, 1991; Vandebosch et al., 2005). Such models thus provide a valuable level of protection against confounding.

Linear structural mean models (Goetghebeur and Vansteelandt, 2005) also remain valid under the null hypothesis in the face of random measurement error, and can be adjusted to account for (known or modeled) average systematic error in measuring compliance. However, when there is a causal effect, the validity of these analyses rests on the assumption that the structural causal model is correct, and the latter is typically not testable based on available data.

It is important to verify the assumptions made in causal models as much as possible, and to assess the sensitivity of the results to plausible deviations from the assumptions. These models allow investigators to predict, under additional assumptions, the expected effects of a given distribution of product exposure within a population, including under full compliance. The models also allow investigators to correct for differential condom use between the study arms, thus allowing estimation of the direct effect of the intervention.

In some settings, investigators compare adherence between participants who become HIV infected and matched controls who do not become infected. A comparison of recent behavior and product exposure could help explain the extent to which seroconverters are nonresponders or noncompliers. However, because such a comparison would be nonrandomized, other factors could confound an observed association. Detailed adherence data obtained retrospectively may also suffer from bias, given that a participant's knowledge that he or she has become HIV infected may change his or her recollection of behavioral details. Investigators could thus complement this retrospective information with simple measures of adherence gathered prospectively, in real time. A substantial difference between prospective (reported by the participant before his or her HIV status is known) and retrospective (reported after the HIV status is known) measures of adherence across study arms may indicate differential measurement error. (See Appendix D for more detail on methods for analyzing adherence data.)

Recommendation 5-6: Investigators should provide data on product adherence and risk behavior results to the data monitoring committee, as this information may influence the committee's views of the relative efficacy and safety of the study arms, and the feasibility of the study.

Recommendation 5-7: Investigators should analyze adherence and behavior as both outcomes in an HIV prevention trial and modifiers of the effect of the biomedical intervention on HIV infection risk.

Recommendation 5-8: Investigators should analyze the potential impact of adherence by doing the following:

- **Perform a stratified analysis when adherence appears similar between study arms. Such analyses aim to provide unbiased comparisons of subpopulations across study arms.**
- **Postulate causal models and perform randomization-based analyses.**
- **Perform matched case-control adherence analyses involving subjects who become HIV infected.**

When reporting model-based analyses of adherence, investigators should clearly state the model's assumptions and discuss their plausibility, as well as the robustness of the analysis to violations of the assumptions.

REFERENCES

Allen, C. F., S. S. Lees, N. A. Desmond, G. Der, B. Chiduo, I. Hambleton, L. Knight, A. Vallely, D. A. Ross, and R. J. Hayes. 2007. Validity of coital diaries in a feasibility study for the microbicides development programme trial among women at high risk of HIV/AIDS in Mwanza, Tanzania. *Sexually Transmitted Infections* [Epub ahead of print].

Amico, K. R., J. J. Harman, and B. T. Johnson. 2006. Efficacy of antiretroviral therapy adherence interventions: A research synthesis of trials, 1996 to 2004. *Journal of Acquired Immune Deficiency Syndromes* 41(3):285-297.

Baer, A., S. Saroiu, and L. A. Koutsky. 2002. Obtaining sensitive data through the web: An example of design and methods. *Epidemiology* 13(6):640-645.

Bangsberg, D. R., F. M. Hecht, E. D. Charlebois, A. R. Zolopa, M. Holodniy, L. Sheiner, J. D. Bamberger, M. A. Chesney, and A. Moss. 2000. Adherence to protease inhibitors, HIV-1 viral load, and development of drug resistance in an indigent population. *AIDS* 14(4):357-366.

Bangsberg, D. R., F. M. Hecht, E. D. Charlebois, M. Chesney, and A. Moss. 2001. Comparing objective measures of adherence to HIV antiretroviral therapy: Electronic medication monitors and unannounced pill counts. *AIDS & Behavior* 5(3):275-281.

Bartley, J. B., D. G. Ferris, L. M. Allmond, E. D. Dickman, J. K. Dias, and J. Lambert. 2004. Personal digital assistants used to document compliance of bacterial vaginosis treatment. *Sexually Transmitted Diseases* 31(8):488-491.

Berg, K. M., and J. H. Arnsten. 2006. Practical and conceptual challenges in measuring antiretroviral adherence. *Journal of Acquired Immune Deficiency Syndromes* 43(Suppl 1): S79-S87.

Bova, C. A., K. P. Fennie, G. J. Knafl, K. D. Dieckhaus, E. Watrous, and A. B. Williams. 2005. Use of electronic monitoring devices to measure antiretroviral adherence: Practical considerations. *AIDS & Behavior* 9(1):103-110.

Chesney, M. A. 2006. The elusive gold standard. Future perspectives for HIV adherence assessment and intervention. *Journal of Acquired Immune Deficiency Syndromes* 43(Suppl 1):S149-S155.

Cramer, J. A., R. D. Scheyer, and R. H. Mattson. 1990. Compliance declines between clinic visits. *Archives of Internal Medicine* 150(7):1509-1510.

Fairley, C. K., A. Permana, and T. R. Read. 2005. Long-term utility of measuring adherence by self-report compared with pharmacy record in a routine clinic setting. *HIV Medicine* 6(5):366-369.

Fogarty, L., D. Roter, S. Larson, J. Burke, J. Gillespie, and R. Levy. 2002. Patient adherence to HIV medication regimens: A review of published and abstract reports. *Patient Education and Counseling* 46(2):93-108.

Friedland, G. H. 2006. HIV medication adherence. The intersection of biomedical, behavioral, and social science research and clinical practice. *Journal of Acquired Immune Deficiency Syndromes* 43(Suppl 1):S3-S9.

Gallo, M. F., F. M. Behets, M. J. Steiner, S. C. Thomsen, W. Ombidi, S. Luchters, C. Toroitich-Ruto, and M. M. Hobbs. 2007. Validity of self-reported "safe sex" among female sex workers in Mombasa, Kenya—PSA analysis. *International Journal of STD and AIDS* 18(1):33-38.

Goetghebeur, E., and S. Vansteelandt. 2005. Structural mean models for compliance analysis in randomized clinical trials and the impact of errors on measures of exposure. *Statistical Methods in Medical Research* 14(4):397-415.

Goggin, K., R. J. Liston, and J. A. Mitty. 2007. Modified directly observed therapy for antiretroviral therapy: A primer from the field. *Public Health Reports* 122(4):472-481.

Gordon, C. M. 2006. Commentary on meta-analysis of randomized controlled trials for HIV treatment adherence interventions. Research directions and implications for practice. *Journal of Acquired Immune Deficiency Syndromes* 43(Suppl 1):S36-S40.

Grossberg, R., Y. Zhang, and R. Gross. 2004. A time-to-prescription-refill measure of antiretroviral adherence predicted changes in viral load in HIV. *Journal of Clinical Epidemiology* 57(10):1107-1110.

Haddad, M., C. Inch, R. H. Glazier, A. L. Wilkins, G. Urbshott, A. Bayoumi, and S. Rourke. 2000. Patient support and education for promoting adherence to highly active antiretroviral therapy for HIV/AIDS. *Cochrane Database of Systematic Reviews* (3):CD001442.

Haug, N. A. and J. L. Sorensen. 2006. Contingency management interventions for HIV-related behaviors. *Current HIV/AIDS Reports* 3:144-149.

Haynes, R. B., X. Yao, A. Degani, S. Kripalani, A. Garg, and H. P. McDonald. 2005. Interventions for enhancing medication adherence [systematic review]. *Cochrane Database of Systematic Reviews* (4).

Hays, M. A., B. Irsula, S. L. McMullen, and P. J. Feldblum. 2001. A comparison of three daily coital diary designs and a phone-in regimen. *Contraception* 63(3):159-166.

Hogarty, K., A. Kasowitz, B. C. Herold, and M. J. Keller. 2007. Assessment of Product Adherence to Product Dosing in a Pilot Microbicide Study. *Sexually Transmitted Diseases* 34(11).

Hufford, M. R. 2002. Paper vs. Electronic diaries: Compliance and subject evaluations. *Applied Clinical Trials* April:38-43.

Jadack, R., G. Willis, and S. M. Rogers. 2001. *Accurate responding to sensitive questions in an STI clinic population: Patient preference for computer-based administration.* Annual Meeting of the Society of Behavioral Medicine, Seattle, Washington.

Kalichman, S. C., C. M. Amaral, H. Stearns, D. White, J. Flanagan, H. Pope, C. Cherry, D. Cain, L. Eaton, and M. O. Kalichman. 2007. Adherence to antiretroviral therapy assessed by unannounced pill counts conducted by telephone. *Journal of General Internal Medicine* 22(7):1003-1006.

Kerr, T., J. Walsh, E. Lloyd-Smith, and E. Wood. 2005. Measuring adherence to highly active antiretroviral therapy: Implications for research and practice. *Current HIV/AIDS Reports* 2(4):200-205.

Lawson, M. L., M. Maculuso, A. Bloom, G. Hortin, K. R. Hammond, and R. Blackwell. 1998. Objective markers of condom failure. *Sexually Transmitted Diseases* 25(8):427-432.

Liu, H., C. E. Golin, L. G. Miller, R. D. Hays, C. K. Beck, S. Sanandaji, J. Christian, T. Maldonado, D. Duran, A. H. Kaplan, and N. S. Wenger. 2001. A comparison study of multiple measures of adherence to HIV protease inhibitors. *Annals of Internal Medicine* 134(10):968-977.

Low-Beer, N., R. Gabe, S. McCormack, V. S. Kitchen, C. J. Lacey, and A. J. Nunn. 2002. Dextrin sulfate as a vaginal microbicide: Randomized, double-blind, placebo-controlled trial including healthy female volunteers and their male partners. *Journal of Acquired Immune Deficiency Syndromes* 31(4):391-398.

Macaluso, M., J. Kelaghan, L. Artz, H. Austin, M. Fleenor, E. W. Hook, 3rd, and T. Valappil. 1999. Mechanical failure of the latex condom in a cohort of women at high STD risk. *Sexually Transmitted Diseases* 26(8):450-458.

Mackinnon, D. P., and J. H. Dwyer. 1993. Estimating mediated effects in prevention studies. *Evaluation Review* 17(2):144-158.

Maher, K., N. Klimas, M. A. Fletcher, V. Cohen, C. M. Maggio, J. Triplett, R. Valenzuela, and G. Dickinson. 1999. Disease progression, adherence, and response to protease inhibitor therapy for HIV infection in an urban veterans affairs medical center. *Journal of Acquired Immune Deficiency Syndromes* 22(4):358-363.

Mannheimer, S. B., E. Morse, J. P. Matts, L. Andrews, C. Child, B. Schmetter, and G. H. Friedland. 2006. Sustained benefit from a long-term antiretroviral adherence intervention. *Journal of Acquired Immune Deficiency Syndromes* 43(1):S41-S47.

Mauck, C. K., and G. F. Doncel. 2007. Biomarkers of semen in the vagina: Applications in clinical trials of contraception and prevention of sexually transmitted pathogens including HIV. *Contraception* 75(6):407-419.

NIMH Collaborative HIV/STD Prevention Trial Group. 2007. The feasibility of audio computer-assisted self-interviewing in international settings. *AIDS* 21(Suppl 2):S49-S58.

Osterberg, L., and T. Blaschke. 2005. Adherence to medication. *New England Journal of Medicine* 353(5):487-497.

Padian, N., A. van der Straten, G. Ramjee, T. Chipato, G. de Bruyn, K. Blanchard, S. Shiboski, E. Montgomery, H. Fancher, H. Cheng, M. Rosenblum, M. van der Loan, N. Jewell, J. McIntyre, and The MIRA Team. 2007. Diaphragm and lubricant gel for prevention of HIV acquisition in southern African women: A randomised controlled trial. *Lancet* 370:251-261.

Pearson, C. R., M. A. Micek, J. A. Simoni, P. D. Hoff, E. Matediana, D. P. Martin, and S. S. Gloyd. 2007. Randomized control trial of peer-delivered, modified directly observed therapy for HAART in Mozambique. *Journal of Acquired Immune Deficiency Syndromes* 46(2):239-244.

Pequegnat, W., M. Fishbein, D. Celentano, A. Ehrhardt, G. Garnett, D. Holtgrave, J. Jaccard, J. Schachter, and J. Zenilman. 2000. NIMH/APPC workgroup on behavioral and biological outcomes in HIV/STD prevention studies: A position statement. *Sexually Transmitted Diseases* 27(3):127-132.

Petersen, M. L., Y. Wang, M. J. van der Laan, D. Guzman, E. Riley, and D. R. Bangsberg. 2007. Pillbox organizers are associated with improved adherence to HIV antiretroviral therapy and viral suppression: A marginal structural model analysis. *Clinical Infectious Diseases* 45(7):908-915.

Pool, R., A. Kamali, and J. A. G. Whitworth. 2006. Understanding sexual behaviour change in rural southwest uganda: A multi-method study. *AIDS Care—Psychological and Socio-Medical Aspects of AIDS/HIV* 18(5):479-488.

Pradier, C., L. Bentz, B. Spire, C. Tourette-Turgis, M. Morin, M. Souville, M. Rebillon, J. G. Fuzibet, A. Pesce, P. Dellamonica, and J. P. Moatti. 2003. Efficacy of an educational and counseling intervention on adherence to highly active antiretroviral therapy: French prospective controlled study. *HIV Clinical Trials* 4(2):121-131.

Raymond, S., and R. Ross. 2000. Electronic subject diaries in clinical trials. *Applied Clinical Trials* (March):48-57.

Remien, R. H., M. J. Stirratt, C. Dolezal, J. S. Dognin, G. J. Wagner, A. Carballo-Dieguez, N. El-Bassel, and T. M. Jung. 2005. Couple-focused support to improve HIV medication adherence: A randomized controlled trial. *AIDS* 19(8):807-814.

Robins, J., and A. Tsiatis. 1991. Adjusting for differential rates of pneumocystis-carinii pneumonia prophylaxis in high versus low-dose AZT treatment arms in an AIDS randomized trial. *American Journal of Epidemiology* 134.

Rogers, S. M., G. Willis, A. Al-Tayyib, M. A. Villarroel, C. F. Turner, L. Ganapathi, J. Zenilman, and R. Jadack. 2005. Audio computer assisted interviewing to measure HIV risk behaviours in a clinic population. *Sexually Transmitted Infections* 81(6):501-507.

Rosen, M. I., K. Dieckhaus, T. J. McMahon, B. Valdes, N. M. Petry, J. Cramer, and B. Rounsaville. 2007. Improved adherence with contingency management. *AIDS Patient Care and STDs* 21(1):30-40.

Rosenberg, Z. F. 2007. *Phase III clinical trial design*. Presentation at the first public meeting for the Committee on Methodological Challenges in HIV Prevention Trials, Washington, DC.

Rueda, S., L. Park-Wyllie, A. M. Bayoumi, A. M. Tynan, T. A. Antoniou, S. B. Rourke, and R. H. Glazier. 2007. Patient support and education for promoting adherence to highly active antiretroviral therapy for HIV/AIDS. *Cochrane Database of Systematic Reviews* (3).

Sankar, A., C. Golin, J. M. Simoni, M. Luborsky, and C. Pearson. 2006. How qualitative methods contribute to understanding combination antiretroviral therapy adherence. *Journal of Acquired Immune Deficiency Syndromes* 43(Suppl 1):S54-S68.

Schroder, K. E. E., M. P. Carey, and P. A. Vanable. 2003a. Methodological challenges in research on sexual risk behavior: I. Item content, scaling, and data analytical options. *Annals of Behavioral Medicine* 26(2):76-103.

Schroder, K. E. E., M. P. Carey, and P. A. Vanable. 2003b. Methodological challenges in research on sexual risk behavior: II. Accuracy of self-reports. *Annals of Behavioral Medicine* 26(2):104-123.

Schroder, K. E. E., C. J. Johnson, and J. S. Wiebe. 2007. Interactive voice response technology applied to sexual behavior self-reports: A comparison of three methods. *AIDS and Behavior* 11(2):313-323.

Shrier, L. A., M. C. Shih, and W. R. Beardslee. 2005. Affect and sexual behavior in adolescents: A review of the literature and comparison of momentary sampling with diary and retrospective self-report methods of measurement. *Pediatrics* 115(5):e573-e581.

Simoes, A. A., F. I. Bastos, R. I. Moreira, K. G. Lynch, and D. S. Metzger. 2006a. Acceptability of audio computer-assisted self-interview (ACASI) among substance abusers seeking treatment in Rio de Janeiro, Brazil. *Drug and Alcohol Dependence* 82(Suppl 1): S103-S107.

Simoes, A. A., F. I. Bastos, R. I. Moreira, K. G. Lynch, and D. S. Metzger. 2006b. A randomized trial of audio computer and in-person interview to assess HIV risk among drug and alcohol users in Rio de Janeiro, Brazil. *Journal of Substance Abuse Treatment* 30(3):237-243.

Simoni, J. M., P. A. Frick, D. W. Pantalone, and B. J. Turner. 2003. Antiretroviral adherence interventions: A review of current literature and ongoing studies. *Topics in HIV Medicine* 11(6):185-198.

Simoni, J. M., C. R. Pearson, D. W. Pantalone, G. Marks, and N. Crepaz. 2006a. Efficacy of interventions in improving highly active antiretroviral therapy adherence and HIV-1 RNA viral load. A meta-analytic review of randomized controlled trials. *Journal of Acquired Immune Deficiency Syndromes* 43(Suppl 1):S23-S35.

Simoni, J. M., A. E. Kurth, C. R. Pearson, D. W. Pantalone, J. O. Merrill, and P. A. Frick. 2006b. Self-report measures of antiretroviral therapy adherence: A review with recommendations for HIV research and clinical management. *AIDS & Behavior* 10(3):227-245.

Simoni, J. M., D. W. Pantalone, M. D. Plummer, and B. Huang. 2007. A randomized controlled trial of a peer support intervention targeting antiretroviral medication adherence and depressive symptomatology in HIV-positive men and women. *Health Psychology* 26(4):488-495.

Skoler, S. 2007. *Population Council: Phase 3 efficacy study of the vaginal gel Carraguard to prevent HIV transmission.* Paper read at the first public meeting for the Committee on Methodological Challenges in HIV Prevention Trials, Washington, DC.

Smith, D. 2007. *CDC PrEP trials.* Presentation at the first public meeting for the Committee on Methodological Challenges in HIV Prevention Trials, Washington, DC.

Tusa, M. G., M. Ladd, M. Kaur, R. Balkrishnan, and S. R. Feldman. 2006. Adapting electronic adherence monitors to standard packages of topical medications. *Journal of American Academy of Dermatology* 55:886-887.

UNAIDS. 2007. *Ethical considerations in biomedical HIV prevention trials.* Geneva, Switzerland: UNAIDS.

Urquhart, J. 1997. The electronic medication event monitor. Lessons for pharmacotherapy. *Clinical Pharmacokinetics* 32(5):345-356.

Van Damme, L., G. Ramjee, M. Alary, B. Vuylsteke, V. Chandeying, H. Rees, P. Sirivongrangson, L. Mukenge-Tshibaka, V. Ettiegne-Traore, C. Uaheowitchai, S. S. Karim, B. Masse, J. Perriens, and M. Laga. 2002. Effectiveness of col-1492, a nonoxynol-9 vaginal gel, on HIV-1 transmission in female sex workers: A randomised controlled trial. *Lancet* 360(9338):971-977.

Van De Wijgert, J., M. Mbizvo, S. Dube, M. Mwale, P. Nyamapfeni, and N. Padian. 2001. Intravaginal practices in Zimbabwe: Which women engage in them and why? *Culture, Health & Sexuality* 3(2):133-148.

Vandebosch, A., E. Goetghebeur, and L. Van Damme. 2005. Structural accelerated failure time models for the effects of observed exposures on repeated events in a clinical trial. *Statistics in Medicine* 24(7):1029-1046.

Vrijens, B. 2007. Presentation at the second meeting for the Committee on Methodological Challenges in HIV Prevention Trials, London, UK.

Vrijens, B., and J. Urquhart. 2005. Patient adherence to prescribed antimicrobial drug dosing regimens. *Journal of Antimicrobial Chemotherapy* 55(5):616-627.

Vrijens, B., A. Belmans, K. Matthys, E. de Klerk, and E. Lesaffre. 2006. Effect of intervention through a pharmaceutical care program on patient adherence with prescribed once-daily atorvastatin. *Pharmacoepidemiology and Drug Safety* 15(2):115-121.

Wallace, A., M. Thorn, R. A. Maguire, K. M. Sudol, and D. M. Phillips. 2004. Assay for establishing whether microbicide applicators have been exposed to the vagina. *Sexually Transmitted Diseases* 31(8):465-468.

Ware, N. C., M. A. Wyatt, D. R. Bangsberg. 2006. Examining theoretic models of adherence for validity in resource limited settings: A heuristic approach. *Journal of Acquired Immune Deficiency Syndromes* 43(1):S18-S22.

Williams, A. B., K. P. Fennie, C. A. Bova, J. D. Burgess, K. A. Danvers, and K. D. Dieckhaus. 2006. Home visits to improve adherence to highly active antiretroviral therapy: A randomized controlled trial. *Journal of Acquired Immune Deficiency Syndromes* 42(3):314-321.

Zenilman, J. M., J. Yuenger, N. Galai, C. F. Turner, and S. M. Rogers. 2005. Polymerase chain reaction detection of Y chromosome sequences in vaginal fluid: Preliminary studies of a potential biomarker for sexual behavior. *Sexually Transmitted Diseases* 32(2):90-94.

6

Design Considerations: Recruitment and Retention

This chapter explores the influence of recruitment and retention on trial design and conduct. As discussed in Chapter 2, late-stage biomedical HIV prevention trials require investigators to enroll several hundred to several thousand participants at one or multiple sites, and often follow them for several years. A slow accrual rate or poor retention of trial participants may result in underpowered or biased results. To ensure confidence in trial outcomes, it is essential for investigators to meet the study's accrual goals and maximize participant retention. Yet meeting each of these goals can be challenging in resource-poor settings with limited infrastructure and highly mobile and diverse populations (Hill, 2004). For example, a recent trial in Tanzania evaluating herpes simplex virus (HSV-2) suppression to reduce HIV infection reported a retention rate of only 60 percent (Watson-Jones et al., 2007).

Despite the critical threat that inadequate recruitment and retention pose to trial validity, there is little empirical data on the effectiveness of alternative recruitment and retention strategies (Lovato et al., 1997; Mapstone et al., 2007; Robinson et al., 2007; Villacorta et al., 2007). Thus, most of what the committee describes below is drawn from publications focusing on practical "lessons learned" from investigators in the field.

RECRUITMENT STRATEGIES

Recruitment of an adequate number of study subjects is critical to the successful completion of a clinical trial. Ideally, participants should be enrolled at a constant rate to minimize uneven or excessive staff workloads and to maintain study power during the follow-up period (Lovato et al., 1997). A slowly accruing trial can prolong the evaluation of a product and thus delay its public heath impact if it is shown to be efficacious.

Participants in HIV prevention trials enroll for a variety of reasons. Reviews have found that people enroll in HIV/AIDS trial for altruistic reasons more than any other disease area (Lovato et al., 1997; Tharawan et al., 2001). Other common reasons for enrolling include access to HIV education, health care services, contraception (which may not be readably accessible in the community), and for financial incentives (Mills et al., 2006; Tolley and Severy, 2006). In some trials, people say they want to enroll because they believe the product or program will personally protect them against HIV. This underscores the need for additional education about the placebo arm and that the test product has unknown efficacy.

Individuals have also cited a number of reasons why they opt not to enroll in HIV prevention trials (Miller et al., 2004; Mills et al., 2006; Newman and Chakrapani, 2006; Suhadev et al., 2006; Tolley and Severy, 2006). Examples include

- fears about contracting HIV from the intervention,
- potential side effects,
- opposition of family or community members,
- fear of discrimination or stigma or being perceived as HIV-infected,
- lack of convenient clinic hours or transportation to clinic,
- fear or dislike of routine procedures (blood draws, pelvic exams),
- migration for work or family; possibility of receiving a placebo,
- appearing to distrust ones partners, and
- distrust of researchers.

Understanding the benefits and barriers of participation is important in identifying potential recruitment strategies and areas for education.

The committee identified two systematic reviews of recruitment strategies (Lovato et al., 1997; Mapstone et al., 2007). Mapstone and colleagues (2007) conducted a review of all randomized and quasi-randomized controlled trials of methods to increase recruitment in research studies. Of the 15 studies that met the criteria for inclusion, five broad types of recruitment strategies were identified. In pre-warning strategies, participants were sent information about the study prior to being approached about enrollment. Extra information strategies provided additional information about the study and discussed the benefits to participation and risks of the disease with the person. Study design strategies examined the impact of study design changes (e.g., having a placebo arm) on participation. Consent change strategies examined how change in the informed consent process affected recruitment. Finally, financial incentive strategies were used. All of the recruitment strategies targeted research participants; no recruitment strategies were targeted at the researcher or ethics committee levels. They found that trials using financial incentives, an additional questionnaire at the enrollment invitation, and providing information about treatment on the consent form were effective. However, due to the heterogeneity of the studies, the authors were unable to quantify the effect of specific strategies on overall participation. They recommend that funders and researchers include evaluation of recruitment strategies in future research studies.

Lovato and colleagues (1997) conducted a qualitative evaluation of recruitment strategies used in clinical prevention and treatment trials across numerous disease areas and published through 1995. The authors found that the most commonly cited reasons for recruitment problems were inadequate planning and monitoring, overestimating the number of participants from a single source, and lack of flexibility or inability to change plans quickly when recruitment strategies failed (Lovato et al., 1997). The review also found that while some trials managed to adhere to the original budget and timeline for recruitment, often investigators underestimated the costs and time needed for recruitment upfront and required time extensions or excessive effort to meet the accrual targets (Lovato et al., 1997).

Based on their review, Lovato and colleagues (1997) identified several key strategies for successful planning and management: (1) establishing an overall recruitment plan including pilot studies of strategies, (2) intensively monitoring that plan and shifting strategies when necessary, and (3) hiring high-quality staff. These are briefly reviewed below.

- *Establishing an Overall Recruitment Plan:* Studies with successful recruitment strategies have sufficient time to plan, establish community awareness and education, and make personal contacts (Lovato et al., 1997). Pilot studies are a critical aspect of this planning process and can help identify the length of the enrollment period, the number of clinical sites, and financial commitments (Lovato et al., 1997). Pilot studies are important to understand individuals' potential willingness to participate in the trial, identify barriers and benefits to participation, and to test specific recruitment strategies (see Chapter 8 for discussion of pretrial research). Such studies have been widely used in the HIV vaccine field and have helped investigators select trial sites and populations and specific retention strategies (see, for example, Dhalla et al., 2007, for a recent review). In addition, investigators should assess local and community beliefs and perceptions about risk behavior, HIV, and clinical research as these can affect community acceptance of clinical trials as well as recruitment and retention strategies (Tolley and Severy, 2006). Understanding these factors can help identify trial design options and education strategies that can mitigate some of the perceived barriers to participation.

In planning a trial, participating sites should also be encouraged to discuss the eligibility requirements and study design with the community to assess the likely screening-to-enrollment ratio that they might realistically expect. The higher the screening-to-enrollment ratio, the more resources are needed to achieve the desired sample size. Regions with high rates of HIV incidence often have high rates of HIV prevalence, so study staff may need to screen many individuals to identify enough eligible uninfected participants, thus increasing the cost of the trial.

- *Monitoring Accrual:* Continuous monitoring of recruitment strategies and enrollment targets is important for identifying areas for improvement and modifying recruitment strategies when needed. If successful recruitment strategies are identified early in the process, more effort can be shifted to those strategies. Furthermore, timely and accurate recruitment monitoring is essential in informing decisions about whether to extend the enrollment period or to add enrollment targets to other sites in order to meet the sample size goals (Lovato et al., 1997). Data tracking systems (e.g., phone logs, interview outcome logs, schedules) are critical for recruitment staff (Lovato et al., 1997). This can be especially important when there is a high screening–to-enrollment ratio. The actual ratio should also be monitored during the enrollment period of the trial. If the ratio is higher than expected, this might indicate whether the eligibility requirements may be too restrictive or whether there is some aspect of the trial that causes some eligible subjects to choose to not enroll.
- *Staffing:* Studies repeatedly cite having high-quality staff as the key to successful recruitment efforts (Lovato et al., 1997; Hill, 2004; Robinson et al., 2007). Having a recruiting coordinator who is responsible for recruitment and who works closely with the principal investigator, data coordinator, and clinic manager in planning strategies can help build success. Laying out recruitment plans well in advance and identifying ways to quickly replace ineffective strategies is important. Ensuring communication across clinic sites and with other clinical trials in the area is important in identifying successful strategies and identifying problems (Lovato et al., 1997). Characteristics of effective staff that have been identified include being flexible, positive, proactive, and having strong problem-solving skills. Volunteer staff (for example, current participants or participants in other trials) can also be extremely useful in recruiting during clinical trial and in helping to maintain visits during follow-up portion of a trial (Lovato et al., 1997).

RETENTION STRATEGIES

Efforts to maximize retention should begin with enrollment and continue throughout the trial. Higher-than-anticipated loss of participants to follow-up (LFU, see Chapters 2 and 9) may result in an underpowered trial, and distorted statistical inferences about the effects of the intervention. When losses are "noninformative" in the sense that the HIV infection risk of those who drop out of the study is the same as those who remain in follow-up, LFUs will not distort either estimates of cumulative HIV infection rates or comparisons of HIV infection risk between intervention arms, but LFUs will reduce the power of the study to detect an intervention effect (Lagakos et al., 1990). Such a loss of power can be addressed by increasing the planned size of the trial to account for anticipated rates of loss to follow-up (Chapter 2). When losses to follow-up are not "noninformative," estimates of cumulative HIV infection and comparisons between intervention arms can be biased and thus not correctable by increasing the sample size of the trial. There is no threshold LFU rate above which a trial's results become uninterpretable. However, in HIV prevention trials, where only a small percentage (often less than 15 percent) of participants become HIV infected during the trial, striving to keep the cumulative number of LFUs that could be informative below this number is prudent, especially if the LFU rates between the intervention arms might differ.

Examples of factors that might affect retention include loss of interest in the study, conflicts in scheduling visits, transportation issues, site location, poor health, familial obligations, financial difficulties, conflicts with jobs, requirements to forego pregnancy throughout the trial, stringent instructions to adhere to study products, mistrust of trial staff or fear a breach of confidentiality, or stigma associated with an HIV-related study (Coday et al., 2005; Mills et al., 2006; Tolley and Severy, 2006).

Investigators and others have also raised concern about whether trials with an unblinded arm would have differential rates of retention across the arms. This situation arose in the recent MIRA diaphragm trial, where participants in the control arm did not have access to the diaphragm plus gel. Investigators were concerned that more women in the control arm than in the intervention arm would drop out of the study. However, dropout rates were low and similar in the intervention and control arms (6 percent and 5 percent, respectively) (Padian et al., 2007).

Researchers have published a number of reviews highlighting promising retention strategies (Hunt and White, 1998; McKenzie et al., 1999; Coday et al., 2005; Robinson et al., 2007; Tansey et al., 2007). As noted, most of these reviews report on lessons learned or identify a common theme among those studies with high rates of retention, but few strategies have been empirically tested. Many of the reviews identify similar themes. However, none were able to correlate specific retention strategies with successful retention rates in trials. Thus, it is unclear which retention strategies work best for whom and under what conditions.

First, Hunt and White (1998) conducted a review of four U.S.-based longitudinal observational cohort studies that provided sufficient information on their procedures to maximize retention. They identified four successful retention strategies: (1) collaborating with community-based organizations, (2) creating effective organizational structures and management, (3) selecting and training motivated field staff, and (4) offering interventions that encourage participants to remain involved (Leonard et al., 2003). They found that successful retention requires motivational systems designed to engage and reward individuals at all levels of the trial including project managers and field staff, participants, and community organizations (Leonard et al., 2003).

In a second review, McKenzie and colleagues (1999) reviewed methods for tracking and follow-up in 15 studies of marginalized populations. They found that the following procedures are helpful in tracking and following participants: collection of contact information, thorough organization of tracking efforts, staff training and support, use of phone and mail follow-up, use of incentives, establishing rapport with participants, assurance of confidentiality, use of agency tracking and field tracking, and attention to safety concerns. However, none of the studies included in the McKenzie et al. (1999) review were from developing countries.

Recent studies show that investigators can achieve retention rates of 84 percent or more in marginalized or "hard to reach" populations over long follow-up periods in resource poor countries (see, for example, Padian et al., 2007; Villacorta et al., 2007), but that these may require different procedures. Tracking individuals in resource-poor settings can be costly and difficult because populations are highly mobile and infrastructure is poor, and formal address systems and population records do not exist (Hill, 2004; Villacorta et al., 2007). A review of 13 studies in developing countries reveals that although tracking participants can be costly, it can reduce attrition up to 45 percent (Hill, 2004). Tracking can be effective if (1) procedures for collecting information on participants' whereabouts are locally appropriate, well planned, and involve the community; and (2) tracking occurs at regular intervals, and interviewers are well trained, supervised, and motivated (Hill, 2004). Some trials have relied on maps of participants' homes—often drawn by participants, sometimes with the help of other community members (Hill, 2004; Watadzaushe, 2007). Soliciting information on a network of "anchoring" friends or family may also help staff members track participants, although they must be careful to maintain participant confidentiality when contacting these sources (Leonard et al., 2003).

In some settings, tracking information may prove difficult to collect and other strategies may be needed. For example, a study with socially marginalized young adults in Peru retained 84 percent of participants after 2 years, even though only 26 percent of the population supplied complete locator information (telephone, address, and names of two friends) (Villacorta et al., 2007). Project staff utilized novel retention strategies because traditional locator information was often unavailable or unreadable. These strategies included conducting preliminary ethnographic research to identify behavior or target groups, methods for developing strong bonds with project staff and participants outside the study setting, and methods to enhance participants' attitudes about the study. Although low-tech, this strategy was labor intensive and may be difficult to replicate (Villacorta et al., 2007).

In some instances, a study participant may become incarcerated, in which case it may be difficult or impossible to continue to follow and evaluate her or him as specified in the study protocol. This is sometimes a problem when working with study populations of commercial sex workers or injecting drug users.

Coday and colleagues (2005) reviewed strategies for retaining study participants in behavioral intervention trials and identified 61 strategies grouped into eight themes:

- Emphasizing the benefits of participation
- Minimizing respondent burden and giving control to participants
- Providing incentives and tokens of appreciation
- Giving tangible support (e.g., transportation expenses)
- Being patient and persistent
- Being flexible
- Enlisting the support of others and providing social support
- Maintaining a good tracking system

Among these, provision of incentives was highly rated as an effective retention strategy. However, there has been considerable debate about giving people financial rewards to participate in research (Coday et al., 2005). For example, during the committee site visit to South Africa, trial staff noted that the government's policy of giving a flat 150 rands per visit (not adjusted for location) may be overly influential in rural areas where income is quite low, but insufficient in some high-cost urban areas. Trials with vulnerable populations must ensure that participants do not perceive incentives that are unduly influential, and local institutional review boards (IRBs) must deem them appropriate.

The review also discussed retention strategies in the context of an ecological model, which recognizes the influence of multiple factors from an interpersonal, intrapersonal, institutional, community, and policy level. They found that few retention strategies have focused on factors external to the participant that may enhance or detract from study participation and suggest future studies consider retention strategies targeting external factors.

Tansey and colleagues (2007) examined review articles and longitudinal studies that focused on practical and clinically relevant attrition lowering strategies. They identified eight narrative reviews that suggested three categories of promising retention strategies. The first theme is respecting patients' ideas and time. They emphasized that developing a positive rapport with study subjects early in the study process (when most participants drop out) was essential. Similar to other reviews, this study identified the importance of collecting comprehensive tracking information at the first visit and updating it frequently. Persistence in follow-up, particularly early on was important. In addition, they identified study personnel as a critical component of effective retention. Key strategies included extensive training of staff, adequate staff support, selection of enthusiastic staff, and frequent meetings to reduce isolation often felt by field workers.

Finally, Robinson and colleagues (2007) recently conducted a systematic review of the literature that included all studies through 2005 that described retention strategies for in-person follow-up and included retention rates. Of 21 studies that met these criteria, the authors identified 368 retention strategies which they grouped into 12 themes (see Table 6-1 for details). Similar to other reviewers, the authors were unable to conduct quantitative analyses or associate the types of strategies most effective in various target populations given the heterogeneity of studies included in their review. The authors conclude that more research is needed to explicitly evaluate the effectiveness of alternative retention and recruitment strategies. In addition, they encourage researchers to report their experiences with retention in actual trials and recommend adopting standard reporting methods for retention.

Overall, investigators and sponsors should anticipate that maintaining timely accrual and high retention rates will be labor intensive and costly throughout a trial. However, these are necessary to maintain internal and external validity. Successful recruitment and retention will require the use of multiple strategies and incentives, the ability to rapidly change procedures when they are not working, and persistence and innovation among staff.

TABLE 6-1 Retention Strategy Themes from Robinson, 2007

Theme	Description	Examples
Community involvement	Involve community in study design, recruitment, and retention.	Present pilot project idea to church leadership and congregation. Create community advisor panel and consult with panel for recommendations regarding protocol and participation.
Study identity	Create study identity for participants.	Create a project identity by using similar colors and fonts on all study materials. Give participants a t-shirt printed with study logo.
Study personnel	Characteristics, training, and management of study personnel.	Assign one primary clinician to each participant. Encourage study personnel to show empathy toward subject's personal situation in scheduling appointments/cancellations.
Study description	Explain study requirements and details, including potential benefits and risks, to participants.	Inform subjects that they will be followed over time and specify the timetable and the methods that will be used to locate them. Offer a copy of a newspaper article or study brochure to each participant.
Contact and scheduling methods	Use systematic method for patient contact, appointment scheduling, and cohort retention monitoring.	Mail a newsletter to participants that includes a message from PI, photos of project staff, and preliminary findings. Obtain multiple contacts for each participant, including two contacts not residing with the participant.
Reminders	Provide reminders about appointments and study participation.	Mail reminder postcards to participants one week before appointment. Visit in-patients before discharge to remind them of out-patient follow-up plan.

TABLE 6-1 Continued

Theme	Description	Examples
Visit characteristics	Minimize participant burden through characteristics and procedures of follow-up study clinic.	Offer flexible clinic appointments (early morning, evenings, and weekends). Provide background music for restful atmosphere in clinic.
Benefits of study	Provide benefits to participants and families that are directly related to the nature of study.	Provide free annual physical examination. Form educational and support groups for families and patients.
Financial incentives	Provide financial incentives or payment.	Provide payment to families in control group (20USD/visit/four visits). Provide pharmacy gift certificate to participant at first follow-up visit ($25).
Reimbursement	Provide reimbursement for research-related expenses or tangible support to facilitate participation.	Provide taxi fare or have staff member pick up study participants. Provide child care during visit.
Nonfinancial incentives	Provide nonfinancial incentives or tokens of appreciation.	Provide an inexpensive token of appreciation (e.g., coffee mug, pen, refrigerator magnet) to participant at each visit. Host holiday parties for study participants.
Special tracking methods	Methods of tracking or dealing with hard-to-find or difficult participants.	Conduct clinic and street outreach for lost to follow-up participants. Identify and address obstacles hindering participation for problem patients.

SOURCE: This table was published in the *Journal of Clinical Epidemiology*, Vol 60 (8), Robinson, K. A., C. R. Dennison, D. M. Wayman, P. J. Pronovost, and D. M. Needham, Systematic review identifies number of strategies important for retaining study participants, 757-765, Copyright Elsevier (2007).

Recommendation 6-1: Investigators should conduct pretrial research to assess the community and individuals' interest in the trial, to pilot test recruitment and retention strategies, and to set a realistic timeline and resource needs for the enrollment period and for retention.

Recommendation 6-2: Because of the loss in study power that can result from inadequate accrual and because the potential biases resulting from losses to follow-up cannot be avoided simply by increasing sample size, investigators should place a high priority on developing effective strategies to achieve accrual rate goals and to minimize losses to follow-up. Specifically, investigators should do the following:

- **Develop a detailed and multifaceted plan for retaining enrolled participants before beginning a study for systematically and frequently monitoring the results, and for modifying the plan if strategies are not working.**
- **Collect as much detailed tracking information as possible on participants.**
- **Develop systems to engage, train, and reward staff for building trust and accountability with participants and within the community, and for meeting recruitment and retention targets.**

Recommendation 6-3: Funders and investigators should include evaluations of the effectiveness of recruitment and retention strategies in future research plans.

REFERENCES

Coday, M., C. Boutin-Foster, T. Goldman Sher, J. Tennant, M. L. Greaney, S. D. Saunders, and G. W. Somes. 2005. Strategies for retaining study participants in behavioral intervention trials: Retention experiences of the NIH Behavior Change Consortium. *Annals of Behavioral Medicine* 29(Suppl):55-65.

Dhalla, S., R. Woods, S. A. Strathdee, D. M. Patrick, and R. S. Hogg. 2007. HIV vaccine preparedness studies in the organization for economic co-operation and development (OECD) countries. *AIDS Care* 19(9):1118-1127.

Hill, Z. 2004. Reducing attrition in panel studies in developing countries. *International Journal of Epidemiology* 33(3):493-498.

Hunt, J. R., and E. White. 1998. Retaining and tracking cohort study members. *Epidemiologic Review* 20(1):57-70.

Lagakos, S. W., L. L. Lim, and J. M. Robins. 1990. Adjusting for early treatment termination in comparative clinical trials. *Statistics in Medicine* 9(12):1417-1424.

Leonard, N. R., P. Lester, M. J. Rotheram-Borus, K. Mattes, M. Gwadz, and B. Ferns. 2003. Successful recruitment and retention of participants in longitudinal behavioral research. *AIDS Education and Prevention* 15(3):269-281.

Lovato, L. C., K. Hill, S. Hertert, D. B. Hunninghake, and J. L. Probstfield. 1997. Recruitment for controlled clinical trials: Literature summary and annotated bibliography. *Controlled Clinical Trials* 18(4):328-352.

Mapstone, J., D. Elbourne, and I. Roberts. 2007. Strategies to improve recruitment to research studies (review). *Cochrane Database of Systematic Reviews* Issue 2, Art. No.: MR000013. DOI: 10.1002/14651858.MR000013.pub3.

McKenzie, M., J. P. Tulsky, H. L. Long, M. Chesney, and A. Moss. 1999. Tracking and follow-up of marginalized populations: A review. *Journal of Health Care for the Poor and Underserved* 10(4):409-429.

Miller, L. C., S. T. Murphy, L. F. Clark, M. Hamburger, and J. Moore. 2004. Hierarchical messages for introducing multiple HIV prevention options: Promise and pitfalls. *AIDS Education and Prevention* 16(6):509-525.

Mills, E., S. Nixon, S. Singh, S. Dolma, A. Nayyar, and S. Kapoor. 2006. Enrolling women into HIV preventive vaccine trials: An ethical imperative but a logistical challenge. *PLoS Medicine* 3(3):e94.

Newman, P. A., and V. Chakrapani. 2006. *Methodological and ethical challenges in research with men who have sex with men in Chennai, India.* Fairfax, VA: Society for Social Work and Research.

Padian, N., A. van der Straten, G. Ramjee, T. Chipato, G. de Bruyn, K. Blanchard, S. Shiboski, E. Montgomery, H. Fancher, H. Cheng, M. Rosenblum, M. van der Loan, N. Jewell, J. McIntyre, and The MIRA Team. 2007. Diaphragm and lubricant gel for prevention of HIV acquisition in southern African women: A randomized controlled trial. *Lancet* 370:251-261.

Robinson, K. A., C. R. Dennison, D. M. Wayman, P. J. Pronovost, and D. M. Needham. 2007. Systematic review identifies number of strategies important for retaining study participants. *Journal of Clinical Epidemiology* 60(8):757-765.

Suhadev, M., A. M. Nyamathi, S. Swaminathan, P. Venkatesan, M. Raja Sakthivel, R. Shenbagavalli, A. Suresh, and J. L. Fahey. 2006. A pilot study on willingness to participate in future preventive HIV vaccine trials. *Indian Journal of Medical Research* 124(6):631-640.

Tansey, C. M., A. L. Matté, D. Needham, and M. S. Herridge. 2007. Review of retention strategies in longitudinal studies and application to follow-up of ICU survivors. *Intensive Care Medicine* 33:2051-2057.

Tharawan, K., C. Manopaiboon, C. Ellertson, K. Limpakarnjanarat, S. Chaikummao, P. H. Kilmarx, K. Blanchard, C. Coggins, T. D. Mastro, and C. Elias. 2001. Women's willingness to participate in microbicide trials in northern Thailand. *Journal of Acquired Immune Deficiency Syndromes* 28(2):180-186.

Tolley, E. E., and L. J. Severy. 2006. Integrating behavioral and social science research into microbicide clinical trials: Challenges and opportunities. *American Journal of Public Health* 96(1):79-83.

Villacorta, V., S. Kegeles, J. Galea, K. A. Konda, J. P. Cuba, C. F. Palacios, and T. J. Coates. 2007. Innovative approaches to cohort retention in a community-based HIV/STI prevention trial for socially marginalized Peruvian young adults. *Clinical Trials* 4(1):32-41.

Watadzaushe, C. 2007. *High cohort retention in a phase III trial of the diaphragm and lubricant gel in southern Africa.* Paper presented at International AIDS Society conference 2007, Sydney, Australia.

Watson-Jones, D., M. Rusizoka, H. Weiss, K. Mugeye, K. Baisley, J. Changalucha, D. Everett, C. Tanton, T. Clayton, D. Ross, and R. Hayes. 2007. *Impact of HSV-2 suppressive therapy on HIV incidence in HSV-2 seropositive women: A randomised controlled trial in Tanzania.* Paper read at Fourth International AIDS Society Conference on HIV Pathogenesis, Treatment and Prevention, Sydney, Australia.

7

Site Preparedness

Once the decision has been made to undertake a late-stage trial to evaluate a biomedical HIV intervention, the next step is to begin developing the study design and protocol. Key components of this effort include selecting appropriate populations and sites for the study, preparing these sites to participate in the study, and involving the community in developing the protocol and facilitating recruitment and interaction with study participants.

In considering potential study sites, investigators must address a number of issues, including (1) whether the community could eventually benefit from the planned intervention if it proves to be effective; (2) whether the goals of the trial are consistent with the long-range needs and priorities of the community and the local and national government; (3) whether there is sufficient community support for hosting a study; and (4) whether the site, with adequate preparation, can identify an appropriate number of participants matching the study's target population, and is likely to meet other criteria, such as a high enrollment-to-screening ratio and a high rate of product adherence and retention.

Once a specific site is selected, it must be readied for participation in the trial. This work includes developing the needed human capacity, physical infrastructure, and regulatory processes, and performing pretrial research—sometimes simultaneously. The costs and resources needed to complete these steps can be substantial. However, sponsors, investigators, and the community must make the necessary investment to prepare sites for a successful trial.

Because the resources required to do so are often enormous, donors, investigators, and communities should discuss long-term plans for the site once a trial is completed. Specifically, they need to consider to what extent the physical infrastructure and human capacity developed at a site can contribute to other research or activities that can bolster the health of the community, and who will help ensure that such long-term plans are realized. This chapter addresses the issues that arise in preparing a site for a late-stage biomedical HIV prevention trial. The published literature on site preparedness focuses largely on HIV vaccine studies and participants' willingness to participate in them (see, for example, Dhalla et al., 2007). Fewer studies address site preparedness methods for nonvaccine biomedical HIV prevention studies.

The committee therefore draws on its collective experiences, information gathered during visits to clinical trial sites in Africa (see Box 7-1), and those of other researchers to outline problems encountered in preparing a site for an HIV prevention trial, solutions devised to address them, and lessons learned to assist sponsors and investigators of new trials (see for example, Francis et al., 2003; Maziak et al., 2004; Cutts et al., 2006; Rerks-Ngarm et al., 2006; Skoler et al., 2006; NIMH Collaborative HIV/STD Prevention Trial Group, 2007a,b,c; Ramjee et al., 2007a,b; UNAIDS and AVAC, 2007; Van den Broeck et al., 2007). (See Chapter 8 for a critical aspect of site preparedness: estimating HIV incidence in a site's catchment area.)

The committee's charge specifically excluded other challenges in site preparedness. These include best practices for engaging community members in preparing for a trial, treatment for participants who become HIV-infected during a trial, compensation for participants who experience trial-related adverse events, and informed-consent procedures. Although this report does not address these complicated and sensitive issues, additional work is needed to reach consensus on how to address them when planning a late-stage HIV prevention trial.

DEVELOPING CAPACITY AND INFRASTRUCTURE

The HIV prevention research agenda requires access to large study populations in settings with the capacity to conduct a wide range of clinical trials. Late-stage HIV prevention trials typically occur in areas with a high incidence of HIV, yet these areas often have the fewest resources and the most limited medical and research infrastructure (Ramjee et al., 2007a). The lack of infrastructure, expertise, and capacity to conduct clinical trials in resource-poor settings has been a significant constraint across many arenas, including testing vaccines for malaria and other diseases, preventing and treating cardiovascular disease, and improving maternal-child health, (Developing country trialists, 2006; Rojas et al., 2007; Stough, 2007).

BOX 7-1
Themes from Committee Site Visits

Committee and staff members conducted informational visits to nine HIV prevention trials in Uganda and South Africa, including those studying microbicides, male circumcision, and HSV-2 suppression. Besides talking with study staff and trial participants at those sites, the committee also consulted other stakeholders, such as community representatives and staff from health ministries.

Study staff noted that they had significantly underestimated the length and cost of the process needed to develop a study protocol and gain approval from an IRB. Investigators also reported that they had underestimated the time required for site preparation and staff training.

Several other recurring themes and observations arose during these discussions (all sites did not raise all issues):

- The involvement of local investigators and staff in developing the research protocol varied by site, and tended to be greater in pre-phase 3 studies, such as feasibility studies. Staff members requested more equal partnerships at all stages of protocol development and trial conduct.
- Staff at several sites discussed the importance of engaging trial participants in social and informational events, such as "town meetings" and peer support groups. Such events provide a forum for airing common concerns, disseminating information, and providing feedback to study staff on trial conduct, and to participants on trial progress. Such events also help empower participants and foster ownership of trial conduct and outcomes.
- Participants' reasons for joining trials include reimbursement, access to better medical care, access to microbicide gel as lubrication and thus better sex, and

Human Capacity

To be successful, late-stage HIV prevention trials require a well-trained and coordinated study team that includes laboratory managers and technicians, pharmacists, data and information technology staff, regulatory personnel, research nurses, HIV counselors, home visitors, social scientists, physicians, and others.

The lack of personnel in developing countries who are trained or experienced in conducting clinical trials is repeatedly cited as a major limitation (Initiative on Public-Private Partnerships for Health, 2002; Vardas et al., 2005; Excler, 2006). Research units often must invest significant resources in developing specially trained personnel to conduct HIV prevention trials (Nchinda, 2002; Lehner et al., 2005).

Senior investigators with the expertise to complete a trial successfully are particularly critical. However, few experienced senior-level investigators

the desire to help prevent HIV. Staff and community representatives expressed concern that participants may overlook potential risks given these benefits.

- Trials must devote significant resources and effort to retain participants. Key factors include developing a trusting relationship with participants and supporting their other nontrial concerns. Providing services such as medical care, counseling, and social support also improves retention.
- Study staff recommend relying on peer leaders to provide support to trial participants, as well as to collect information on their sexual behavior and adherence, as participants may be more likely to give truthful responses to peers than to health professionals.
- Providing family-planning services onsite reduces pregnancy rates. Shorter follow-up of participants would enable trials to decrease pregnancy rates, as it is difficult for young women to delay getting pregnant for several years. Staff members expressed concern that providing hormonal contraception might encourage participants to stop using condoms. Many couples use condoms primarily as a mechanism for family planning, and not to protect themselves from HIV infection. Community members and staff at some sites also expressed concern about excluding women who become pregnant.
- Given the large number of clinical trials under way in close proximity, study staff expressed concern that participants will enroll in multiple studies. Some potential participants lack enough information to distinguish different HIV prevention trials. Media play an important role in disseminating both correct and incorrect information. Trials need to appoint a community liaison to educate people about the trial and correct misinformation. Community members, media, and government officials alike need more research literacy. Health ministries need research and assistance in translating effective trial results into larger-scale programs.

may be available in an area, and they may be overburdened with other responsibilities. Successful trials therefore require the full-time commitment of junior investigators, who may have more time to dedicate to a trial even if they lack some experience (Initiative on Public-Private Partnerships for Health, 2002). A training and mentoring system that enables junior investigators to learn from more senior investigators—onsite and internationally—will help expand the local capacity for independent investigation (Nchinda, 2002; Maziak et al., 2004).

Several successful programs have targeted medical and postgraduate students for training to build research capacity. These programs mentor such students by involving them in small studies, allowing them to learn basic research skills and potentially motivating them to perform research during their careers (Maziak et al., 2004; Wallis et al., 2007). Developing and supporting a culture of research at local universities and medical and nursing schools can provide the basis for further training.

Given the limited number of physicians available in many settings, greater use of research nurses to perform a wide variety of activities, including coordinating a study, may be an efficient and cost-effective approach. However, nursing programs in the developing world may not routinely train students to conduct research or address research ethics. Only a few trials and training programs now train nurses to coordinate research (Edwards and Roelofs, 2007).

Developing countries often lack personnel with training and experience in data management and analysis and information technology (Acosta et al., 2007; Van den Broeck et al., 2007). This is particularly true for well-trained, experienced biostatisticians, who are critical to designing clinical trials, writing study protocols, and analyzing results. Given the growing complexity of electronic media and database management, training site personnel in setting up and maintaining computer hardware and software, database management, including designing instruments for collecting data, and quality control systems is also essential.

Even if large, multicenter trials rely on offsite data management centers, investigators must develop the capacity of local personnel to track participant visits, identify missing participants for immediate tracing, track specimens, monitor lab test results, manage pharmacy systems, and manage an administrative database and financial accountability. These efforts must be compliant with Good Clinical Practices, include the requisite documentation, and require oversight by well-trained personnel.

Establishing and maintaining a trial site also requires additional administrative and coordination expertise (Chandiwana and Ornbjerg, 2003; Maziak et al., 2004; Lehner et al., 2005). This expertise includes personnel trained in project administration, finance and grant management, human resources, and facilities management. The National Institute of Child Health and Development's International Extramural Associates Program provides training and support in some of these areas.

A comprehensive approach to training is required to build the long-term, sustainable, and independent research capacity to rapidly mount large-scale HIV prevention trials in developing countries. One example of such a training program is the National Institutes of Health's Fogarty International Center, which builds the capacity of low- and middle-income countries to conduct research in a variety of health arenas (Kupfer et al., 2004). Links between Fogarty AIDS International Training and Research Programs and in-country HIV research units have allowed trainees to immediately use their skills to benefit research units at home (Orem et al., 2005). This one program, however, only meets a fraction of the need for training.

Creating long-term research capacity in developing countries will require investing in master's and doctoral training programs (Nchinda, 2002; Maziak et al., 2004). Regional programs—such as "summer institutes" in epidemiology, training provided during clinical trials, and south-to-south training, wherein research units or institutions in developing countries train and mentor less experienced units—can also be effective in enhancing human capacity (Nchinda, 2002; Maziak et al., 2004).

Public-private partnerships and research networks have also provided some local, regional, and international training in areas such as Good Laboratory Practices, Good Clinical Practices, ethics, managing investigational products, and laboratory procedures (Nchinda, 2002). Such efforts include the International AIDS Vaccine Initiative, European and Developing Countries Clinical Trials Partnership, and the clinical trial networks created by the Division of AIDS of the National Institute of Allergy and Infectious Diseases.

Physical Infrastructure

Physical infrastructure includes adequate facilities for recruiting, screening, and following study participants; providing pharmacy services for the trial interventions and concomitant care; ensuring reliable laboratory services; and managing data. New research sites usually require significant up-front investment in all of these areas.

Sites also need the transportation capacity to travel to the homes of participants who miss visits to the study clinic (Nchinda, 2002; Cutts et al., 2006; Van den Broeck et al., 2007). Sites that enroll a large number of participants from a large catchment area may need to establish satellite clinics, in addition to the main clinic, to facilitate study visits for study participants from far away.

Clinics should have enough private, comfortable space to allow participants to speak freely during HIV testing and counseling sessions, as well as during sensitive discussions of risk behavior. Inadequate attention to the space available will lead to overcrowded clinics with long waiting times, which may discourage participants from returning for scheduled visits.

Research budgets often overlook or do not support the significant costs of providing basic services to a trial site, such as installing and maintaining a stable supply of electricity and water, phone services, plumbing facilities that can adhere to sanitation standards, a system for safely disposing of biohazard wastes, and security. For example, U.S. federal funding for studies abroad does not cover the costs of running a facility, although it does fund a site's efforts to comply with public policies, such as those that ensure ethical treatment of human subjects. If local institutions cannot reliably provide these services, sponsors and investigators must include the substantial costs of providing them in their research budgets.

Another critical component of physical infrastructure is a research pharmacy that can handle blinded study products according to Good Clinical Practices (GCP), with enough space to store and maintain the products in a temperature-controlled setting. In areas of unstable power, this includes access to continuous power backup and stabilization, and a system of alarms that will alert study staff to a temperature problem 24 hours a day (Cutts et al., 2006).

Most HIV prevention trials require laboratory tests to evaluate primary endpoints such as HIV status, and to monitor the toxicity of the study product. Yet adequate labs that use Good Laboratory Practices, and have the ability to provide testing that meets those standards, are commonly limited or unavailable at potential sites (Lehner et al., 2005). Deficiencies in laboratory performance can lead to unreliable results, an inability to analyze or use data, or even suspension of the trial or site (Shetty et al., 2003; Peterson et al., 2007). Investigators therefore need to consider the proximity of a capable laboratory to the research clinic, and its ability to rapidly process tests of participants' HIV status and overall health.

Trials also need capacity to store laboratory reagents and large numbers of study specimens (Lehner et al., 2005), a computerized system for identifying and tracking specimens (Van den Broeck et al., 2007), and a reliable system for specimen shipping according to International Air Transport Association guidelines, as well as appropriate material transfer agreements.

Bringing local laboratories up to the standards required for clinical trials often requires significant initial and continued technical assistance and oversight. The ideal approach is to develop high-quality laboratories that are self-sustaining through income from tests, and that are capable of supporting a wide range of research and care, both locally and regionally (Chandiwana and Ornbjerg, 2003).

Modern information technology and data management capabilities, including computer resources and Internet links, are also essential for late-stage HIV prevention trials, to ensure effective communication and the ability to rapidly and accurately enter, analyze, and transmit data and report adverse events (Nchinda, 2002; Lehner et al., 2005; Van den Broeck et al., 2007). In many developing countries, Internet services may be limited, unreliable, or, if present, costly to establish and maintain. Research budgets need to reflect the resources required to set up and sustain these services.

Efforts to fulfill these demanding requirements are usually costly and time and labor intensive, regardless of whether investigators rely on infrastructure at a separate research facility or upgrade local public health facilities to take on these activities (van de Wijgert and Jones, 2006). For a study to succeed, any infrastructure investments must occur up front, as part of site preparation.

Regulatory Infrastructure

Trials also need infrastructure beyond the specific study site. For example, investigators must assess the capacity and regulations of local organizations such as institutional review boards (IRBs), ethics committees (ECs), national drug authorities, ministries of health, universities, and other scientific and research advisory bodies. Studies funded by the U.S. government must ensure that a local IRB registers with the Office of Human Research Protections of the U.S. Department of Health and Human Services, and that the IRB adheres to international standards of study review.

IRBs and ECs must have formal systems for conducting an initial comprehensive review of the research protocol, annual reviews, and real-time reviews of serious adverse events, and for documenting those reviews. The local IRB/EC must also have the proper membership, training in research ethics, regulations, and methodology, and adequate support to conduct these activities in a timely fashion.

Trials may further require an institutional biosafety committee (IBC), depending on the product being investigated and the funding agency. Few developing countries have an existing IBC with the capacity to oversee human trials. Both IRBs/ECs and IBCs must include members who are familiar with the local setting and represent the communities from which the trials are recruiting. The lack of a knowledgeable and suitable IRB/EC can significantly delay or even prevent HIV prevention research, as has occurred at several research sites in developing countries (Vardas et al., 2005; Kass et al., 2007).

If a potential site lacks this regulatory infrastructure, investigators may consider several options. An approach that usually provides the greatest long-term benefit to the community and country is to provide training and resources to enable an existing IRB to meet international review standards. If that is not possible, investigators should explore alternatives, such as creating or using a central IRB with representatives from countries involved in the trial, or inviting members of the local lay and scientific communities to join an existing IRB or IBC of the sponsoring institution or country.

Other agencies may also regulate the conduct of clinical trials, including the U.S. Food and Drug Administration (FDA) or European and in-country drug authorities (e.g., the Medicines Control Council in South Africa). Assessment of the site infrastructure must therefore include an evaluation of a site's ability to meet all the requirements of these agencies. This often presents a challenge and can cause significant delays for multicenter trials with multiple layers of review in each participating country (NIMH Collaborative HIV/STD Prevention Trial Group, 2007a).

Recommendation 7-1: Donors and investigators should invest in the human capacity and physical infrastructure needed to ensure successful HIV prevention trials in resource-poor settings. These efforts should include a comprehensive and realistic assessment of how to prepare a site, a training plan for staff, and a mentoring plan for inexperienced investigators.

Recommendation 7-2: If the regulatory infrastructure of a planned study site is insufficient, study sponsors, funding agencies, research organizations, and other stakeholders should assist local IRBs in developing the ability to provide comprehensive and timely oversight of clinical trials according to international standards.

PROTOCOL DEVELOPMENT

Developing a trial's protocol requires an extensive process to address scientific, regulatory, and logistical issues. These include creating informed-consent documents, procedures for screening and enrolling subjects, counseling strategies, case report forms, study evaluations, and visit schedules.

Because the sociocultural context influences participants' behavior and willingness to participate in trials, it is vital that investigators and sponsors work collaboratively with local researchers and other members of the community in developing the protocol (McCoy et al., 2005; Rerks-Ngarm et al., 2006). Investigators should engage community members as early as possible in the protocol planning process. As the 2007 UNAIDS and AVAC report *Good Participatory Practice Guidelines for Biomedical HIV Prevention Trials* notes, "Best practices build in mechanisms for input from both local investigators and communities prior to trial protocol finalization and for participation of local investigators and community representatives on the protocol team" (UNAIDS and AVAC, 2007, p. 23).

Protocol development is even more complex when prevention trials include multiple sites within one country, or sites in multiple countries (Excler, 2006). Because sociocultural beliefs, attitudes, and practices vary within and among regions and countries, investigators of multisite trials have the added challenge of recognizing and adapting to these differences across sites while maintaining the integrity of the study design. All these factors require obtaining substantial input from local investigators and community leaders in the regions where a trial will be conducted (McCoy et al., 2005; NIMH Collaborative HIV/STD Prevention Trial Group, 2007a,b).

Another challenge for multicenter, multicountry trials is that local IRBs and ECs may require or request information on how investigators will conduct the trial at their site. This information may include details about the study team, the specific population to be studied, how and where populations will be recruited, what local laboratories the study will use, and what incentives participants will receive. For one protocol, sites may enroll different populations at different sites (e.g., discordant couples at one site and sexually active women at another), requiring different approaches to recruiting and protecting study participants. Local IRBs need this site-specific information to properly evaluate the protocol in their setting. However, protocols for multicenter HIV prevention trials often do not contain this level of detail on each study site.

Some studies have addressed this gap by creating template protocols with common features but allowing each site to insert unique information into particular sections, thus allowing site-specific protocols. In other cases, a single common protocol contains site-specific addenda that provide more detailed information. When only one protocol for a study is allowed, such as for U.S. government-funded projects conducted under a U.S. FDA Investigational New Drug (IND) application, another option is to submit a separate site-specific implementation plan in addition to a common protocol for local IRB review. This can allow for more rapid and thorough local review of multicenter protocols.

Particularly for multicenter trials involving multiple IRBs, investigators may revise a study protocol numerous times before obtaining final approval (Musil et al., 2004). This process requires accurate and culturally appropriate translation of informed-consent forms and other participant materials, with the assistance of a trial-specific community advisory board or with outreach to other community groups. In some countries, IRB and other regulatory reviews may take 6 to 9 months (Maggon, 2004).

Recommendation 7-3: Sponsors and investigators from outside the trial region should solicit meaningful input from local investigators and community representatives as they develop the study protocol, and throughout the trial. The trial should itself promote equal partnerships between outside and local investigators.

PRETRIAL RESEARCH

Qualitative pretrial research is critical in developing culturally relevant adaptations of interventions, informed consent, and study procedures; facilitating site selection; and in working closely with a community (Corneli et al., 2007; NIMH Collaborative HIV/STD Prevention Trial Group, 2007b; Vallely et al., 2007). Qualitative research can provide key insights into participants' behavior and the sociocultural context and other factors that shape it.

Investigators have used numerous strategies to collect qualitative data before, during, and after clinical trials, including one-on-one interviews with research participants, interviews with key informants outside the study, case studies, focus groups, exercises to map the location of potential participants, direct observation, and rapid ethnographic assessment methods (Corneli et al., 2007; NIMH Collaborative HIV/STD Prevention Trial Group, 2007b). Without such research, investigators would have overlooked important aspects of many trials and jeopardized their implementation (Corneli et al., 2007).

Pretrial research can also be critical to more accurately determining key attributes of study participants, and thus the power and interpretability of the trial results. For example, pretrial studies can estimate HIV incidence in the study population (see Chapter 8), likely product adherence, pregnancy rates, and accrual and retention rates (see Chapter 2). Failure to accurately estimate these factors can lead to failed trials, or trials that yield equivocal results. Researchers have found pretrial research to gain more precise estimates of these factors critical in overcoming some of the challenges of conducting microbicide and other clinical trials in developing countries (Ramjee et al., 2000).

Preparedness studies can also be useful in refining a number of processes important to a successful study. Such studies can be used to identify gaps in staffing or training, to develop procedures for running the research clinic smoothly, to improve the informed-consent process and materials, and to evaluate product acceptability. Investigators could use a similar approach to test their system for monitoring and reporting adverse events, and to gauge the capacity of the IRB to perform timely reviews.

Recommendation 7-4: Donors should fund and investigators should undertake extensive pre-trial research to develop accurate estimates of HIV incidence, participant accrual, retention, and pregnancy rates, and to develop and evaluate logistical and regulatory processes to be used during the trial.

ENSURING SUSTAINABILITY

In light of the extensive efforts required to prepare a site for an HIV prevention trial, and the need for further HIV prevention trials in any given study area, funders and investigators need to consider sustaining site capacity beyond the needs of a given prevention trial. In most cases it is cost inefficient and not in the community's best interest if investigators go to great lengths to prepare a site for a trial, only to shut down the site after completion of the trial.

Creating a sustainable research infrastructure that can be used for other studies can provide long-term benefits to the community even if the current trial fails to show a protective benefit (Nchinda, 2002; Lehner et al., 2005;

McCoy et al., 2005). Long-term research units may provide HIV testing and counseling services as they determine whether people are eligible to participate in a trial, expand the number of local health care personnel, and establish laboratory and radiological services accessible to the whole community.

Unfortunately, some trial sites have been shut down after a single trial. The result is a substantial loss of knowledge and experience. More important, this can be very discouraging to investigators and staff who have invested considerable time and effort in conducting a trial, as well as to the participants and the community. This type of disappointment may jeopardize community support for other HIV prevention trials and types of research. Advance planning, and the flexibility to address other questions in the context of an HIV prevention trial, may decrease the need to shut down a new research unit in the face of negative results.

Recommendation 7-5: When considering a new trial site that requires extensive preparation, investigators, sponsors, and community leaders should discuss and carefully consider how the site could be sustained after completion of the trial.

If investigators or donors do not expect the human capacity and site infrastructure to continue beyond the planned trial, the committee questions the value to the community of the investment in preparing a new site.

Sponsors have established many HIV-related research networks and local cohorts of potential trial participants over the last decade, with the goal of expanding the capacity to conduct HIV prevention and treatment trials in both the developed and developing world (Brown and Nitayaphan, 2004). The expected benefits of such "pluripotent" research sites include consolidation of resources and shared efficiencies across trials (Nchinda, 2002; Lehner et al., 2005).

The creation of research centers of excellence—with the infrastructure and capacity to conduct studies across disciplines and diseases—is an ideal mechanism to leverage financial support from a variety of sources, take full advantage of an investment in site development, provide job security for investigators and staff (who can then commit to careers as "clinical trialists"), and maintain community support (Nchinda, 2002; Chandiwana and Ornbjerg, 2003; Lehner et al., 2005).

Recommendation 7-6: Given limited funding and the extensive investment required to prepare research sites, donors and investigators should explore creative and flexible collaborations with HIV and non-HIV trial networks, health organizations, and local research units that have

access to suitable study populations or existing research infrastructure, with cost sharing benefiting both partners.

REFERENCES

Acosta, C. J., C. M. Galindo, R. L. Ochiai, M. C. Danovaro-Holliday, A. Laure-Page, V. D. Thiem, Y. Jin, M. I. Khan, S. M. Sahito, H. B. Hamza, J. K. Park, H. Lee, H. Bock, R. A. Elyazeed, M. J. Albert, C. Ascaso, T. Q. Robles, M. Ali, P. Ngai, M. K. Puri, Y. M. Koo, M. D. Agtini, R. Soeharno, D. Bai-qing, D. Kohl, Z. Y. Xu, B. Ivanoff, L. Jodar, T. Pang, Z. Bhutta, and J. D. Clemens. 2007. Implementation of good clinical practice guidelines in vaccine trials in developing countries. *Vaccine* 25(15):2852-2857.

Brown, A. E., and S. Nitayaphan. 2004. Foundations for a Phase III human immunodeficiency virus vaccine trial: A decade of Thai-U.S. Army collaborative research. *Military Medicine* 169(8):588-593.

Chandiwana, S., and N. Ornbjerg. 2003. Review of north-south and south-south cooperation and conditions necessary to sustain research capability in developing countries. *Journal of Health, Population and Nutrition* 21(3):288-297.

Corneli, A. L., E. G. Piwoz, M. E. Bentley, A. Moses, J. R. Nkhoma, B. C. Tohill, L. Adair, B. Mtimuni, Y. Ahmed, A. Duerr, P. Kazembe, and C. van der Horst. 2007. Involving communities in the design of clinical trial protocols: The ban study in Lilongwe, Malawi. *Contemporary Clinical Trials* 28(1):59-67.

Cutts, F. T., G. Enwere, S. M. Zaman, and F. G. Yallop. 2006. Operational challenges in large clinical trials: Examples and lessons learned from the Gambia pneumococcal vaccine trial. *PLoS Clinical Trials* 1(3):e16.

Developing country trialists are key for malaria vaccine goals. 2006. *Lancet* 368(9554): 2185.

Dhalla, S., R. Woods, S. A. Strathdee, D. M. Patrick, and R. S. Hogg. 2007. HIV vaccine preparedness studies in the organization for economic co-operation and development (OECD) countries. *AIDS Care* 19(9):1118-1127.

Edwards, N. C., and S. Roelofs. 2007. Strengthening nurses' capacity in HIV policy development in sub-Saharan Africa and the Caribbean: An international program of research and capacity building. *Canadian Journal of Nursing Research* 39(3):187-189.

Excler, J. L. 2006. AIDS vaccine efficacy trials: Expand capacity and prioritize. *Expert Review of Vaccines* 5(2):167-170.

Francis, D. P., W. L. Heyward, V. Popovic, P. Orozco-Cronin, K. Orelind, C. Gee, A. Hirsch, T. Ippolito, A. Luck, M. Longhi, V. Gulati, N. Winslow, M. Gurwith, F. Sinangil, and P. W. Berman. 2003. Candidate HIV/AIDS vaccines: Lessons learned from the world's first Phase III efficacy trials. *AIDS* 17(2):147-156.

Initiative on Public-Private Partnerships for Health. November 2002. *Workshop on clinical trials capacity in low-and middle-income countries: Experiences, lessons learned and priorities for strengthening*, Arusha, Tanzania.

Kass, N. E., A. A. Hyder, A. Ajuwon, J. Appiah-Poku, N. Barsdorf, D. E. Elsayed, M. Mokhachane, B. Mupenda, P. Ndebele, G. Ndossi, B. Sikateyo, G. Tangwa, and P. Tindana. 2007. The structure and function of research ethics committees in Africa: A case study. *PLoS Medicine* 4(1):e3.

Kupfer, L., K. Hofman, R. Jarawan, J. McDermott, and K. Bridbord. 2004. Roundtable: Strategies to discourage brain drain. *Bulletin of the World Health Organization* 82(8):616-619; discussion 619-623.

Lehner, T., M. Hoelscher, M. Clerici, F. Gotch, L. Pedneault, J. Tartaglia, C. Gray, J. Mestecky, Q. Sattentau, J. van de Wijgert, C. Toure, S. Osmanov, R. E. Schmidt, P. Debre, M. Romaris, A. Hoeveler, and S. Di Fabio. 2005. European Union and EDCTP strategy in the global context: Recommendations for preventive HIV/AIDS vaccines research. *Vaccine* 23(48-49):5551-5556.

Maggon, K. 2004. Investigator and site selection and performing GCP clinical studies in India. *Controlled Clinical Trials* 25(4):366-377.

Maziak, W., K. D. Ward, T. Eissenberg, R. C. Klesges, and U. Keil. 2004. The Syrian center for tobacco studies: A model of international partnership for the creation of sustainable research capacity in developing countries. *Promotion and Education* 11(2):93-97, 116, 134.

McCoy, C. B., R. Achi, H. P. Wolfe, and L. A. Crandall. 2005. The CDRC principles of international health research. *Journal of Urban Health* 82(3 Suppl 4):iv5-iv8.

Musil, C. M., J. Mutabaazi, M. Walusimbi, J. G. Okonsky, Y. Biribonwa, S. Eagan, M. A. Dimarco, S. Mbaballi, and J. J. Fitzpatrick. 2004. Considerations for preparing collaborative international research: A Ugandan experience. *Applied Nursing Research* 17(3):195-200.

Nchinda, T. C. 2002. Research capacity strengthening in the south. *Social Science and Medicine* 54(11):1699-1711.

NIMH (National Institute of Mental Health) Collaborative HIV/STD Prevention Trial Group. 2007a. Methodological overview of a five-country community-level HIV/sexually transmitted disease prevention trial. *AIDS* 21(Suppl 2):S3-S18.

NIMH (National Institute of Mental Health) Collaborative HIV/STD Prevention Trial Group. 2007b. Design and integration of ethnography within an international behavior change HIV/sexually transmitted disease prevention trial. *AIDS* 21(Suppl 2).

NIMH (National Institute of Mental Health) Collaborative HIV/STD Prevention Trial Group. 2007c. Selection of populations represented in the NIMH collaborative HIV/STD prevention trial. *AIDS* 21(Suppl 2):S19-S28.

Orem, J., M. W. Otieno, C. Banura, E. Katongole-Mbidde, J. L. Johnson, L. Ayers, M. Ghannoum, P. Fu, E. G. Feigal, J. Black, C. Whalen, M. Lederman, and S. C. Remick. 2005. Capacity building for the clinical investigation of AIDS malignancy in East Africa. *Cancer Detection and Prevention* 29(2):133-145.

Peterson, L., K. Nanda, B. K. Opoku, W. K. Ampofo, M. Owusu-Amoako, A. Y. Boakye, W. Rountree, A. Troxler, R. Dominik, R. Roddy, and L. Dorflinger. 2007. SAVVY® (C31G) gel for prevention of HIV infection in women: A phase 3, double-blind, randomized, placebo-controlled trial in Ghana. *PLoS ONE* 2(12):e1312.

Ramjee, G., N. S. Morar, M. Alary, L. Mukenge-Tshibaka, B. Vuylsteke, V. Ettiegne-Traore, V. Chandeying, S. A. Karim, and L. Van Damme. 2000. Challenges in the conduct of vaginal microbicide effectiveness trials in the developing world. *AIDS* 14(16):2553-2557.

Ramjee, G., S. Kapiga, S. Weiss, L. Peterson, C. Leburg, C. Kelly, and B. Masse. 2007a. The value of site preparedness studies for future implementation of phase 2/IIb/III HIV prevention trials: Experience from the HPTN 055 study. *Journal of Acquired Immune Deficiency Syndromes* 47(1):93-100.

Ramjee, G., R. Govinden, N. S. Morar, and A. Mbewu. 2007b. South Africa's experience of the closure of the cellulose sulphate microbicide trial. *PLoS Medicine* 4(7):e235.

Rerks-Ngarm, S., A. E. Brown, C. Khamboonruang, P. Thongcharoen, and P. Kunasol. 2006. HIV/AIDS preventive vaccine "prime-boost" phase III trial: Foundations and initial lessons learned from Thailand. *AIDS* 20(11):1471-1479.

Rojas, M. A., J. M. Lozano, and M. X. Rojas. 2007. International collaborative research. A Colombian model that promotes infant health and research capacity. *Journal of Perinatology* 27(12):808.

Shetty, A. K., H. M. Coovadia, M. M. Mirochnick, Y. Maldonado, L. M. Mofenson, S. H. Eshleman, T. Fleming, L. Emel, K. George, D. A. Katzenstein, J. Wells, C. C. Maponga, A. Mwatha, S. A. Jones, S. S. Abdool Karim, and M. T. Bassett. 2003. Safety and trough concentrations of nevirapine prophylaxis given daily, twice weekly, or weekly in breast-feeding infants from birth to 6 months. *Journal of Acquired Immune Deficiency Syndromes* 34(5):482-490.

Skoler, S., L. Peterson, and W. Cates, Jr. 2006. Our current microbicide trials: Lessons learned and to be learned. *Microbicide Quarterly* 4(1):6.

Stough, W. G., F. Zannad, B. Pitt, and S. Goldstein. 2007. Globalization of cardiovascular clinical research: The balance between meeting medical needs and maintaining scientific standards. *American Heart Journal* 154(2):232-238.

UNAIDS and AVAC. 2007. *Good participatory practice guidelines for biomedical HIV prevention trials: Discussion draft.* Geneva, Switzerland: UNAIDS.

Vallely, A., C. Shagi, S. Kasindi, N. Desmond, S. Lees, B. Chiduo, R. Hayes, C. Allen, and D. Ross. 2007. The benefits of participatory methodologies to develop effective community dialogue in the context of a microbicide trial feasibility study in Mwanza, Tanzania. *BMC Public Health* 7:133.

van de Wijgert, J., and H. Jones. 2006. Challenges in microbicide trial design and implementation. *Studies in Family Planning* 37(2):123-129.

Van den Broeck, J., M. Mackay, N. Mpontshane, A. Kany Kany Luabeya, M. Chhagan, and M. L. Bennish. 2007. Maintaining data integrity in a rural clinical trial. *Clinical Trials* 4(5):572-582.

Vardas, E., S. Butto, R. Glashoff, M. S. Malnati, G. Poli, and M. Clerici. 2005. Preparing for phase II/III HIV vaccine trials in Africa. *Microbes and Infection* 7(14):1436-1444.

Wallis, A. B., R. Chereches, F. Oprescu, A. Brinzaniuc, and C. I. Dungy. 2007. An international model for staffing maternal and child health research: The use of undergraduate students. *Breastfeeding and Medicine* 2(3):139-144.

8

Estimating HIV Incidence

One of the most important aspects of site preparation is accurately estimating the HIV incidence rate in the trial population. As Chapter 2 notes, studies are powered based on the number of HIV infections investigators expect to occur during the trial. Small errors in estimates of HIV incidence can have a significant impact on study power and sample size.

Overestimating HIV incidence can have particularly disastrous effects. For example, several recent late-stage microbicide and PrEP studies were stopped prematurely because HIV incidence was much lower than originally estimated. In the Savvy microbicide trials in Ghana and Nigeria, estimated HIV incidence at both sites was 5 percent, while observed incidence was 1.9 percent and 1 percent, respectively. Other multisite trials (HPTN 035, CS-CONRAD) have closed some individual sites because HIV incidence was lower than expected. Canceling trials or closing individual sites because of lower-than-expected incidence ultimately delays the ability to identify effective agents, wastes scarce resources, and disrupts the local community (van de Wijgert and Jones, 2006). These experiences underscore the need to accurately estimate HIV incidence before a trial starts.

Although HIV prevalence—the proportion of people who are infected at a single point in time—can be measured through cross-sectional studies, estimating HIV incidence, or the number of people who become infected with HIV over a given amount of time, is much more difficult, because HIV infection is a silent event. There are three major approaches for estimating HIV incidence for the purpose of designing a trial: direct longitudinal follow-up of populations; biomarkers that indicate recent infection on cross-sectional samples; and mathematical models that rely on serial prevalence data.

Other indirect methods used in the past to estimate HIV incidence are not appropriate for estimating incidence for trial design. Back-calculation—a method that infers HIV incidence from AIDS case-reporting data and the distribution of "incubation periods" (the time from initial infection to the onset of AIDS) (Brookmeyer and Gail, 1986; Brookmeyer, 1991; Bacchetti et al., 1993)—is less relevant for several reasons. First, back-calculation requires an accurate and complete AIDS case-reporting system, which is not available in most resource-poor settings. Second, with the advent of effective therapies, the incubation period has been difficult to predict, making this approach unusable in areas where antiretroviral therapy is available (McDougal et al., 2005). Third, while back-calculation methods can be used to estimate past HIV incidence, they cannot provide statistically reliable estimates of current HIV incidence rates, because recent HIV infections are not reflected in AIDS case data because of the long incubation period.

Surrogate markers and behavioral risk factors have sometimes been used to indirectly infer information about HIV incidence rates during the pretrial period. For instance, high incidence of reported bacterial sexually transmitted infections (STIs), such as syphilis or gonorrhea, can suggest geographical areas and groups in which sexual transmission of HIV may be occurring. Similarly, high incidence of hepatitis B and hepatitis C (or, more likely, high prevalence in the case of hepatitis C) in injection drug users can suggest where parenteral transmission of HIV may be occurring. Behavioral surveys may also help guide investigators to geographical areas, demographic groups, or risk groups with an elevated likelihood of HIV transmission. However, although surrogate markers and behavioral risk factors can be used to target further investigations of HIV incidence, they cannot provide quantitative estimates of HIV incidence, and they should not substitute for direct measurement of HIV incidence in trial design.

DIRECT LONGITUDINAL FOLLOW-UP: COHORT STUDIES

A method often used to estimate HIV incidence is a prospective cohort study, in which a well-defined cohort of at-risk, uninfected individuals is followed over time and serially tested for HIV infection to identify seroconversions. Cohort studies may follow individuals in the same geographic area as a planned trial, or they may employ a run-in design, in which the population or a subset of individuals selected for the trial is followed in the period leading up to the trial. Cohort studies are advantageous in that they can provide a direct and unbiased measure of HIV incidence at or near the trial site. As discussed in Chapter 7, a run-in design also has other advantages, in that it simulates the conditions of the trial and can provide valuable information about factors such as adherence, retention, and pregnancy.

The drawbacks of cohort studies are that they are costly, time consuming, and can be logistically difficult to implement. Also, while cohorts provide unbiased results, cohort studies must have large sample sizes to obtain a tight confidence interval (CI) on the true HIV incidence rate. For example, if the true incidence rate were 5 percent, a 1-year cohort study would require about 1,900 subjects to provide a 95% CI of width 2 percent (for example, 4–6 percent). If the cohort study were based on 500 subjects, the CI width would be 4 percent (for example, 3–7 percent), with an underlying 5 percent incidence rate, which would likely be too wide for confidently planning a randomized trial.

Another drawback is that estimates of HIV incidence from cohort studies may not necessarily reflect the HIV incidence that would occur during a prevention trial. The differences could result from differences in study populations, participation rates, follow-up rates, or secular changes in incidence (Brookmeyer and Quinn, 1995; McDougal et al., 2005). Furthermore, as trial participants are exposed to repeated prevention counseling and education over time, HIV incidence could decline within the study population itself. If secular changes in incidence are occurring in the community apart from the trial itself, HIV estimates could misrepresent actual incidence. Researchers need to assess such factors, though it recognizes that such an assessment may in part be qualitative.

BIOMARKERS OF RECENT INFECTION

A second approach that has been investigated since the 1990s entails using laboratory-based assays, which can distinguish recent from long-standing HIV infections based on virologic or immunologic markers of HIV disease progression, to estimate population-level HIV incidence (Brookmeyer and Quinn, 1995).[1] The development of an accurate biomarker of recent infection that could be used to estimate incidence would be a major advance. The key advantage of this approach is that investigators can estimate incidence by testing blood samples at a single point in time from a cross-sectional sample, thus avoiding the problems of recruitment, follow-up bias, or secular changes in incidence, and reducing the cost and time required in cohort studies.

In practice, this method involves a two-stage process. First, antibody status of blood samples collected through surveillance studies is determined by using standard HIV-1 serological tests. A second assay is then

[1]This section does not address the use of laboratory assays for testing and diagnosing acute HIV infection in individuals.

applied to the HIV-1-positive samples (or seronegative samples depending on the specific tests used and the testing algorithm) to determine if they represent "recent" or "established" infections based on defined parameters (McDougal et al., 2005). Incidence is then calculated using standard epidemiological relationships between prevalence and mean duration. In this case, mean duration refers to the mean duration of the "window" period—the time it takes newly infected individuals to pass from "recent" infection to "established" infection according to the biomarkers. The window periods are not the same for all samples; rather, there is inherent variability. The window periods are random and have a probability distribution. The mean window period is the average of these window periods, which represents the "typical" duration of time it takes to move from recent to established infection, as shown in Equation 1 below (Quinn et al., 2000; McDougal et al., 2005).

$$\text{Incidence} = \text{prevalence/mean duration of the window period} \qquad (1)$$

The accuracy of the incidence estimate depends on the accuracy of both factors: prevalence and mean duration of the window period (McDougal et al., 2005). Prevalence is calculated as the proportion of those identified as recent infections divided by the number of individuals in the susceptible (uninfected) population. As a result, the sensitivity and specificity of the tests designed to identify recent infection are important factors in the accuracy of prevalence.

The mean window period is needed in order to convert the data collected from a cross-sectional sample into an incidence rate. The mean window period is assessed in advance based on serological panels of known seroconverters (obtained from cohort or other studies) who are serially tested over time. All else equal, tests with longer window periods will provide more statistically stable and reliable HIV incidence estimates (McDougal et al., 2005).

The biomarker-based assays used in algorithms to detect recent infection can be classified into two groups: viral tests and antibody tests.

Viral Tests

Viral tests can detect HIV infection in individuals who are acutely infected but who have not yet seroconverted. Although individuals with acute infection will not test positive for antibodies, markers of HIV replication, such as RNA and DNA will generally begin to appear during the second week following exposure. Estimating incidence using viral tests involves a two-stage algorithm that first tests all samples for antibodies and then tests all antibody negative samples with a viral preseroconversion test, such as an HIV-1 RNA assay (nucleic acid amplification test or RNA PCR test) or the HIV-1 antigen (p24) assay. Those who are negative on the antibody test but positive on the viral test are classified as recent infections.

Although viral preseroconversion tests are used in the United States and abroad for blood bank screening and clinical testing algorithms (see, for example, Pilcher et al., 2002), these tests are not practical for use in estimating HIV incidence in resource-constrained settings for two reasons. First, the mean duration of the window period—the period of time from the appearance of viral products to the development of antibodies—is very short (on the order of one to two weeks). Thus very large sample sizes are required to estimate incidence with any statistical precision. Second, the viral tests are expensive and must be performed on all antibody-negative samples. Identifying and testing large cohorts of seronegative individuals can be costly and logistically difficult, particularly in resource-constrained settings with high HIV prevalence.

Antibody Tests

Antibody tests can be used to estimate incidence by distinguishing antibody responses in recently infected individuals from antibody responses in those with established infection. The two most commonly used antibody based methods are: the Serological Testing Algorithm for Recent HIV Seroconversion (STARHS) (Janssen et al., 1998) and BED capture enzyme immunoassay (BED-CEIA) (Parekh et al., 2002).

The STAHRS algorithm involves testing blood samples drawn from a cross-sectional population for HIV antibodies using standard antibody tests. In a second step, researchers test those samples that were positive for antibodies in the first test with a less sensitive or "detuned" assay (Janssen et al., 1998). Those samples that test positive on the first antibody test, but negative on the second test, are classified as recent infections (Parekh et al., 2002).

The BED-CEIA can be used to estimate HIV incidence by measuring increasing levels of HIV-1-specific immunoglobulin (IgG) as a proportion of total IgG following seroconversion (Parekh et al., 2002). Following seroconversion, the proportion of HIV-specific IgG to total IgG rises over the first year of seroconversion. Both the United States and South Africa have used BED to develop national estimates of HIV incidence for surveillance purposes (Rehle et al., 2005; Lee and McKenna, 2007) but not for trial design.

Because these antibody assays have a longer window period than the viral assays (p24 antigen or RNA tests), they are theoretically more suitable for use in estimating HIV incidence (McDougal et al., 2005). However, these assays have three major limitations. First, the STAHRS was developed and optimized for estimating the incidence of subtype B HIV-1, using sero-samples from the Americas, Australia, Japan, the Caribbean, and Europe. These assays do not perform as well when applied to other HIV subtypes, such as those found in sub-Saharan Africa (A, C, D, E), India (C), and South East Asia (C, E) (McDougal et al., 2006). As a result, they need to be recalibrated using seropanels of other subtypes.

A concern with both the BED-CEIA, along with LS-EIA, is that it misclassifies as recent infections some individuals with longer-term infections (more than 1 year), individuals with AIDS, and individuals receiving antiretrovirals (McDougal et al., 2006; Karita et al., 2007; Sakarovitch et al., 2007).[2] Furthermore, because BED-CEIA is based on the proportion of anti-HIV immunoglobulins (IgG) to total IgG,[3] misclassification may be greater in areas with high HIV prevalence and high chronic coinfection that can result in elevated background rates of IgG. The concern is that these false positives lead researchers to overestimate HIV incidence.

To correct for this overestimation, at least two different statistical adjustments have been proposed. McDougal and colleagues (2006) incorporate various misclassification rates that provide sensitivity and specificity corrections.

Hargrove and colleagues (2006) proposed a second, simpler statistical adjustment. Using data from a study in Zimbabwe, Hargrove et al. estimate that the BED assay would classify 5.2 percent of persons who have been infected for 12 or more months as recent infections. He uses this number to correct the incidence estimates by essentially subtracting 5.2 percent of all HIV positives from the number identified as recent infections by the BED assay.

Some empirical studies indicated that these adjustments performed well in specific settings. Nevertheless, the committee identified some theoretical questions regarding these adjustments. Equation 1 relies on the mean or average window duration. For example, the reported 160-day mean window for the BED assay (Parekh et al., 2002) included people who have windows much longer than 160 days as well as people with windows much shorter than 160 days. As such, the calculation is already accounting for persons with very long windows periods. Thus, theoretically, no other statistical adjustments should be needed, so the theoretical foundation for the adjustments is unclear.

An alternative approach to enhancing the performance of the BED assay is to improve the accuracy of the mean window period in Equation

---

[2]In Sakarovitch et al., 2007, most of the specimens that were misclassified as incident cases were from individuals infected longer than 6 months but less than 1 year.

[3]The BED-CEIA detects levels of anti-HIV IgG relative to total IgG and is based on the observation that the ratio of anti-HIV IgG to total IgG increases with time after HIV infection.

1. That improvement could eliminate the need for any additional ad hoc statistical adjustments. The BED test could be useful in estimating HIV incidence for prevention trials, provided that scientists adequately adjust for uncertainty in the window period.

MacDougal et al. (2006) have also proposed another potential method for reducing false positives in sequential testing algorithms. This approach involves taking specimens that BED classifies as recent infections and retesting them with a different assay for recent infection. The specimen must be classified as recent infection by both assays to be considered positive for recent infection.

McDougal and colleagues (2006) applied such a sequential testing algorithm—using the BED assay followed by the avidity assay—to specimens obtained from a longitudinal cohort study, the AIDSVAX B/B vaccine trial, which had a direct measure of HIV incidence. Although the sequential testing algorithm reduced false positives by 41 percent, it also slightly decreased (by 11 percent) the number of true positives that registered as recent. Sequential testing algorithms using a different combination of tests may further reduce misclassification (McDougal et al., 2006).

Overall, researchers' efforts to identify better biomarker-based methods of incidence have been limited by inadequate understanding of antibody formation and insufficient numbers of specimens to test new approaches. To understand the generation of immune responses, a massive cross-sectional population screening program is required, which would recruit subjects pre-seroconversion and follow them for at least 2 years. The CHAVI 001 protocol (CHAVI, 2005) is one example of work in this field that is designed to address some of the current shortcomings in the development of antibody formation. CHAVI 001 is a multicenter, prospective, observational, cohort study that will collect biological specimens for up to 1300 enrollees followed for 2 years to study the HIV-1 virus, the host response, the genetic factors that determine HIV transmission, and viral set point. Although this effort is primarily directed at vaccine discovery and characterization, this type of research could potentially support discovery of markers of acute infection.

Overall, these methods can provide quick and inexpensive estimates of HIV incidence rates. However, the results are not only imprecise but may also be biased. Further validation studies are under way to address concerns that the BED test may produce biased estimates of HIV incidence.

MATHEMATICAL MODELS

A third approach to estimating HIV incidence in study populations relies on mathematical models of serial cross-sectional data on HIV prevalence. Although this method for estimating incidence can be relatively inexpensive and quick, it is the least direct of the three approaches, and the most uncertain, because it requires input parameters for which there is sometimes relatively little information.

Mathematical models have been most often used to estimate population-level trends in the HIV epidemic. For example, UNAIDS and the World Health Organization use modeling to produce annual country-specific estimates of adult HIV prevalence, incidence, and mortality (Walker et al., 2003). These groups use a two-step process to estimate incidence. First, the UNAIDS/WHO Estimation and Project Package (EPP) develops prevalence curves by modeling HIV data collected over time from national surveillance systems and ad hoc research studies (Walker et al., 2003). Second, Spectrum software (Stover, 2002) estimates incidence by applying assumptions (such as survival time after HIV infection and sex ratio of HIV prevalence) to the EPP prevalence curves (Walker et al., 2003).

The quality of these and other model estimates is affected by the availability, quality, and representativeness of the underlying data. For example, one of the major weaknesses of the EPP model is its reliance on prevalence data from national surveillance systems, which vary in quality. Countries with generalized HIV epidemics[4] base prevalence estimates among all adults on sentinel surveillance of pregnant women tested at prenatal clinics. Assumptions are required to translate prevalence among pregnant women to prevalence in the adult population. In addition, much of the information is collected in urban locations and little in rural settings (Walker et al., 2003).

More complex models incorporate many input parameters in an effort to more closely mirror reality. However, the data for those parameters may be so unreliable that a more complex model is actually less reflective of reality than a simple model. As a result, it is important to understand the source and validity of the data, the methods used to develop estimates, and how well those estimates match reality.

Overall, while incidence estimates derived from mathematical models can be particularly useful in tracking changes in the HIV epidemic at the population level (partly because the relative change rather than the absolute estimate is important), such models do not have enough precision to estimate HIV incidence for a prevention trial. Investigators should use them only as a corroborating source of evidence.

In sum, each of the three methods for estimating HIV incidence has strengths and weaknesses. The methods can be broadly classified into those that involve the direct longitudinal follow-up of individuals, and those that indirectly infer incidence rates using other methods. The latter include

[4]Countries with generalized epidemics are those where HIV prevalence in pregnant women is greater than 1 percent.

those based on biomarkers of recent infection derived from cross-sectional samples and mathematical models of serial prevalence data.

Recommendation 8-1: Investigators should base their estimate of HIV incidence on at least one source of data from the direct longitudinal follow-up of individuals in the trial setting. Given the importance of accurate estimates and the inherent uncertainties of any single approach, the direct estimate of HIV incidence should be corroborated by at least one other source.

This corroborating source could be based on any of a number of approaches, including direct longitudinal follow-up in the proposed setting, follow-up in related populations in another setting, or any of the indirect approaches. Researchers should also critically assess factors that could change estimates of HIV incidence, such as the impact of sustained counseling and education on a cohort or trial participants, secular changes in incidence as the epidemic evolves, and attrition rates that vary by risk level of HIV infection.

Recommendation 8-2: Donors and appropriate U.S. and international agencies should make development of a reliable, accurate biomarker-based test for recent HIV infection that can be run with blood from a single draw a high priority. They should provide the necessary funding and laboratory resources to conduct a substantial cross-sectional screening program. This will require recruiting subjects from countries with low-level, concentrated, and generalized epidemics during the pre-seroconversion period and following them for several years.

Recommendation 8-3: Although further validation studies are being conducted to examine concerns that the STAHRS and BED tests may produce biased estimates of HIV incidence, investigators should not rely solely at this time on these or other biomarker assays of recent infection to estimate HIV incidence for the specific purpose of designing a prevention trial.

REFERENCES

Bacchetti, P., M. Segal, and N. Jewell. 1993. Backcalculation of HIV infection rates. *Statistics in Medicine* 8(2):82-101.

Brookmeyer, R. 1991. Reconstruction and future trends of the AIDS epidemic in the United States. *Science* 253(5015):37-42.

Brookmeyer, R., and M. H. Gail. 1986. Minimum size of the acquired immunodeficiency syndrome (AIDS) epidemic in the United States. *Lancet* 2(8519):1320-1322.

Brookmeyer, R., and T. C. Quinn. 1995. Estimation of current human immunodeficiency virus incidence rates from a cross-sectional survey using early diagnostic tests. *American Journal of Epidemiology* 141(2):166-172.

CHAVI (Center for HIV/AIDS Vaccine Immunology). 2005. *CHAVI 001: Acute HIV-1 infection prospective cohort study*. Bethesda, MD: NIAID.

Hargrove, J. K., J. Humphrey, and K. Mutasa. 2006. *Back to BED: Resurrecting a method for estimating HIV incidence from a single cross-sectional survey*. Paper presented at STARHS workshop in association with the 16th International Conference on AIDS, Toronto, Canada.

Janssen, R. S., G. A. Satten, S. L. Stramer, B. D. Rawal, T. R. O'Brien, B. J. Weiblen, F. M. Hecht, N. Jack, F. R. Cleghorn, J. O. Kahn, M. A. Chesney, and M. P. Busch. 1998. New testing strategy to detect early HIV-1 infection for use in incidence estimates and for clinical and prevention purposes. *Journal of the American Medical Association* 280(1):42-48.

Karita, E., M. Price, E. Hunter, E. Chomba, S. Allen, L. Fei, A. Kamali, E. J. Sanders, O. Anzala, M. Katende, and N. Ketter. 2007. Investigating the utility of the HIV-1 BED capture enzyme immunoassay using cross-sectional and longitudinal seroconverter specimens from Africa. *AIDS* 21(4):403-408.

Lee, L. M., and M. T. McKenna. 2007. Monitoring the incidence of HIV infection in the United States. *Public Health Reports* 122(Suppl 1):72-79.

McDougal, J. S., C. D. Pilcher, B. S. Parekh, G. Gershy-Damet, B. M. Branson, K. Marsh, and S. Z. Wiktor. 2005. Surveillance for HIV-1 incidence using tests for recent infection in resource-constrained countries. *AIDS* 19(Suppl 2):S25-S30.

McDougal, J. S., B. S. Parekh, M. L. Peterson, B. M. Branson, T. Dobbs, M. Ackers, and M. Gurwith. 2006. Comparison of HIV type 1 incidence observed during longitudinal follow-up with incidence estimated by cross-sectional analysis using the BED capture enzyme immunoassay. *AIDS Research and Human Retroviruses* 22(10):945-952.

Parekh, B. S., M. S. Kennedy, T. Dobbs, C. P. Pau, R. Byers, T. Green, D. J. Hu, S. Vanichseni, N. L. Young, K. Choopanya, T. D. Mastro, and J. S. McDougal. 2002. Quantitative detection of increasing HIV type 1 antibodies after seroconversion: A simple assay for detecting recent HIV infection and estimating incidence. *AIDS Research and Human Retroviruses* 18(4):295-307.

Pilcher, C. D., J. T. McPherson, P. A. Leone, M. Smurzynski, J. Owen-O'Dowd, A. L. Peace-Brewer, J. Harris, C. B. Hicks, J. J. Eron, Jr., and S. A. Fiscus. 2002. Real-time, universal screening for acute HIV infection in a routine HIV counseling and testing population. *Journal of the American Medical Association* 288(2):216-221.

Quinn, T. C., R. Brookmeyer, R. Kline, M. Shepherd, R. Paranjape, S. Mehendale, D. A. Gadkari, and R. Bollinger. 2000. Feasibility of pooling sera for HIV-1 viral RNA to diagnose acute primary HIV-1 infection and estimate HIV incidence. *AIDS* 14(17):2751-2757.

Rehle, T., O. Shisana, V. Pillay, and K. Zuma. 2005. National HIV incidence measures—new insights into the South African epidemic. *South African Medical Journal* 95(3):6.

Sakarovitch, C., F. Rouet, G. Murphy, A. K. Minga, A. Alioum, F. Dabis, D. Costagliola, R. Salamon, J. V. Parry, and F. Barin. 2007. Do tests devised to detect recent HIV-1 infection provide reliable estimates of incidence in Africa? *Journal of Acquired Immune Deficiency Syndromes* 45(1):115-122.

Stover, J. 2002. *AIM: A computer program for making HIV/AIDS projections and examining the social and economic impacts of AIDS*. Produced for USAID by the POLICY Project. Washington, DC.

van de Wijgert, J., and H. Jones. 2006. Challenges in microbicide trial design and implementation. *Studies in Family Planning* 37(2):123-129.

Walker, N., K. A. Stanecki, T. Brown, J. Stover, S. Lazzari, J. M. Garcia-Calleja, B. Schwartlander, and P. D. Ghys. 2003. Methods and procedures for estimating HIV/AIDS and its impact: The UNAIDS/WHO estimates for the end of 2001. *AIDS* 17(15):2215-2225.

9

Interim Monitoring and Analysis of Results

Randomized clinical trials often take several years to complete subject enrollment, or accrual, and follow-up. That means that information about the risks and benefits of the intervention becomes available during the trial, sometimes from the trial itself and sometimes from external sources such as other trials.

This information provides a scientific basis for monitoring the interim results of the trial—and indeed the ethical necessity to do so—to assess whether the trial should be modified in some way, or possibly terminated, given those results. During interim reviews of the trial, as well as after it has been completed, investigators must analyze the results in valid ways that reflect the trial's design and protocol. This chapter explores the challenges entailed in performing interim monitoring and analyzing the results of HIV prevention trials.[1]

ENSURING EFFECTIVE INTERIM MONITORING

The evolving interim results of phase 3 and some phase 2 randomized trials are typically monitored by a data monitoring committee (DMC) (also known as a data and safety monitoring board, or a data monitoring board). Such a committee is composed of independent experts appointed by the study investigators or sponsor to ensure that the best interests of study participants are met during the trial (Ellenberg et al., 2002).

[1]For more on reporting trial results, see the CONSORT guidelines at http://www.consort-statement.org/index.aspx?o=1030.

For example, the DMC monitors whether randomly assigning participants to intervention and control groups is still ethical given interim results, and whether subjects who are already enrolled should continue to receive their assigned interventions. The DMC also tracks a study's evolving results to determine whether the trial still has the potential to achieve its scientific goals. The DMC may also recommend modifications to the trial design based on interim results, including changing the target period for enrolling or following subjects, or modifying the criteria for enrolling subjects.

Though not the focus of this chapter, another function of the DMC is to evaluate the quality of the study conduct. In particular, the DMC usually reviews investigators' compliance with data management and operating procedures. For example, the DMC may monitor the accuracy and completeness of the data collected, the trial's compliance with restrictions on the eligibility of some potential participants, the adequacy of their accrual rates, and the trial's adherence to drug distribution policies. If it detects problems, the DMC may suggest changes to procedures (Ellenberg et al., 2002).

After reviewing a trial's interim results, a DMC could recommend terminating the trial for a number of reasons, including the following:

- The intervention and control arms are convincingly different (that is, the intervention is efficacious), or, in the case of a noninferiority trial, the study arms are convincingly similar.
- One or more of the study arms produces unacceptable side effects or toxicity.
- Accrual of participants is so slow that completion of the trial in a reasonable time period is no longer feasible.
- Information from other studies with related goals and similar intervention arms makes continuation of the trial unnecessary or unethical.

This section reviews key aspects of interim monitoring of randomized HIV prevention trials, including the composition of DMCs and the typical format of their meetings, the importance of access to complete information, challenges in monitoring trial assumptions, safety, efficacy, and futility, and the use of information from sources external to the trial.

DMC Composition and Meetings

The DMC for an HIV prevention trial typically includes statisticians and clinicians and often other scientists such as a virologist or someone with expertise in a key diagnostic test, an ethicist, and a lay participant—all appointed by the study's investigators or sponsors (Ellenberg et al., 2002; Fleming et al., 2002). Because of the central role of behavior in biomedical

HIV prevention studies, their DMCs should usually also include an individual with expertise in behavioral or social sciences.

HIV prevention trials are often designed and sponsored by investigators and organizations based outside the countries where the trials occur, such as pharmaceutical companies, governments, or nonprofit foundations. If that is the case, including representatives of local communities on the DMC is critical. For example, in the late-1990s, two mother-to-child HIV prevention trials were undertaken in Thailand, supported by the U.S. government and designed primarily by non–Thai scientists (Shaffer et al., 1999; Lallemant et al., 2000). Although both trials demonstrated significant declines in mother-to-child transmission, the trial that compared a shortened AZT (antiretroviral) regimen to no treatment had a DMC with minimal representation from the host country. That fact helped spark considerable ethical debate about the use of a placebo group when the efficacy of AZT had been established elsewhere (Angell, 1997).

Recommendation 9-1: The data monitoring committees of trials with sponsors and scientific leaders from outside the host country should include multiple representatives from the host country. These members—who should compose at least one-third of the committee—should include scientists, ethicists, and lay people familiar with the community and local norms.

DMC Meetings

A key consideration for DMCs is how often they should meet. A trial's protocol for interim monitoring should include guidelines for determining the frequency of meetings—typically expressed as a measure of information, such as the number of observed HIV infections. For example, a trial design might call for an interim efficacy analysis when 25, 50, and 75 percent of the anticipated number of HIV infections in the control group have occurred. The protocol should also specify how the trial should "spend" the overall type I error (say, 5 percent) among its interim and final analyses. (See more on this below, and, for example, Ellenberg et al., 2002.)

As noted, DMCs also meet to monitor participant accrual, HIV incidence rates, attrition, and adherence, and to assess safety—sometimes while also assessing efficacy. It is common, and advisable, to require that a DMC meet at least once a year to perform such monitoring.

The DMC typically holds open sessions at which it discusses the progress of a trial with key investigators, including the sponsors. This information—usually presented in an "open" report—may include the rates at which the trial is enrolling subjects, their baseline characteristics, the completeness of the data that the trial is collecting, and its ability to retain subjects, all aggregated across study arms. The committee also reviews a "closed" report—typically prepared by the study's statistician—in a closed session, usually attended only by DMC members and the study statistician. This report usually includes summaries of safety, efficacy, adherence, and attrition by blinded study arm.

Most DMCs have the authority to unblind the study arms—that is, to find out which arm the data are from—if they feel that doing so is important to determining whether to modify or continue a trial. For example, a nonsignificant trend in trial results favoring the control arm could convince the DMC to recommend ending a trial, but a similar trend favoring the experimental arm would typically convince the committee to continue the trial. If the former situation potentially exists, DMC members should unblind themselves, to determine whether the trial should end on the grounds that the experimental arm is not helping subjects as much as the control arm.

In some instances, DMCs have operated under criteria that members will remain unblinded unless interim analyses comparing efficacy among a trial's arms demonstrate a significant result. For example, Van Damme and colleagues (2002) report that the DMC for the N-9 microbicide trial had planned to remain unblinded unless results from the study arms became significantly different at the $P = 0.001$ level.

The committee fails to see the rationale behind such criteria in trials comparing a new intervention to a control group because the threshold for stopping a trial due to a higher risk of HIV infection in the intervention group should be lower than the threshold for stopping the trial because of a lower risk of infection in the intervention group. For example, a nonsignificant trend suggesting increased HIV risk in the intervention group would usually mean that there is a real concern that the participants are being harmed and also that the trial would be unlikely to demonstrate a significantly lower HIV infection risk in the intervention group if the trial were completed as planned. This was the motivation for the recent termination of the Merck STEP trial (http://www.avac.org/pdf/STEP_data_release.7Nov.pdf). The committee believes that DMCs should always have the option of unblinding study arms, if they believe that doing so is in the best interests of the participants.

Recommendation 9-2: The data monitoring committees for HIV prevention trials should always have the option of unblinding interim results if they believe that doing so might lead them to recommend that the trial be modified or terminated, or lead to other actions that are in the best interests of the trial participants. In particular, when the efficacy data show nonsignificant trends favoring one of the blinded

arms, a DMC should unblind itself as this might reflect an intervention that may be harming patients.

Deciding Whether a Trial Remains Feasible

In most randomized clinical trials, the DMC monitors the assumptions used to determine a trial's sample size and planned duration to ensure that it remains feasible. Ideally, a charter prepared prior to the start of a trial details the tasks the DMC will perform and the criteria it will use. In HIV prevention trials, these assumptions include the following:

- Assumed versus actual rates of subject accrual, and the demographics of enrolled subjects
- Assumed versus actual HIV infection rates
- Assumed versus actual adherence of subjects to study interventions
- Assumed versus actual retention of subjects, including rates of loss to follow-up, and missing data
- Assumed versus actual rates of pregnancy and other reasons for discontinuing the product

Enough information is usually available during a trial to estimate participant accrual, adherence, behavior, and retention rates precisely. (An important consideration is whether adherence and behavior can be measured in an unbiased fashion—see Chapter 5.) However, HIV incidence rates are typically so low that the DMC may have trouble obtaining sufficiently precise estimates to determine whether the incidence rate used to determine the sample size and study duration is accurate. And as Chapter 2 noted, an overly optimistic estimate of HIV incidence in the control group could mean that a trial is underpowered, and thus that it is unable to achieve its goals.

For example, if a study has assumed that the annual HIV incidence rate in the control arm will be 4 percent, the width of the 95 percent confidence interval (CI) for the rate estimated from trial results is about $0.8/\text{sqrt}(n \times f)$, where n denotes the number of subjects on which the estimate is based, and f denotes their average follow-up time.

Thus, if investigators conduct an interim analysis after enrolling 500 subjects (250 per arm), with an average follow-up time of 1 year per subject, the width of the 95 percent CI for the true incidence rate is about 5 percent. That is, an observed HIV incidence rate of 3 percent would still be consistent with the assumed rate of 4 percent used to power the study, yet it would also be consistent with a rate that would indicate insufficient power. This underscores the need to adequately justify a study's assumed

HIV incidence rate, and to be conservative in using it to determine the sample size and duration of follow-up of enrolled subjects.

Many randomized trials either do not provide guidelines and criteria that the DMC will use to recommend modifying the sample size or duration of follow-up, or do so only in vague terms. Such modifications would not change the statistical validity of a trial if they were not based on comparative analyses of the interim data. For example, a DMC could recommend increasing a trial's sample size based on the HIV incidence rate in a placebo group or across study arms. Such recommendations should be based on specific criteria set forth in the protocol, such as the pooled HIV incidence rate versus the incidence rate in the control group. However, a recommendation to continue accruing subjects because of "interesting trends" in HIV infections across study arms could be problematic, as this will tend to inflate the false positive rate (type I error) in standard analyses of the results.

Recommendation 9-3: Investigators should clearly describe in the study protocol the basis and criteria for any recommendation by the data monitoring committee to modify a trial's size or duration. If such changes are implemented, the protocol should also specify how investigators should evaluate the trial results.

Monitoring for Safety, Efficacy, and Futility

To determine whether to stop or modify a trial based on its interim results, the DMC monitors emerging data on the safety and efficacy of a study's interventions. In HIV trials, this information includes

- safety data,
- differences in HIV infection rates between study arms, and
- differences in other measures of efficacy between study arms.

Trials usually include more structured rules for modifying or stopping them in two instances: when they demonstrate the efficacy or noninferiority of a new intervention, and when they demonstrate its futility. The criteria for terminating or modifying a trial may also include unexpected side effects.

Safety

The side effects of interventions could be minor (such as rash or soreness) or more serious (greater susceptibility to other infections).

Side effects of products used in HIV prevention studies could also include behavioral changes. For example, participants could be more likely to engage in risky sexual behavior—this is known as disinhibition, or risk compensation (Cassell et al., 2006)—if they believe the product being tested provides partial or complete protection against HIV infection.

Demonstrating Benefit

Conducting multiple statistical tests comparing a new and control intervention increases the rate of a false positive result (type I error) (Pocock, 1974). Because a DMC usually reviews a study's interim results on several occasions, statistical analyses need to account for this inflated risk (Turnbull, 2006). That is, the criteria for achieving statistical significance at each interim analysis must be chosen to cap the overall chance of a false positive at some predefined level—typically 5 percent (or 0.05).

Multiple ways of "spending" this type I error among interim analyses are available. Pocock suggested using the same criteria for each analysis, selected to give the desired overall type I error (see, for example, O'Brien and Fleming, 1979). However, most trials employ a more conservative rule, such as the O'Brien-Fleming spending function (O'Brien and Fleming, 1979), which requires early analyses to reach higher thresholds (that is, smaller *P* values) for statistical significance, and allows the final analysis to reach a lower threshold.

For example, for a trial with three interim analyses and one final analysis, investigators could achieve an overall type I error rate of 5 percent by using a Pocock spending function requiring a *P* value of 0.016 or less at each analysis. Or investigators could achieve that error rate by using an O'Brien-Fleming approach requiring *P* values of 0.000005, 0.013, and 0.0228 at the first, second, and third interim analyses, and 0.0417 at the final analysis. However, although both approaches would yield an overall type I error rate of 5 percent, the O'Brien-Fleming boundaries are less likely to end a trial early than the Pocock boundaries. If an interim analysis does not prompt termination, the O'Brien-Fleming boundaries are also more likely to have a lower threshold for demonstrating that the treatment has made a significant difference at the final analysis. (For an example of early stopping of an HIV treatment trial for efficacy, see Hammer et al., 1997.)

In HIV prevention studies, where subjects' adherence and behavior are important determinants of an intervention's effect, investigators must also consider whether the intervention sustains that effect. For example, a microbicide that reduces the risk of HIV infection for 6 months—but not thereafter, because users do not adhere to the regimen—is unlikely to have an important impact in controlling the HIV epidemic. Thus terminating an effectiveness trial of such a microbicide based on a short-term effect at an interim analysis (say, after 6 months) may be unwise. However, an efficacy trial designed specifically to assess whether the intervention has some protective ability might well use a 6-month effect on HIV infection as a primary endpoint (see Chapter 2).

One way to attempt to incorporate this consideration into the design of a monitoring plan is to use a conservative spending function, as noted. However, a better approach is to define the endpoint used in an interim analysis to reflect a sustained effect, such as the difference between intervention and control arms in cumulative HIV incidence at 2 years. One recently completed trial of the efficacy of male circumcision in preventing HIV infection used such a criterion (Bailey et al., 2007).

> **Recommendation 9-4: For effectiveness trials, guidelines for stopping HIV prevention trials based on positive interim results should require evidence of a sustained impact on cumulative HIV incidence.**

Demonstrating Futility

Interim analyses may suggest stopping a trial because of futility—that is, because the trial is highly unlikely to show that a new intervention is superior, given current evidence and the added information that would become available if the trial continued. In an HIV prevention trial, "futility" need not refer only to evidence of a complete lack of benefit in preventing HIV infection, but also to evidence that the protective efficacy is less than some minimal amount (such as 40 percent), or that the intervention does not produce a sustained drop in HIV infection rates. Or, an effectiveness trial might include a stopping rule for futility if the interim data rule out a short-term effect on HIV infection (say, 6 months after randomization).

A trial of an intervention that reaches such a futility criterion would typically prompt the study's investigators to pursue no further testing. For example, Hall et al. evaluated the value of intravenous and intrathecal cytarabine for prolonging the survival of HIV-infected people with progressive multifocal leukoencephalopathy (1998). At the time of the second interim analysis, when 57 of the scheduled 90 subjects had enrolled, 14 deaths had occurred in each of the cytarabine arms, as well as in the placebo arm, and cytarabine was associated with significant side effects. The chances that the study would show a significant survival benefit with cytarabine if the trial were completed were exceedingly small, given those results and the fact that only 33 more subjects would be enrolled. Thus the DMC recommended ending the trial for futility.

More recently, in October 2007, the DMC for an HIV vaccine trial recommended terminating the trial based on an interim analysis, concluding that the vaccine could neither prevent HIV infection nor reduce the amount of virus in people who became infected (National Institute of Allergy and

Infectious Diseases, 2007). Soon afterward, the DMC for a companion vaccine trial recommended terminating that trial also. The sponsors of the STEP trial have since announced that participants would be notified whether they received placebo or vaccine (see http://www.hvtn.org/media/pr/STEPStudyOC.pdf).

Terminating a trial for futility can prevent the inefficient use of resources. However, there is also an ethical basis for stopping a trial when the likelihood is low that it will achieve a definitive result. In the cytarabine example, early termination avoided exposing study participants to a therapy that appeared unlikely to help them but that does have serious side effects. In the HIV vaccine examples, the possibility that a vaccine might increase the risk of HIV infection could not be excluded based on the interim data, providing an ethical basis for terminating the trial. However, even if a new intervention does not have side effects and does not seem to increase risk, an ethical case could be made that participants would incur an opportunity cost by remaining in a trial, if by doing so they could not seek other options. This underscores the need for a detailed informed-consent process that alerts people to both the risks and benefits of participating in a trial.

Rules that encourage investigators to terminate a study based on a low likelihood that the intervention will show adequate efficacy can play an important role in HIV prevention trials. Designing a phase 3 effectiveness trial with carefully constructed futility criteria could mimic a strategy of following a phase 2B trial with a phase 3 trial only if the 2B results were encouraging. Such a strategy would avoid the ethical problems of pursuing a phase 3 trial after finding promising results in a phase 2B trial.

In some instances, there may be advantages to continuing a trial even when the interim data suggest that an intervention is unlikely to be superior to the control regime. For example, if a trial compares a group that receives a common but unproven intervention with an untreated control group, interim evidence that the intervention is unlikely to produce a better response may not be sufficient grounds for terminating the trial owing to futility, because of the value of showing that the intervention is not very effective.

Using Information from Similar Trials or Other Sources

Information that affects the equipoise between risks and benefits of a trial's study arms sometimes becomes available from sources outside the trial. For example, after public disclosure of interim results from the Thai PHPT trial on preventing mother-to-child transmission of HIV, the DMC for a Botswana trial recommended terminating one of four study arms that was similar to the terminated arm of the Thai trial (Talawat et al., 2002; Shapiro et al., 2006).

Other examples have occurred with other diseases. For example, a recent meta-analysis (Nissen and Wolski, 2007) that raised questions about the cardiovascular side effects of rosiglitazone in diabetics led the investigators of a randomized trial of the drug's safety to convene an unscheduled interim analysis (Home et al., 2007). Because of inconsistencies between their results and those of the meta-analysis, the investigators chose to continue their trial.

These examples illustrate that DMCs need to be aware of emerging results from similar trials and other sources. They also suggest that investigators consider including guidelines on whether and how they might use information that becomes available from related trials in interim monitoring.

Dixon and Lagakos (2000) have cautioned against having the DMCs for similar contemporaneous trials share efficacy results, as that would raise serious questions about the appropriate publication of the findings, and detract from the long-standing desire for trials to yield reproducible results. Terminating a trial based on the unplanned pooling of efficacy data from another trial undermines the prespecified study criteria. As such, this approach represents a post hoc analysis, as the methods used to undertake such pooling and interpret the results are not part of the study design. This is a very different matter from terminating an arm of a trial, or ending a trial altogether, based on external data, as occurred when investigators terminated the African Phambili trial (HVTN 503) of a Merck HIV vaccine based on the findings of the international STEP trial (HVTN 502).

Different studies may also use different criteria for assessing or defining endpoints, and for including or excluding subjects, and set different schedules for subject visits, further complicating the interpretation of interim information based on post hoc pooling. Finally, if two trials were stopped based on post hoc pooling of efficacy data, many researchers would insist that the results be published as a single paper, because any conclusion that the intervention had a positive effect would stem from the combined data. This would introduce other complications.

However, because DMCs use less formal criteria to assess the safety of a new product than they use to document efficacy, sharing safety information from concurrent trials is acceptable and can be informative, especially for less frequent adverse events. One recent proposal—perhaps motivated by recent safety problems with microbicides (N-9 and cellulose sulfate), but applicable to any HIV biomedical prevention—is to create a "super DMC" that would monitor several microbicide trials with one or more intervention arms in common (Nunn, 2007). The basic idea is that DMCs would agree to share a core set of safety data, and that participating investigators would be notified of any emerging safety problems. Such an idea is intriguing. However, implementing it would require careful planning to avoid arbitrary decisions on when to notify individual DMCs of overall results, and on which results each participating DMC should see. For example, if two three-arm trials had one common experimental arm and a common control arm, would the DMCs share safety information about all three arms?

Also important are details about the procedures for capturing safety data, as trials may differ in the method, frequency, and completeness with which they collect safety information. There may also be ethical or regulatory considerations, including whether the informed-consent process must be changed in such circumstances, as well as scientific issues, such as whether and when participating trials should release a single publication on the main trial results, as opposed to separate publications for each trial.

To the committee's knowledge, very little has been written about how best to share safety information among DMCs, yet the committee sees value in doing so in an appropriate manner. Nor has anyone discussed whether DMCs should share safety information routinely, or only if a possible concern is raised.

Recommendation 9-5: Investigators, donors, and regulatory agencies should encourage research on how to combine safety information from concurrent trials of similar products, including the scientific advantages and disadvantages of sharing information, the timing and logistics of doing so, ethical concerns (such as how such information might affect the informed-consent process), and how to report the results from such trials.

ANALYZING TRIAL RESULTS

Analyzing the results of HIV prevention trials is particularly challenging, for several reasons:

- HIV infection is a "silent" event—that is, it is not directly observable—and the tests used to diagnose infection are imperfect.
- When pregnancies occur during a trial, women are often taken off the study product.
- Participants in such trials may not adhere to the study interventions.
- Investigators need to account for the impact of HIV exposure on trial outcomes—which is determined by both HIV prevalence and the behavior of participants—while also addressing the challenges of obtaining accurate information on behavior.
- Investigators need to assess the relationships among interventions, adherence, exposure, and the risk of HIV infection.

The Silence of HIV Infection and the Imperfections of Diagnostic Tests

In contrast to "time-to-event" endpoints such as mortality and progression of HIV, as measured by a biomarker such as viral load, determining HIV infection requires a diagnostic test such as EIA, RNA-PCR, or a more recently developed rapid test. Repeated testing of subjects in an HIV prevention trial leads to "interval-censored" observations of the time to HIV infection, rather than an exact date. That is, periodic testing brackets an individual's time of infection between the last negative and first positive diagnostic test.

The situation is further complicated by the fact that the diagnostic tests used to detect HIV infection are not perfect. For example, RNA-PCR can have a low sensitivity when used within 2 weeks of HIV infection (Balasubramanian and Lagakos, 2003), leading to false negatives. Similarly, EIA does not usually detect HIV infection in persons who have not yet developed HIV antibodies (that is, those who have not yet seroconverted).

These features imply that some participants who enroll in HIV prevention trials may already be infected, and that some participants who become infected during a trial may not be diagnosed. Investigators need to take those possibilities into account when analyzing trial results.

Excluding Subjects Who Were HIV Infected When Enrolled from Analysis

HIV prevention trials have used different approaches in analyzing results from participants who are later suspected of having been HIV infected at the time of enrollment. One approach has been to use postenrollment diagnostic tests to avoid counting subjects believed to have been infected at the time of randomization. If investigators could identify and exclude all subjects already infected when they are randomized, and no others, estimates of the relative efficacy of an intervention, and tests of the null hypothesis, would improve in several ways (Balasubramanian and Lagakos, 2004):

- Estimates of product efficacy or effectiveness would be less biased.
- The type I error of tests comparing study arms with respect to HIV infection rates would remain valid.
- The power of the trial to detect a real difference in efficacy between arms would increase.

However, despite these potential advantages of excluding subjects who are already infected at the time of randomization, the impact of doing so is often minimal because the number of such exclusions is small. On the other hand, postrandomization exclusions can introduce biases and distort comparisons of the intervention and control arms, if they do not exclude all subjects infected at the time of randomization, or if they incorrectly exclude some subjects who were uninfected at enrollment, differentially among the intervention arms. This could occur, for example, if the post hoc testing of baseline samples is triggered by positive HIV test occurring shortly after randomization (say, at 3 months), since this could be influenced by a differential intervention effect.

Biases can also occur if the criteria for determining which participants to exclude are not identical in the intervention and control arms, or if the patterns of participants' clinic visits are not identical in each arm. Thus, investigators must carefully weigh the potential gains from excluding individuals who may have been infected at enrollment against the possibility that doing so will introduce bias into the comparison of study arms. Even if investigators could theoretically justify the post hoc exclusion of subjects, critics might question the face validity of results from trials that exclude more subjects from the intervention arm than from the control arm.

Recommendation 9-6: Investigators should base their primary analysis of the efficacy of an intervention on all randomized subjects. Secondary sensitivity analyses that exclude subjects believed to have been HIV infected when they were randomized can be useful. However, investigators should not substitute such analyses for the primary analysis, unless such exclusions (and nonexclusions) can confidently be made without error.

Recommendation 9-7: Investigators of trials evaluating an intervention that is believed to have a delayed impact may find it efficient to exclude people found to be HIV infected after randomization but before a given follow-up time. If so, the trial protocol should specify and justify such an approach, and investigators should use it only if follow-up of subjects and assessment and confirmation of HIV infection during this period is identical in all study arms. Investigators should undertake secondary analyses based on all randomized subjects.

Confirming HIV Infections

Subjects who test HIV positive typically undergo confirmatory tests. Some of the initial results turn out to be true positives, while some are false positives. In theory, some of the true positives might not be confirmed because of the imperfect sensitivity of the confirmatory test—that is, these subjects would be considered negative when they are actually positive—thus increasing the number of false positives.

Given that tests to detect HIV infection are imperfect, a trial protocol should set clear criteria for confirming that subjects are indeed infected. Although such confirmation could increase the number of false negatives, it would decrease the number of false positives and lead to more confidence that the observed endpoints are "real." It is critical that investigators develop criteria for assessing endpoints that are applied equally in the intervention and control arms.

Analyzing Time to Infection

Standard methods for analyzing the amount of time that elapses between randomization and HIV infection assume that investigators know the exact time of infection. These methods include the log-rank test, Kaplan-Meier estimator, and Cox's model. To account for the interval-censored nature of information on HIV infection in prevention trials, and the imperfection of the tests, investigators could use modified versions of these methods (Richardson and Hughes, 2000; Balasubramanian and Lagakos, 2004; Gupte et al., 2007; Zhang and Lagakos, in press).

These standard methods provide valid tests of the efficacy of an intervention if subjects are evaluated based on the same schedule of clinic visits in each study arm, and if the sensitivity and specificity of the diagnostic test does not depend on the study arm. In that case, similar periodic results would be expected to occur in the study arms under the null hypothesis of no intervention effect. Under these circumstances the following occurs:

- Standard Kaplan-Meier estimates of cumulative HIV infection rates are valid at the scheduled visit times. However, these cumulative rates cannot be estimated for times between visits, so the curves should not be displayed in the usual way as step functions.
- In practice, participants are often not evaluated according to the exact visit schedule. In such cases, the Kaplan-Meier estimator, log-rank test, and Cox model should use the scheduled visit time rather than the actual time. That is because the tests depend on the magnitudes of the observed times only through their relative ranks (that is, they are "rank invariant"), and thus small differences in the time of visits can have a big impact on the results.
- Investigators should include information from unscheduled visits in the analyses only if they can safely assume that such visits do not depend on subjects' infection status. Otherwise, investigators should base their analyses only on results from scheduled visits.

In some studies, such as in newborns and infants, a nonnegligible proportion of subjects may die before being detected as HIV infected. In such settings, investigators should use methods for analyzing competing risks, or use HIV-free survival rather than HIV infection as the endpoint (see, for example, Richardson and Hughes, 2000).

Effects of Product Discontinuation and Loss to Follow-Up

Participants may stop using an intervention during a trial for several reasons, most commonly adverse treatment effects, an inability to continue the treatment or lack of interest in doing so, or, in some HIV prevention studies, pregnancy. In some trials, investigators stop tracking participants who discontinue their randomized intervention prematurely. It is well known that this can lead to distorted statistical inferences about intervention effects (Lagakos et al., 1990) because subjects who discontinue their intervention, including placebo, can have different risks of becoming infected than those that do not. For example, Hughes et al. (1994) noted that HIV patients with more rapidly declining CD4+ cell counts were more likely to discontinue treatment than other patients. Another example is the Coronary Drug Project (Canner et al., 1986). In that trial, death rates in patients randomized to receive Clofibrate were 18 percent for compliers compared with 25 percent for noncompliers, suggesting that the drug might be beneficial. However, the corresponding death rates for the placebo group were 15 percent and 28 percent, indicating that something about being noncompliant was associated with a poorer outcome (Snapinn et al., 2004). For both examples, if the rates of discontinuation differed among the intervention groups and analyses were based only on outcome events that occurred prior to discontinuation (sometimes referred to as "as treated" analyses), the comparisons of outcome events among the interventions would be biased. Thus, the accepted practice is to continue to follow participants for the study endpoint regardless of whether or not they prematurely discontinue their randomized intervention, and to use all outcome events in the analysis of the data, and not just those that precede discontinuation of the intervention; such analyses are called intention-to-treat analyses. As noted in Chapter 2, the power of intention-to-treat analyses will, in general, be reduced by product discontinuation. Chapter 5 discusses several ways in which the effect of persistence and more generally adherence and behavior on HIV incidence can be meaningfully analyzed.

Handling Pregnancies During Follow-Up

If a pregnancy that occurs during a trial does not trigger a modification of the intervention, then analyses of time to HIV infection will not change. However, if a product is temporarily or permanently discontinued when a woman is found to be pregnant, the more general discussion of product discontinuation described in the previous paragraph applies. Thus, it is important that investigators continue to follow pregnant women for HIV infection after they discontinue a product owing to pregnancy and, when analyzing results, use intention-to-treat analyses that utilize outcome events for the duration of follow-up, and not just those occurring prior to the pregnancy.

An alternative method of analysis is to "censor" a woman's time of infection when she is found to be pregnant and discontinues the product. That is, investigators would regard this woman's time of infection as being "at least *x*," where *x* is the time from randomization until she is found to be pregnant and taken off the product. This convention is sometimes referred to as an "as-treated" analysis. As with other forms of discontinuation, such analyses could lead to biased estimates of the cumulative risk of HIV infection if pregnancy represented a type of "informative censoring"—that is, if the risk of (subsequent) HIV infection in a pregnant woman is different from that of a nonpregnant women with equal follow-up. Although the evidence for a differential risk of HIV infection during infection is limited and thus somewhat controversial, there have been reports of increased HIV risk in pregnant women (Taha et al., 1998; Gray et al., 2005; Morrison et al., 2007). The impact of pregnancy on "as-treated" statistical tests comparing intervention groups is somewhat different. Here, if the rates of pregnancy do not differ among the intervention arms, and if the risk of HIV infection for a pregnant woman does not depend on the product she had been taking, at-treated tests that censor a woman at the time of pregnancy will lead to valid comparisons. However, when planning a trial, investigators usually cannot be assured of either of these assumptions; thus, it is prudent to continue to follow women who become pregnant for the study's outcome events and to analyze the resulting data using intention-to-treat methods.

Recommendation 9-8: In all trials, investigators should continue to follow women who become pregnant for HIV infection, regardless of whether they discontinue their study intervention. In addition, intention-to-treat analyses should be the primary basis for comparing intervention groups with respect to HIV infection and other efficacy endpoints. Investigators can include as-treated analyses as secondary analyses, but should interpret them cautiously, because of the possibility that such discontinuations represent a type of informative censoring.

REFERENCES

Angell, M. 1997. The ethics of clinical research in the third world. *New England Journal of Medicine* 337(12):847-849.

Bailey, R. C., S. Moses, C. B. Parker, K. Agot, I. Maclean, J. N. Krieger, C. F. Williams, R. T. Campbell, and J. O. Ndinya-Achola. 2007. Male circumcision for HIV prevention in young men in Kisumu, Kenya: A randomised controlled trial. *Lancet* 369(9562):643-656.

Balasubramanian, R., and S. W. Lagakos. 2003. Estimation of a failure time distribution based on imperfect diagnostic tests. *Biometrika* 90(1):171-182.

Balasubramanian, R., and S. W. Lagakos. 2004. Analyzing time-to-event data in a clinical trial when an unknown proportion of subjects has experienced the event at entry. *Biometrics* 60(2):335-343.

Canner, P. L., K. G. Berge, N. K. Wenger, J. Stamler, L. Friedman, R. J. Prineas, and W. Friedewald. 1986. Fifteen-year mortality in coronary drug project patients: Long-term benefit with niacin. *Journal of the American College of Cardiology* 8(6):1245-1255.

Cassell, M. M., D. T. Halperin, J. D. Shelton, and D. Stanton. 2006. Risk compensation: The Achilles heel of innovations in HIV prevention? *BMJ* 332(7541):605-607.

Dixon, D. O., and S. W. Lagakos. 2000. Should data and safety monitoring boards share confidential interim data? *Controlled Clinical Trials* 21(1):1-6; discussion 54-55.

Ellenberg, S., P. L. Fleming, and D. L. DeMets. 2002. *Data monitoring committees in clinical trials: A practical perspective.* Edited by S. Senn and V. Barnett. West Sussex, UK: John Wiley & Sons Ltd.

Fleming, T. R., S. Ellenberg, and D. L. DeMets. 2002. Monitoring clinical trials: Issues and controversies regarding confidentiality. *Statistics in Medicine* 21(19):2843-2851.

Gray, R. H., X. Li, G. Kigozi, D. Serwadda, H. Brahmbhatt, F. Wabwire-Mangen, F. Nalugoda, M. Kiddugavu, N. Sewankambo, T. C. Quinn, S. J. Reynolds, and M. J. Wawer. 2005. Increased risk of incident HIV during pregnancy in Rakai, Uganda: A prospective study. *Lancet* 366(9492):1182-1188.

Gupte, N., R. Brookmeyer, R. Bollinger, and G. Gray. 2007. Modeling maternal-infant HIV transmission in the presence of breast-feeding with an imperfect test. *Biometrics* 63(4):1189-1197.

Hall, C. D., U. Dafni, D. Simpson, D. Clifford, P. E. Wetherill, B. Cohen, J. McArthur, H. Hollander, C. Yainnoutsos, E. Major, L. Millar, and J. Timpone. 1998. Failure of cytarabine in progressive multifocal leukoencephalopathy associated with human immunodeficiency virus infection. AIDS Clinical Trials Group 243 Team. *New England Journal of Medicine* 338(19):1345-1351.

Hammer, S. M., K. E. Squires, M. D. Hughes, J. M. Grimes, L. M. Demeter, J. S. Currier, J. J. Eron, Jr., J. E. Feinberg, H. H. Balfour, Jr., L. R. Deyton, J. A. Chodakewitz, and M. A. Fischl. 1997. A controlled trial of two nucleoside analogues plus indinavir in persons with human immunodeficiency virus infection and cd4 cell counts of 200 per cubic millimeter or less. AIDS Clinical Trials Group 320 Study Team. *New England Journal of Medicine* 337(11):725-733.

Home, P. D., S. J. Pocock, H. Beck-Nielsen, R. Gomis, M. Hanefeld, N. P. Jones, M. Komajda, and J. J. McMurray. 2007. Rosiglitazone evaluated for cardiovascular outcomes—an interim analysis. *New England Journal of Medicine* 357(1):28-38.

Hughes, M. D., D. S. Stein, H. M. Gundacker, F. T. Valentine, J. P. Phair, and P. A. Volberding. 1994. Within-subject variation in cd4 lymphocyte count in asymptomatic human immunodeficiency virus infection: Implications for patient monitoring. *Journal of Infectious Diseases* 169(1):28-36.

Lagakos, S. W., L. L. Lim, and J. M. Robins. 1990. Adjusting for early treatment termination in comparative clinical trials. *Statistics in Medicine* 9(12):1417-1424.

Lallemant, M., G. Jourdain, S. Le Coeur, S. Kim, S. Koetsawang, A. M. Comeau, W. Phoolcharoen, M. Essex, K. McIntosh, and V. Vithayasai. 2000. A trial of shortened zidovudine regimens to prevent mother-to-child transmission of human immunodeficiency virus type 1. Perinatal HIV prevention trial (Thailand) investigators. *New England Journal of Medicine* 343(14):982-991.

Morrison, C. S., J. Wang, B. Van Der Pol, N. Padian, R. A. Salata, and B. A. Richardson. 2007. Pregnancy and the risk of HIV-1 acquisition among women in Uganda and Zimbabwe. *AIDS* 21(8):1027-1034.

NIAID (National Institute of Allergy and Infectious Diseases). 2007. Statement: Immunizations are discontinued in two HIV vaccine trials. Bethesda, MD: NIAID. http://www3.niaid.nih.gov/news/newsreleases/2007/step_statement.htm (accessed November 2007).

Nissen, S. E., and K. Wolski. 2007. Effect of rosiglitazone on the risk of myocardial infarction and death from cardiovascular causes. *New England Journal of Medicine* 356(24):2457-2471.

Nunn, A. 2007. *Issues in microbicide trial design, monitoring, and analysis*. Paper read at the second public meeting for the Committee on Methodological Challenges in HIV Prevention Trials, April 19, London, UK.

O'Brien, P. C., and T. R. Fleming. 1979. A multiple testing procedure for clinical trials. *Biometrics* 35(3):549-556.

Pocock, S. J. 1983. *Clinical trials: A practical approach*. Chichester, UK: John Wiley & Sons, Inc.

Richardson, B. A., and J. P. Hughes. 2000. Product limit estimation for infectious disease data when the diagnostic test for the outcome is measured with uncertainty. *Biostatistics* 1(3):341-354.

Shaffer, N., R. Chuachoowong, P. A. Mock, C. Bhadrakom, W. Siriwasin, N. L. Young, T. Chotpitayasunondh, S. Chearskul, A. Roongpisuthipong, P. Chinayon, J. Karon, T. D. Mastro, and R. J. Simonds. 1999. Short-course zidovudine for perinatal HIV-1 transmission in Bangkok, Thailand: A randomised controlled trial. Bangkok Collaborative Perinatal HIV Transmission Study Group. *Lancet* 353(9155):773-780.

Shapiro, R. L., I. Thior, S. Gilbert, C. Lockman, C. Wester, L. Smeaton, S. J. Stevens, K. Heymann, K. McIntosh, S. Ndung'u, V. Gaseitsiwe, T. Novitsky, S. Peter, E. Kim, C. Widenfelt, P. Moffat, P. Ndase, P. Arimi, P. Kebaabetswe, P. Mazonde, R. Lee, J. Marlink, J. Makhema, S. Lagakos, and M. Essex. 2006. A randomized comparison of strategies for adding single-dose nevirapine to zidovudine to prevent mother-to-child HIV transmission in Botswana. *AIDS* 20:1281-1288.

Snapinn, S. M., Q. Jiang, and B. Iglewicz. 2004. Informative noncompliance in endpoint trials. *Current Controlled Trials in Cardiovascular Medicine* 5(1):5.

Taha, T. E., G. A. Dallabetta, D. R. Hoover, J. D. Chiphangwi, L. A. Mtimavalye, G. N. Liomba, N. I. Kumwenda, and P. G. Miotti. 1998. Trends of HIV-1 and sexually transmitted diseases among pregnant and postpartum women in urban Malawi. *AIDS* 12(2):197-203.

Talawat, S., G. J. Dore, S. Le Coeur, and M. Lallemant. 2002. Infant feeding practices and attitudes among women with HIV infection in northern Thailand. *AIDS Care* 14(5):625-631.

Turnbull, B. 2006. Group sequential tests. In *Encyclopedia of Statistical Science*. New York: John Wiley & Sons, Inc.

Van Damme, L., G. Ramjee, M. Alary, B. Vuylsteke, V. Chandeying, H. Rees, P. Sirivongrangson, L. Mukenge-Tshibaka, V. Ettiegne-Traore, C. Uaheowitchai, S. S. Karim, B. Masse, J. Perriens, and M. Laga. 2002. Effectiveness of COL-1492, a nonoxynol-9 vaginal gel, on HIV-1 transmission in female sex workers: A randomised controlled trial. *Lancet* 360(9338):971-977.

Zhang, P., and S. W. Lagakos. In press. Analysis of time to a silent event whose occurrence is monitored with error, with application to mother-to-child HIV transmission. *Statistics in Medicine*.

10

Alternative Designs

Late-stage biomedical HIV prevention trials have mostly used superiority designs to compare a new biomedical intervention, such as a PrEP antiretroviral or a microbicide gel, to a control arm—often a placebo—with subjects in both arms receiving risk-reduction counseling. Such trials aim to advance the field by assessing whether the new intervention is superior to a standard prevention method, with the expectation that if the trial is positive, it might change practice.

This approach is commonly used to evaluate new interventions in a wide variety of prevention and treatment trials. However, the committee believes that use of alternative types of superiority trials as well other types of trial designs, which also have been used in other settings, can offer important advantages for certain nonvaccine biomedical HIV prevention studies.

First, product adherence and risk behavior are important determinants of the effectiveness of a biomedical HIV prevention intervention, but these factors can vary substantially across populations and individuals (see Chapter 5). This variability can complicate the interpretation of prevention studies using a superiority design, because the "average" intervention effect may not apply to different subpopulations with different risk behaviors and adherence patterns. This argues for studies that can identify improved ways of improving adherence and/or reducing high-risk behavior, or tailor an individual's intervention to provide the maximal amount of protection against HIV infection that is available with current interventions.

Similarly, although investigators conducting late-stage biomedical HIV prevention trials are ethically required to provide all participants with risk-reduction counseling and other prevention interventions (e.g., access to free condoms), there is limited experimental evidence on the relative effectiveness of behavioral risk-reduction interventions in many of the settings where biomedical trials are conducted (see Chapter 3). One way to advance knowledge in this area is to incorporate evaluations of behavioral risk-reduction interventions into the design of biomedical HIV prevention trials.

In addition, no single preventive intervention is likely to have a substantial and sustained protective effect. Designs that allow investigators to determine optimal combinations of interventions—including both biomedical and behavioral components—therefore hold greater promise for slowing the epidemic, even though using different combinations in one trial can complicate the evaluation process.

The "optimal" intervention is also likely to vary among individuals based on the nature of their exposure to HIV. For example, some women may have difficulty negotiating certain forms of prevention, such as condom use. Designs that allow access to alternative forms of protection could be more effective in reducing the risk for these individuals.

Finally, given the complex dynamics among members of a community in the transmission of HIV, some intervention trials, such as trials involving behavioral risk-reduction interventions, might be better suited to randomizing groups of subjects rather than individuals. And further, when feasible, there can be important advantages to designs that enroll HIV-discordant couples to assess the protective effectiveness of interventions in settings where the main, and sometimes sole, HIV exposure of the uninfected partner is known.

The committee believes that these considerations suggest the need for investigators to explore alternative study designs that test multiple preventive interventions, including multiple behavioral risk-reduction interventions and strategies to improve product adherence. Ideally these strategies could be individualized to reflect changes in people's behavior and adherence over time. This chapter reviews the advantages and disadvantages of several alternatives to the traditional superiority design including factorial and other multiarm designs, noninferiority designs, discordant couple designs, cluster randomization designs, and dynamic designs.

FACTORIAL AND OTHER MULTIARM DESIGNS

Treatment trials commonly use factorial designs to investigate the value of two or more types of interventions. To illustrate, consider a 2×2 factorial design with two types of interventions, for example A and B, each of which can be given at one of two levels (e.g., A1 or A2 and B1 or B2).

Subjects are randomized to one of the four (2×2) combinations of interventions; that is, to A1 + B1, A1 + B2, A2 + B1, or A2 + B2. For example, if the levels of A (or B) include getting intervention A (or intervention B) versus getting a placebo for intervention A (or B), the arms of the trial would be as follows:

Arm 1: A1 + B1 = Intervention A combined with Intervention B
Arm 2: A1 + B2 = Intervention A combined with Placebo B
Arm 3: A2 + B1 = Intervention B combined with Placebo A
Arm 4: A2 + B2 = Placebo A combined with Placebo B

This design need not necessarily involve a placebo alternative to each factor. Thus, the A component could entail offering some participants a biomedical intervention and no other intervention (without a placebo), while B could entail offering some participants a more intense behavioral risk-reduction intervention and offer others standard risk-reduction counseling, in which case subjects would be unblinded with respect to both their biological and behavioral interventions.

Or, in A, some participants may receive a biomedical intervention while others receive a placebo of this intervention, as in the original example, while some subjects in B might receive either a new behavioral risk-reduction intervention while others receive standard risk-reduction counseling. Here, subjects will be blinded to their biological intervention but not to their behavioral risk-reduction intervention. This is called a partially blinded factorial design. Although this example focuses on intervention strategies to reduce risk-taking behavior, the designs also apply to evaluating and comparing strategies aimed at improving adherence.

Factorial designs are motivated by an assumption of "no interaction" between the two interventions. Simply put, this means that the relative benefit of intervention A in the absence of intervention B is the same as the relative benefit of intervention A in the presence of intervention B. In the above example, if the intervention effect is measured by relative risk (RR), the assumption of no interaction means that the RR of intervention A to placebo A in subjects who receive placebo B is the same as the RR of intervention A to placebo A in subjects who receive intervention B. That is, the incremental benefit of adding intervention A (in this example measured by RR) is the same in the presence or absence of intervention B. For example, if the risk of becoming HIV infected is 0.10 or 0.02, depending on whether intervention B is or is not used, and the RR of A is 0.5, then the risk of becoming infected is 0.01 (0.5×0.02) if both A and B are used, and is 0.05 (0.5×0.10) if only A is used.

Quantitative vs. Qualitative Interactions

Interactions are sometimes classified as quantitative versus qualitative. In a quantitative interaction, receiving intervention A is better than not receiving it for each level of B, but the magnitude of the benefit varies. For example, intervention A might reduce the risk of HIV infection by 30 percent in individuals receiving intervention B, but reduce it by 50 percent in subjects who do not receive intervention B.

Quantitative interactions might be expected to occur in a trial where A represents a biomedical intervention or its placebo, and B represents two behavioral risk-reduction strategies. The basis for anticipating that there would be either no interaction or a quantitative interaction in this setting is based on the fact that the biological intervention is blinded to study subjects. Thus, while the two intervention strategies could modify risk behavior and thus HIV infection risk in different ways, the "better" behavioral risk-reduction intervention strategy would not depend on whether a subject is receiving A or its placebo. If the biomedical intervention were efficacious, one would expect it to be effective, though possibly by different amounts, in subjects receiving either of the behavioral risk-reduction interventions.

In contrast, an example of a qualitative interaction is one in which receiving intervention A is better than not receiving it for one level of B but worse for the other level of B. For example, when A denotes a biomedical intervention and B denotes two behavioral risk-reduction interventions, a qualitative interaction would occur if intervention A reduced risk in subjects who receive one behavioral risk-reduction intervention but increased risk in subjects receiving the other behavioral intervention. Such outcomes may not be implausible when A is an unblinded comparison (for example, of receiving intervention A versus not receiving intervention A), as knowledge of whether a participant is receiving A could affect her or his response to the different behavioral risk-reduction interventions.

For example, if B denotes intense versus standard risk-reduction counseling, disinhibition might occur in subjects who receive standard counseling. The result could be that subjects who receive a marginally efficacious biomedical intervention (A) have a higher HIV infection rate than subjects who do not receive A. Meanwhile subjects who receive more of an intensive behavioral risk-reduction intervention may have no disinhibition, so subjects receiving A have a lower infection rate than those not receiving A. The interpretation of a trial with a qualitative interaction is usually more complicated than when there is no interaction or only a quantitative interaction.

Sample Size and Analysis of Factorial Designs

If the assumption of no interaction holds, the attractiveness of a 2 × 2 factorial design is that it can evaluate two different interventions (e.g., microbicide versus placebo gel and enhanced versus standard counseling) with the same sample size as a trial investigating only one of the interventions (e.g., microbicide versus placebo gel). The benefit of intervention A is assessed by comparing the combined results from arms 1 (A1 + B1) and 2 (A1 + B2) to the combined results from arms 3 (A2 + B1) and 4 (A1 + B2), with stratification by the level of intervention Fawzi et al. (1999) and Thior et al. (2006) provide examples of factorial designs in mother-to-child HIV prevention trials.

To illustrate how investigators might use a factorial design to assess a new microbicide gel, but also to compare two behavioral intervention strategies, suppose subjects are counseled for condom use and other risk-reducing behaviors at one of two levels (e.g., new behavioral risk-reduction intervention versus standard risk-reduction counseling). Then a 2 × 2 factorial design aiming to assess the benefits of the microbicide as well as the type of behavioral risk-reduction intervention would have the following arms:

Arm 1: Microbicide gel plus standard risk-reduction counseling
Arm 2: Microbicide gel plus enhanced behavioral risk-reduction intervention
Arm 3: Placebo gel plus standard risk-reduction counseling
Arm 4: Placebo gel plus enhanced behavioral risk-reduction intervention

This is a partially blinded design because subjects would know if they are receiving an enhanced behavioral risk-reduction intervention versus standard risk-reduction counseling, but they would not know whether they are receiving the microbicide or placebo gel. The assumption of no interaction means that the incremental value (e.g., relative risk) of the microbicide relative to placebo is the same for subjects who receive enhanced behavioral risk-reduction intervention versus standard counseling. This is equivalent to saying that the relative benefit of the enhanced behavioral risk-reduction intervention (compared with standard counseling) is the same regardless of whether a subject receives the microbicide or placebo. A quantitative interaction would mean that the direction of the effect of A (or B) is the same regardless of the level of the other factor, but that the effect differs in magnitude.

The advantage of a factorial design lies in the fact that if there is no interaction, this design would have about the same power as an equally sized trial comparing microbicide to placebo in subjects receiving a single type of counseling. Yet this design could assess the added value of the microbicide as well as the difference in effectiveness between the enhanced behavioral risk-reduction intervention and standard counseling. If there is a quantitative interaction, the trial would have about the same power as an equally sized trial comparing microbicide to placebo in subjects receiving a single type of counseling whose effect is, loosely speaking, equal to the average effect of the two types of behavioral risk-reduction interventions in the factorial design.

When investigators analyze a factorial trial, the first step is to assess whether the assumption of no interaction or a quantitative interaction is consistent with the data. If it is, then the full data can be used to separately assess each intervention. If there is a qualitative interaction, the levels of each intervention (e.g., A1 versus A2) would be compared separately for the levels (B1 and B2) of the other intervention. As a result, the power to detect differences between the levels of each intervention is reduced because comparisons are based on half the sample size.

As noted above, a partially blinded 2 × 2 factorial design that involves a placebo-controlled biomedical intervention and an unblinded comparison of two behavioral interventions may often be expected to have no interaction or a quantitative interaction. When a qualitative interaction may still be plausible in such a setting, it may be prudent to size the factorial trial to have reasonable power (e.g., 70 percent) if a qualitative interaction is found. For example, a factorial trial with equal allocation of subjects to each arm, a 5 percent type I error rate, and 90 percent power to detect a reduction in HIV incidence from 3 percent to 1.5 percent would require a total of 4,286 subjects, each followed for 1 year, if there were no interaction. If this sample size were increased by 17 percent to 5,036, the power would rise to 94 percent, and the power to test each subgroup separately, assuming a qualitative interaction was found, would be 70 percent. Thus the use of factorial designs with augmented sample sizes offers some protection against an unexpected interaction.

Variations on Standard Factorial Design

The 2 × 2 factorial design discussed above is intended to provide an example of the potential benefits of a factorial design in a setting where a qualitative interaction is unlikely. The ideas can apply to any two interventions that might be used simultaneously, and to two nonzero levels of each intervention, such as two doses or schedules of a microbicide, rather than the presence or absence of the microbicide.

In a multisite trial conducted in different sociocultural settings, it may be possible to evaluate multiple behavioral risk-reduction interventions if an endpoint other than HIV infection could be confidently used to compare the behavioral interventions. For example, suppose a trial were being planned to evaluate a new microbicide gel (versus placebo gel) at three sites, and with 1,000 subjects per site. Suppose also that the behavioral interventions could be reliably compared based on reported condom use rather than on the acquisition of HIV. Then, within each site, each of the 1,000 subjects could be randomized to microbicide gel (A1) versus placebo gel (A2), as well as to either intensive or standard counseling. That is, the design would be as follows:

Site 1: A1 + S1 vs. A1 + S2 vs. A2 + S1 vs. A2 + S2
Site 2: A1 + S3 vs. A1 + S4 vs. A2 + S3 vs. A2 + S4
Site 3: A1 + S5 vs. A1 + S6 vs. A2 + S5 vs. A2 + S6

Here S1, S3, and S5 refer to the more intensive counseling strategies used at the three sites, while S2, S4, and S6 refer to the standard counseling strategies used at the three sites. With this sample size (250 in each of the four resulting arms), the study may have adequate power to enable investigators to compare different pairs of counseling strategies at each of the three sites if this is based on reported condom use instead of HIV infection rates, while still using all 3,000 subjects to evaluate the efficacy of the microbicide based on HIV infection rates. Investigators would need to carefully examine the details of such designs in specific settings. The key point is that with the use of endpoints other than HIV infection to evaluate the behavioral risk-reduction interventions, it may be possible to tailor behavioral interventions and comparisons to different study sites, and evaluate these in a trial of a biomedical intervention without a substantial increase in sample size or duration. However, when an alternative endpoint cannot be reliably used, the behavioral interventions should be based on the endpoint of HIV infection, which implies that the number of distinct behavioral interventions would typically be the same as the number of biomedical intervention arms.

Incomplete Factorial Designs

In settings where investigators plan to assess more than one intervention, but all combinations of the interventions are not of interest, they can realize economies of scale by using a single trial with a common control group. For example, suppose investigators wish to assess each of two microbicide gels used with either enhanced behavioral risk-reduction intervention versus standard risk-reduction counseling. Rather than comparing the gel plus standard risk-reduction counseling to the gel plus the enhanced risk-reduction counseling in one trial, and comparing the gel plus standard risk-reduction counseling with standard counseling in a different trial, the investigators could combine these into a single trial with three arms to reduce the needed sample size, because they could use the same control group (gel plus standard counseling) for both assessments. Such a design can be viewed as an incomplete factorial design because it contains 3 of the 4 possible arms used in the 2 trials.

The Breast-feeding, Antiretroviral, and Nutrition (BAN) study now under way in Malawi is using an incomplete factorial design to study the prevention of mother-to-child transmission. In that study, all mothers and infants are given a standard peripartum HIVNET 012 NVP and ZDV/3TC regimens. Mother-infant pairs are randomized to one of three arms: (1) additional maternal-only antiretroviral therapy (ART) versus (2) additional infant-only ART versus (3) no additional infant or mother ART (beyond the NVP and ZDV/3TC standard). Women are also randomized to receive nutritional supplements versus no nutritional supplements.[1] The study is an incomplete factorial because the investigators are not evaluating all possible combinations.

Recommendation 10-1: Investigators planning late-stage randomized trials of biomedical interventions are encouraged to utilize partially blinded factorial designs in order to also evaluate the relative effectiveness of different behavioral intervention strategies. Factorial designs can provide valuable information about both types of interventions with the same sample size as a trial evaluating only the biomedical intervention.

DISCORDANT COUPLE DESIGNS

Most late-stage HIV prevention trials of biomedical interventions have used designs which enroll at-risk subjects and follow them for HIV infection, without direct knowledge of their exposures to HIV. An implicit assumption in such studies is that the types and frequencies of HIV exposures of participants may vary, but that the randomized intervention groups have similar distributions ("mixes") of exposures, so that a comparison of the cumulative incidence of HIV infection rates between the intervention arms reflects the relative effectiveness of these interventions in preventing HIV infection.

An alternative approach is to conduct what is commonly called a "discordant couples" study, in which HIV-discordant couples are identified and one (typically the uninfected member) is randomized to one of the intervention arms. In HIV, discordant-couple designs were initially used to estimate

---

[1] See http://www.id.unc.edu/malawi/studies_research.htm#unccdc.

the per-contact transmission risk of HIV. However, they also can be used to evaluate a new intervention. As with traditional designs, the results of such a study can be analyzed by comparing the cumulative incidence rates of HIV infection in the different intervention arms. Despite offering counseling on HIV prevention, trials enrolling such couples have recorded HIV infection rates as high as 8–12 per 100 person-years (Quinn et al., 2000; Hugonnet et al., 2002; Allen et al., 2003; Coldiron et al., 2007). However, because more is known about the primary (and sometimes sole) source of exposure of the participants, discordant-couple designs can have several advantages to traditional designs.

Efficiency

A traditional randomized trial evaluating a new biomedical intervention enrolls subjects who are expected to be exposed to HIV because of their behavior. Given the types and frequency of risky behaviors participants engage in, investigators estimate their potential exposure to HIV. However, some subjects in each study arm will not be exposed to HIV because any risky behaviors they undertake would be with HIV-uninfected people. This would attenuate any effect of the intervention. For others, their HIV exposure in each sexual act is not known. For example, a commercial sex worker might be able to convince 75 percent of her partners to use a condom, but investigators do not know how many times those who are HIV infected do or do not use a condom.

In contrast, in discordant couples, investigators know the actual HIV exposure of the uninfected partner based on the types and frequency of risky behaviors with the infected partner. (See, for example, Jewell and Shiboski, 1990; Kim and Lagakos, 1990; Jewell and Shiboski, 1992; Magder and Brookmeyer, 1993.) As a result, if the susceptibility of subjects were similar in both types of trials, a study with discordant couples would require a smaller sample size to achieve the same power. Discordant couples could thus be a valuable population for efficacy studies.

More Intervention Options

Uninfected partners could be randomized to receive an intervention (e.g., a microbicide gel) versus a control (e.g., a placebo gel). Or, the intervention could be directed at the infected partner, to try to reduce the transmissibility of HIV. For example, HPTN 052, a study of 1,750 discordant couples, is investigating the efficacy of ART treatment of the infected partner in preventing transmission of HIV to the uninfected partner (www.hptn.org). The Partners in Prevention study is investigating the efficacy of acyclovir suppression of HSV-2 on HIV acquisition in HIV/HSV-2 discordant couples (Celum and Wald, 2005).

Social Support and Adherence

As noted, a trial involving individuals in known discordant couples may enlist both partners in the prevention process rather than just individuals. Such a trial could educate both the infected and uninfected partner on the product regimen, and give both partners social support and HIV prevention tools. In discordant couples in which the woman is HIV-negative, involving both partners in the study can increase the likelihood that they will adhere to condoms, family-planning services, and the study product (Hugonnet et al., 2002; Allen et al., 2003).

Scientific Insights

Partner studies also facilitate research on other pressing scientific concerns, such as the transmission efficiency of certain subtypes of HIV-1, including mutations that confer resistance—a topic of considerable interest in vaccine trials (see, for example, Gilbert, 2001), but also in studies of other biomedical interventions. As the HIV prevention armamentarium expands to include antiretroviral agents such as microbicides and PrEP, involving both partners in clinical trials could advance research on the potential effect of these products on HIV-infected partners.

Despite these potential advantages, discordant-couples designs are sometimes not feasible because of challenges in identifying a sufficient number of discordant couples for participation in a trial (Coldiron et al., 2007). In addition, there sometimes are concerns that substantial numbers of couples would break up once they became aware of their discordant status. However, this is not always the case and several studies have not encountered that problem (Allen et al., 2003). With regard to recruitment, the Partners in Prevention Study has successfully enrolled and followed more than 3,000 HIV/HSV discordant couples in an HSV suppression trial in seven countries over a two-year period (Celum, 2007). In endemic areas, such as sub-Saharan Africa, with a high prevalence of HIV infection in both genders, the potential exists to identify discordant couples and enroll the uninfected partner into an HIV prevention trial. Thus, in light of the potential advantages of using discordant couples in late-stage HIV prevention trials of biomedical interventions, the committee believes that their feasibility should be assessed in the early stages of the planning of such trials.

Recommendation 10-2: When feasible and consistent with the scientific goals of a late-stage HIV prevention trial, investigators are encour-

aged to consider discordant couple designs because of their advantages over designs in which the actual HIV exposures of participants are unknown.

NONINFERIORITY DESIGNS

Padian et al. recently evaluated the use of a diaphragm plus lubricant gel for preventing HIV in a two-arm superiority trial (Padian et al., 2007). The trial randomized sexually active women to the intervention plus counseling for condom use versus just counseling for condom use. The treatment arms were unblinded.

Overall, the study failed to show that the use of a diaphragm reduced the risk of HIV infection. However, reported condom use was substantially lower (54 percent versus 85 percent) in the subjects who received the intervention.

Suppose that what actually happened in this trial is that women assigned to the intervention felt that it offered an effective alternative to condoms in protecting against HIV infection, and that they preferred the alternative because they could avoid confrontations with their sexual partners over condom use. In that case, another view of the trial results is that an alternative strategy to condom use—namely, "use condoms where possible, but if that is inconvenient, use the diaphragm plus lubricant"—may be equally effective in preventing HIV infection as a simple recommendation that women use condoms. However, the former might be preferable because it gives women a choice. Investigators cannot reliably make such an inference based on the simple trial results in Padian et al. (2007), since this is not how the interventions were administered. Nevertheless, the example shows it might sometimes make sense to assess whether one intervention strategy is as good as another, rather than the traditional superiority design in which one seeks to determine whether a particular strategy is superior in efficacy than another.

Traditionally, investigators use a noninferiority (sometimes called equivalence) design to compare a new intervention with an established intervention, in settings where the new intervention is expected to have some inherent advantages (such as lower cost or fewer side effects) but similar efficacy. For example, a woman who might find it difficult to convince a male partner to use a condom might choose to use a diaphragm. For this woman, a strategy of encouraging her to "use condoms where feasible, but use a diaphragm otherwise" might have equal or better efficacy than a strategy of encouraging only condom use. Yet, even if the efficacy of the first strategy were equal to that of the condom-only strategy, the woman might strongly prefer the diaphragm/condom strategy because it gives her greater control over her HIV infection risk. Here a noninferiority trial might address the scientific goals better than a superiority trial. Noninferiority designs have been used in HIV and in a wide variety of other diseases. An early HIV example is a Thai trial (Lallemant et al., 2000) that was initiated after it had been demonstrated in several studies that antepartum/intrapartum administration of AZT was shown to dramatically reduce mother-to-infant transmission of HIV. Lallemant and colleagues (2000) sought to determine whether a shorter course of AZT could provide similar protective efficacy as the standard course, on the grounds that if it did, it would be less expensive, and perhaps safer, and thus preferable, especially in a resource-limited setting. For a general methodological discussion of noninferiority designs, see D'Agostino et al. (2003).

Once initial advances are made for specific types of biomedical interventions for HIV, such as microbicides or PrEP, noninferiority designs might be naturally employed to assess whether a similar preparation or alternative mode of delivery is about as effective as the original, especially if the new product has other advantages, such as lower cost, ease of delivery, or fewer side effects.

However, noninferiority designs might also be useful in settings seeking to identify more choices of prevention strategies, and where the specific scientific interest is in whether an alternative approach to prevention of HIV transmission is approximately as effective as a more standard approach, in part because of a change in behavior that would be expected to occur with the availability of the new approach, and where the alternative approach may be advantageous in other respects, for example, as in the discussion of the Padian et al. study. Such trials might thus intentionally be unblinded because use of a placebo might not lead to behavior changes typical of what would occur in a real-world setting.

CLUSTER RANDOMIZATION

This chapter has so far focused on trials in which each individual is randomly assigned to one of the intervention arms. An alternative approach is cluster randomization, in which a group of subjects (e.g., from a specific community) rather than individuals is randomized to each study arm.

Clusters can be defined in a number of different ways, depending on the research question. For example, they can be catchment populations at vaccination centers or schools. For a phase 3 microbicide trial, one strategy could be to define clusters as communities served by different health centers, and randomize all the women in a given community to receive either the microbicide gel or the placebo.

Investigators have used cluster randomization most often to evaluate interventions normally delivered to groups or communities, such as controls on sexually transmitted diseases (Grosskurth et al., 1995; Wawer et al., 1999) or school-based education (Hayes et al., 2005). Some phase 3 vaccine trials have also used the approach (Moulton et al., 2001; Barreto et al., 2002; O'Brien et al., 2003). Investigators prepared for one trial of a pneumococcal vaccine by comparing the advantages of individual and community randomization (Jaffar et al., 1999).

In individually randomized trials, subjects from both study arms usually live side by side and receive the intervention and control from the same clinic or other setting. This approach might not resemble what would occur if the intervention were introduced into the community. An advantage of cluster-randomized trials is that they mimic real life more closely, as entire communities receive either the intervention or the control strategy. However, migration can be high in many regions, including areas in Africa, and communities receiving the control strategy would need to provide it to individuals who move into their area from intervention communities, and vice versa.

A potential advantage of cluster randomization is that it can allow investigators to estimate individual plus community-level protection against infectious disease. This is known as "herd immunity" (Jaffar et al., 1999). For example, in a trial of a vaccine for pneumonia or malaria, vaccinating all children in a community could reduce exposure by reducing the overall number of infections in that community. If vaccination leads to herd immunity, a cluster-randomized trial could provide a truer estimate of the effectiveness of the vaccine when used in a normal setting posttrial. In an individually randomized trial, no more than half the target population is usually randomized to the intervention, so vaccinated individuals would be more likely to mix with nonvaccinated individuals, thus increasing their exposure and reducing the possibility of herd immunity.

However, herd immunity is unlikely to develop during the relatively short course of a randomized trial. For example, in trials of a vaccine for pneumonia or malaria, the vaccinees—young children—are only a small proportion of the population, and many young children could become infected from adults or children who are not part of the trial. Thus the reduction in exposure that would result from using cluster randomization rather than individual randomization would usually be minimal (Jaffar et al., 1999).

Cluster randomization is a natural approach when an intervention includes educational efforts best conducted at the group level. For example, Project Accept (HPTN 043) is the first randomized, controlled phase 3 trial to determine the efficacy of a behavioral/social science intervention with an HIV incidence endpoint in the developing world (NIMH, 2007). The study involves randomizing 34 communities in Africa (in South Africa, Tanzania, and Zimbabwe) and 14 communities in Thailand to receive either community-based voluntary counseling and testing (VCT) in addition to standard clinic-based VCT, or standard clinic-based VCT alone. The primary objective of this study is to test the hypothesis that communities receiving 3 years of the community-based intervention in addition to the standard services will have lower prevalence of recent HIV-1 infection.

Trials involving microbicides and PrEP could be individually or cluster randomized, and in some cases could mix features of each approach. For a trial evaluating a microbicide, with HIV incidence among women as the primary endpoint, a microbicide would need to protect women to reduce HIV infections in men in the community. Reducing the number of HIV-infected men will then reduce the risk to women in the trial and provide an added benefit (herd effect). For a trial of male circumcision, with HIV incidence among men as the primary outcome, a trial would need to protect men to reduce HIV infections in women in the community. Reducing the number of HIV-infected women will then reduce the risk to men in the trial and provide an added benefit.

Because trials usually last no more than 2 or 3 years, an appreciable herd effect is unlikely to develop, except in populations where partner change is high, HIV incidence is rising rapidly, and the source of new infections is localized within each community. There are probably relatively few settings where such conditions exist, and even fewer where reliable information on HIV incidence and the source of infections is well known, or investigators can collect that information quickly and accurately enough to design community-randomized trials of microbicides. A possible exception is polygamous societies where entire households form clusters for randomization. In general populations, no evidence suggests that providing microbicides or PrEP would lead to a herd effect in a cluster-randomized trial.

In a partially blinded factorial design aimed at evaluating a new biological intervention as well as comparing two behavioral counseling strategies (see Chapter 5), the behavioral component might involve counseling at the group level. In such a setting, concerns about biases that can occur from cluster randomization with a small number of clusters would not generally apply. However, if a "group effect" in behavioral change occurs, investigators might need to make some adjustment to the standard analysis of individual-randomized studies. Further research into the analysis of such mixed designs is warranted.

As noted, cluster randomization can be disadvantageous when the number of clusters is too small. Several large cluster-randomized trials have fewer than 10 clusters per arm (Grosskurth et al., 1995; Wawer et al., 1999; Kamali et al., 2003). When there is heterogeneity among the clusters and the number of clusters is not sufficiently large, randomization of the clusters can more easily result in chance differences between those assigned to the different interventions than in individually randomized trials with a similar number of subjects.

For example, in the widely cited trial of sexually transmitted disease control in Mwanza, Tanzania (Grosskurth et al., 1995), 12 large communities (i.e., clusters) were randomized to either the intervention or the control. A cohort of 1,000 subjects was evaluated in each community. The baseline HIV prevalence was 3.8 and 4.4 percent, respectively, in the two arms. In a similar-sized cluster-randomized trial of mass syndromic treatment for sexually transmitted diseases in Rakai, Uganda (Wawer et al., 1999), baseline HIV prevalence in the intervention and control arms was 16.1 and 15.5 percent, respectively. Investigators can adjust their estimates of the efficacy of an intervention to help account for such baseline imbalances, but only for known confounders they can measure accurately.

Properly designed phase 3 trials that are individually randomized, in contrast, usually have near-perfect control of both known and unknown confounders. For example, in a recent trial of diaphragm and lubricant gel involving just over 5,000 women (Padian et al., 2007)—less than half the number of subjects as in the Mwanza and Rakai trials—baseline indicators such as proportion married, proportion circumcised, and reported condom use were almost identical in the intervention and control arms. The randomized trials of male circumcision in South Africa, Kenya, and Uganda (Auvert et al., 2005; Bailey et al., 2007; Gray et al., 2007) were of similar size as the trial of diaphragm and lubricant gel (Padian et al., 2007) and also achieved excellent balance between the intervention and control arms.

Because of the potential for imbalance between arms in cluster-randomized trials, investigators should ensure that there are an adequate number of clusters, but also collect data on known potential confounders, so they can also adjust the statistical analysis to account for any differences between arms. This adds complexity to the trial. In a microbicide trial, study staff would need to collect data on all potential risk factors for HIV incidence, such as the frequency and nature of risky sexual behavior. Collecting such data can be a substantial undertaking and require more time from subjects. In contrast, individually randomized trials usually collect minimal data on confounding factors.

Cluster-randomized trials may also have less statistical power than individually randomized trials for the same number of individuals. The loss of power can be substantial, depending on the variation in outcomes between clusters, such as HIV incidence. This is known as the "intraclass coefficient of variation" (Guittet et al., 2005). Importantly, power is difficult to estimate accurately before a trial begins, as the intraclass coefficient is not known in advance and is often difficult to estimate. Estimates of the intraclass coefficient in large HIV-prevention trials evaluating controls on sexually transmitted disease have varied widely (Grosskurth et al., 1995; Wawer et al., 1999; Kamali et al., 2003; Todd et al., 2003).

Blinding can be essential to an unbiased assessment of a trial's outcomes. However, blinding might be difficult in community-randomized trials if the product has a major effect on HIV incidence. If HIV incidence drops noticeably in intervention communities and not in control communities, it could become evident which group is receiving the treatment.

Overall, cluster randomization has a potentially useful role in HIV prevention studies, especially where some interventions, such as certain counseling or educational interventions, are easier to give to groups rather than individuals. However, such interventions must be used critically to ensure that biases do not result from differences among clusters or a lack of blinding.

DYNAMIC DESIGNS

More long-term treatments for chronic disease or prevention, as well as a call for more individualized medicine, have spurred growing interest in so-called dynamic intervention strategies. A dynamic regime consists of a sequence of decision rules for how to vary interventions over time according to subject-specific measurements. Although in the early stages of development, dynamic trial designs acknowledge that one intervention may not apply equally well to all people. This is especially true when an intervention aims to change behavior (Carroll and Rounsaville, 2007; Dawson et al., 2007).

Consider a young woman who has enrolled in an HIV prevention trial. When she begins the study, she requires HIV protection only when her partner, a migrant worker, returns home every three months. The partner does not want to use condoms and would like to have a child. During this time, the woman may prefer a female-controlled product without contraceptive properties. In the middle of the study, the partner returns from extended work abroad. This same woman may now require a different form of HIV protection. Her partner may demand sexual intercourse without advance warning and without the use of a condom, making it difficult to use a coitally dependent product. During this time the woman may prefer a daily protection method. By the end of the study, the protective needs of the woman have changed yet again. She is now pregnant and requires a product that will protect her from HIV infection and that is safe to use during pregnancy.

Dynamic designs aim to adapt to individuals' changing needs and opportunities based on predetermined rules. For example, some HIV treatment trials prescribe changes in individual treatments when resistance emerges on when his or her viral load is no longer suppressed. HIV prevention trials could also offer multiple interventions based on a sequence of predetermined decision rules.

To compare two dynamic strategies in a standard parallel design, investigators would assign one dynamic strategy to one arm and a reference strategy to another. However, to help determine how best to adapt an intervention strategy to become part of a sequence of interventions and responses, sequentially multiple assignment randomized (SMAR) trials have recently been introduced (Murphy, 2005; Murphy et al., 2007). At several stages during such studies, subjects are randomized over a number of possible interventions, which depend on the interventions and responses to that point. In designing sequentially randomized trials or evaluating dynamic intervention strategies, investigators need to consider what observed event might spur a change in intervention, and therefore trigger another randomization.

In the context of an HIV prevention trial, at least two types of events might trigger a change in preventive treatment: pregnancy and nonadherence to the treatment.

As discussed in Chapter 4, despite counseling on use of condoms and providing access to contraceptives, the incidence of pregnancy in many biomedical HIV prevention trials is very high. Trials typically require women who become pregnant to stop using the product during pregnancy, which can reduce study power. As an alternative to this practice, investigators could accept that women in this age range are likely to become pregnant, especially when the trial has a long follow-up period, and regard the dynamic intervention as a total package. If the best course of action for pregnant women is unclear, investigators could take the opportunity to learn how best to protect pregnant women from HIV infection, and randomize them at that point over a set of prevention options such as remaining on product versus discontinuing product and initiating intense counseling for ways of preventing HIV infection during pregnancy versus discontinuing product without initiating any additional form of preventive intervention. This approach could yield valuable information for future practice, even if a single trial does not have the power to establish a definitive course of action.

A dynamic strategy could also be implemented that would give individuals who are poor adherers to the product regimen an alternative prevention strategy. For example, investigators could consider at least two different courses of action for participants who cross a predefined adherence threshold considered to be unacceptable. First, they could randomize individuals to different interventions to increase it, or second, they could offer the participant an alternative prevention product that is perhaps better suited to the participant.

Recommendation 10-3: Investigators should consider the potential merits of using noninferiority, cluster randomization, and dynamic designs in future biomedical HIV prevention trials.

REFERENCES

Allen, S., J. Meinzen-Derr, M. Kautzman, I. Zulu, S. Trask, U. Fideli, R. Musonda, F. Kasolo, F. Gao, and A. Haworth. 2003. Sexual behavior of HIV discordant couples after HIV counseling and testing. *AIDS* 17(5):733-740.

Auvert, B., D. Taljaard, E. Lagarde, J. Sobngwi-Tambekou, R. Sitta, and A. Puren. 2005. Randomized, controlled intervention trial of male circumcision for reduction of HIV infection risk: The ANRS 1265 trial. *PLoS Medicine* 2(11):e298.

Bailey, R. C., S. Moses, C. B. Parker, K. Agot, I. Maclean, J. N. Krieger, C. F. Williams, R. T. Campbell, and J. O. Ndinya-Achola. 2007. Male circumcision for HIV prevention in young men in Kisumu, Kenya: A randomised controlled trial. *Lancet* 369(9562): 643-656.

Barreto, M. L., L. C. Rodrigues, S. S. Cunha, S. Pereira, M. A. Hijjar, M. Y. Ichihara, S. C. de Brito, and I. Dourado. 2002. Design of the Brazilian BCG-revac trial against tuberculosis: A large, simple randomized community trial to evaluate the impact on tuberculosis of BCG revaccination at school age. *Controlled Clinical Trials* 23(5):540-553.

Carroll, K. M., and B. J. Rounsaville. 2007. A vision of the next generation of behavioral therapies research in the addictions. *Addiction* 102(6):850-862; discussion 863-859.

Celum, C. 2007. *Phase III Randomized Placebo-Controlled Trial of HSV-2 Suppression to Prevent HIV Transmission among HIV-Discordant Couples.* Presentation at the second public meeting for the Committee on Methodological Challenges in HIV Prevention Trials, London, UK.

Celum, C., and A. Wald. 2005. *Phase III randomized placebo-controlled trial of HSV-2 suppression to prevent HIV transmission among HIV-discordant couples*, Protocol Version 4.1.1.

Coldiron, M. E., R. Stephenson, E. Chomba, C. Vwalika, E. Karita, K. Kayitenkore, A. Tichacek, L. Isanhart, S. Allen, and A. Haworth. 2007. The relationship between alcohol consumption and unprotected sex among known HIV-discordant couples in Rwanda and Zambia. *AIDS Behavior.* http://www.springerlink.com/content/v5kn5371165761xv/fulltext.html (accessed March 25, 2008).

D'Agostino, R. B., Sr., J. M. Massaro, and L. M. Sullivan. 2003. Non-inferiority trials: Design concepts and issues—the encounters of academic consultants in statistics. *Statistics in Medicine* 22(2):169-186.

Dawson, R., P. W. Lavori, J. L. Luby, N. D. Ryan, and B. Geller. 2007. Adaptive strategies for treating childhood mania. *Biological Psychiatry* 61(6):758-764.

Fawzi, W. W., G. I. Msamanga, D. Spiegelman, E. J. Urassa, and D. J. Hunter. 1999. Rationale and design of the Tanzania vitamin and HIV infection trial. *Controlled Clinical Trials* 20(1):75-90.

Gilbert, P. B. 2001. Interpretability and robustness of sieve analysis models for assessing HIV strain variations in vaccine efficacy. *Statistics in Medicine* 20(2):263-279.

Gray, R. H., G. Kigozi, D. Serwadda, F. Makumbi, S. Watya, F. Nalugoda, N. Kiwanuka, L. H. Moulton, M. A. Chaudhary, M. Z. Chen, N. K. Sewankambo, F. Wabwire-Mangen, M. C. Bacon, C. F. Williams, P. Opendi, S. J. Reynolds, O. Laeyendecker, T. C. Quinn, and M. J. Wawer. 2007. Male circumcision for HIV prevention in men in Rakai, Uganda: A randomised trial. *Lancet* 369(9562):657-666.

Grosskurth, H., F. Mosha, J. Todd, E. Mwijarubi, A. Klokke, K. Senkoro, P. Mayaud, J. Changalucha, A. Nicoll and G. ka-Gina. 1995. Impact of improved treatment of sexually transmitted diseases on HIV infection in rural Tanzania: Randomised controlled trial. *Lancet* 346(8974):530-536.

Guittet, L., B. Giraudeau, and P. Ravaud. 2005. A priori postulated and real power in cluster randomized trials: Mind the gap. *BMC Medical Research Methodology* 5:25.

Hayes, R. J., J. Changalucha, D. A. Ross, A. Gavyole, J. Todd, A. I. Obasi, M. L. Plummer, D. Wight, D. C. Mabey, and H. Grosskurth. 2005. The MEMA kwa Vijana project: Design of a community randomised trial of an innovative adolescent sexual health intervention in rural Tanzania. *Contemporary Clinical Trials* 26(4):430-442.

Hugonnet, S., F. Mosha, J. Todd, K. Mugeye, A. Klokke, L. Ndeki, D. Ross, H. Grosskurth, and R. Hayes. 2002. Incidence of HIV infection in stable sexual partnerships: A retrospective cohort study of 1802 couples in Mwanza region, Tanzania. *Journal of Acquired Immune Deficiency Syndromes* 30(1):73-80.

Jaffar, S., A. Leach, A. J. Hall, S. Obaro, K. P. McAdam, P. G. Smith, and B. M. Greenwood. 1999. Preparation for a pneumococcal vaccine trial in the Gambia: Individual or community randomisation? *Vaccine* 18(7-8):633-640.

Jewell, N. P., and S. C. Shiboski. 1990. Statistical analysis of HIV infectivity based on partner studies. *Biometrics* 46(4):1133-1150.

Jewell, N. P., and S. C. Shiboski. 1992. The design and analysis of partner studies of HIV transmission. In *Methodological issues of AIDS behavioral research*, edited by D. Ostrow and R. Kessler. New York: Plenum.

Kamali, A., M. Quigley, J. Nakiyingi, J. Kinsman, J. Kengeya-Kayondo, R. Gopal, A. Ojwiya, P. Hughes, L. M. Carpenter, and J. Whitworth. 2003. Syndromic management of sexually transmitted infections and behaviour change interventions on transmission of HIV-1 in rural Uganda: A community randomised trial. *Lancet* 361(9358):645-652.

Kim, M. Y., and S. W. Lagakos. 1990. Estimating the infectivity of HIV from partner studies. *Annals of Epidemiology* 1(2):117-128.

Lallemant, M., G. Jourdain, S. Le Coeur, S. Kim, S. Koetsawang, A. M. Comeau, W. Phoolcharoen, M. Essex, K. McIntosh, and V. Vithayasai. 2000. A trial of shortened zidovudine regimens to prevent mother-to-child transmission of human immunodeficiency virus type 1. Perinatal HIV prevention trial (Thailand) investigators. *New England Journal of Medicine* 343(14):982-991.

Magder, L., and R. Brookmeyer. 1993. Analysis of infectious disease data from partner studies with unknown source of infection. *Biometrics* 49(4):1110-1116.

Moulton, L. H., K. L. O'Brien, R. Kohberger, I. Chang, R. Reid, R. Weatherholtz, J. G. Hackell, G. R. Siber, and M. Santosham. 2001. Design of a group-randomized Streptococcus pneumoniae vaccine trial. *Controlled Clinical Trials* 22(4):438-452.

Murphy, S. A. 2005. An experimental design for the development of adaptive treatment strategies. *Statistics in Medicine* 24(10):1455-1481.

Murphy, S. A., D. W. Oslin, A. J. Rush, and J. Zhu. 2007. Methodological challenges in constructing effective treatment sequences for chronic psychiatric disorders. *Neuropsychopharmacology* 32(2):257-262.

NIMH (National Institute of Mental Health). 2007. Project Accept: A phase III randomized controlled trial of community mobilization, mobile testing, same-day results, and post-test support for HIV in sub-Saharan Africa and Thailand. More information available at www.cbvct.med.ucla.edu/overview.html.

O'Brien, K. L., L. H. Moulton, R. Reid, R. Weatherholtz, J. Oski, L. Brown, G. Kumar, A. Parkinson, D. Hu, J. Hackell, I. Chang, R. Kohberger, G. Siber, and M. Santosham. 2003. Efficacy and safety of seven-valent conjugate pneumococcal vaccine in American Indian children: Group randomised trial. *Lancet* 362(9381):355-361.

Padian, N., A. van der Straten, G. Ramjee, T. Chipato, G. de Bruyn, K. Blanchard, S. Shiboski, E. Montgomery, H. Fancher, H. Cheng, M. Rosenblum, M. van der Loan, N. Jewell, J. McIntyre, and The MIRA Team. 2007. Diaphragm and lubricant gel for prevention of HIV acquisition in southern African women: A randomised controlled trial. *Lancet* 370:251-261.

Quinn, T. C., R. Brookmeyer, R. Kline, M. Shepherd, R. Paranjape, S. Mehendale, D. A. Gadkari, and R. Bollinger. 2000. Feasibility of pooling sera for HIV-1 viral RNA to diagnose acute primary HIV-1 infection and estimate HIV incidence. *AIDS* 14(17):2751-2757.

Thior, I., S. Lockman, L. M. Smeaton, R. L. Shapiro, C. Wester, S. J. Heymann, P. B. Gilbert, L. Stevens, T. Peter, S. Kim, E. van Widenfelt, C. Moffat, P. Ndase, P. Arimi, P. Kebaabetswe, P. Mazonde, J. Makhema, K. McIntosh, V. Novitsky, T. H. Lee, R. Marlink, S. Lagakos, and M. Essex. 2006. Breastfeeding plus infant zidovudine prophylaxis for 6 months vs. formula feeding plus infant zidovudine for 1 month to reduce mother-to-child HIV transmission in Botswana: A randomized trial: The Mashi study. *Journal of the American Medical Association* 296(7):794-805.

Todd, J., L. Carpenter, X. Li, J. Nakiyingi, R. Gray, and R. Hayes. 2003. The effects of alternative study designs on the power of community randomized trials: Evidence from three studies of human immunodeficiency virus prevention in East Africa. *International Journal of Epidemiology* 32(5):755-762.

Wawer, M. J., N. K. Sewankambo, D. Serwadda, T. C. Quinn, L. A. Paxton, N. Kiwanuka, F. Wabwire-Mangen, C. Li, T. Lutalo, F. Nalugoda, C. A. Gaydos, L. H. Moulton, M. O. Meehan, S. Ahmed, and R. H. Gray. 1999. Control of sexually transmitted diseases for AIDS prevention in Uganda: A randomised community trial. *Lancet* 353(9152):525-535.

Appendix A

Public Committee Meeting Agendas

Committee on Methodological Challenges in HIV Prevention Trials

MEETING ONE

February 6–7, 2007
Washington, DC

February 6, 2007

10:15–10:20 a.m.	**Welcome and Overview**
	Stephen Lagakos, Ph.D. (Chair) *Professor of Biostatistics* *Department of Biostatistics* *Harvard School of Public Health*
10:20–10:35 a.m.	**Charge to the Committee**
	Renee Ridzon, M.D. *Senior Program Officer* *HIV, TB, and Reproductive Health* *Bill & Melinda Gates Foundation*
10:35–11:05 a.m.	**Overview of Methodological Challenges in HIV Prevention Trials**
	Sten Vermund, M.D., Ph.D. *Amos Christie Chair in Global Health* *Director, Institute for Global Health* *School of Medicine* *Vanderbilt University*

11:05–11:20 a.m.	**Quick Working Group Activities**
	Polly Harrison, Ph.D. *Director, Alliance for Microbicide Development*
11:20–11:35 a.m.	**Break**
11:35–11:45 a.m.	**NIH Microbicide Trial Network**
	Sharon Hillier, Ph.D. *Director, Reproductive Infectious Disease Research* *Magee-Womens Hospital* *Professor, Department of Obstetrics, Gynecology, and Reproductive Sciences* *University of Pittsburgh*
11:45 a.m.–Noon	**Biomedical Intervention for HIV Prevention Project: The Forum for Collaborative HIV Research**
	Veronica Miller, Ph.D. *Director, Forum for Collaborative HIV Research* *Associate Research Professor* *The George Washington University*
Noon–1:00 p.m.	**Lunch**
1:00–1:30 p.m.	**Incidence Estimation in Microbicide Trials**
	Salim Abdool Karim, M.B.Ch.B., Ph.D. *Director, Centre for the AIDS Program of Research in South Africa (CAPRISA)* *Pro Vice-Chancellor for Research* *University of KwaZulu-Natal, Durban, South Africa*

Late-Stage Microbicide Efficacy Trials

1:30–2:05 p.m.	**CONRAD: Phase 3 Trial of 6% Cellulose Sulfate Gel and the Effect on Vaginal HIV Transmission (multiple countries, ongoing)** **FHI: Phase 3 Trial of Cellulose Sulfate Gel to Prevent HIV Infection (Nigeria, ongoing)** *Doug Taylor, Ph.D.* *Director of Biostatistics* *Family Health International (FHI)*
2:05–2:35 p.m.	**Population Council: Phase 3 Efficacy Study of the Vaginal Gel Carraguard to Prevent HIV Transmission (South Africa, ongoing)** *Stephanie Skoler, M.P.H.* *Study Manager, Microbicides Program* *Population Council*
2:35–3:05 p.m.	**HPTN 035: Phase II/IIB Safety and Effectiveness Study of Vaginal Micobicides Buffergel and 0.5% PRO2000/5 GEL (P) for the Prevention of HIV in Women (multiple countries, ongoing)** *Benoît Mâsse, Ph.D.* *Associate Member, Statistical Center for HIV/AIDS Research & Prevention (SCHARP) Fred Hutchinson Cancer Research Center* *Affiliate Associate Professor, Biostatistics* *School of Public Health and Community Medicine* *University of Washington*
3:05–3:25 p.m.	**FHI: Phase 3 Trial of SAVVY Vaginal Gel to Prevent HIV Infection (Ghana, closed in 2005)** **FHI: Phase 3 Trial of SAVVY Vaginal Gel to Prevent HIV Infection (Nigeria, closed in 2006)**

	Leigh Peterson, Ph.D. *Senior Scientist, Clinical Research Department* *Family Health International (FHI)*
3:25–3:40 p.m.	**Break**
3:40–4:05 p.m.	**IPM: Phase III Trial of Dapivirine Gel Referred to as IPM 009 (multisite, planned)**
	Zeda Rosenberg, Sc.D. *Chief Executive Officer* *International Partnership for Microbicides (IPM)*
4:05–4:25 p.m.	**CAPRISA: Phase 2/2B trial of Tenofovir/PMPA Gel, Referred to as CAPRISA 004 (South Africa, planned)**
	Salim Abdool Karim, M.B.Ch.B., Ph.D. *Pro Vice-Chancellor, Research* *University of KwaZulu-Natal, Durban, South Africa* *Director, Centre for the AIDS Program of Research in South Africa (CAPRISA)*
4:25–6:00 p.m.	**Q&A with Microbicide Investigators**
6:00 p.m.	**Adjourn**

February 7, 2007

8:30–9:00 a.m.	**MRC: Phase 3 Trial to Evaluate the Efficacy and Safety of 0.5% and 2% PRO 2000/5 Gels for the Prevention of Vaginally Acquired HIV Infection (multiple countries, ongoing)**
	Sheena McCormack, M.B.B.S., M.Sc., F.R.C.P. (by conference call) *Clinical Epidemiologist* *Medical Research Council (MRC)*

Late-Stage Pre-Exposure Prophylaxis (PrEP) Efficacy Trials

9:00–9:50 a.m.	**CDC: Phase 3 Safety and Efficacy Trial of Tenofovir Plus Emtricitabine (Truvada) to Prevent HIV Infection (Botswana, planned; TDF trial, closing)** **CDC: Phase 2/3 Safety and Efficacy Trial of Tenofovir to Prevent HIV Infection (Thailand, ongoing)** *Dawn Smith, M.D., M.P.H., M.S.* *Medical Epidemiologist and Acting Associate Branch Chief for Science in the Epidemiology Branch* *Division of HIV/AIDS Prevention* *National Center for HIV, STD, and TB Prevention* *Centers for Disease Control and Prevention (CDC)* *Ramses Sadek, Ph.D.* *Lead Mathematical Statistician* *Division of HIV/AIDS Prevention* *National Center for HIV, STD, and TB Prevention* *Centers for Disease Control and Prevention (CDC)*
9:50–10:20 a.m.	**NIH: Phase 3 Safety and Efficacy Trial of Tenofovir Plus Emtricitabine (Truvada) to Prevent HIV Infection (Peru, planned)** *Robert M. Grant, M.D., M.P.H., M.S.* *Associate Investigator* *Gladstone Institute of Virology and Immunology* *Associate Professor of Medicine* *University of California, San Francisco* *David V. Glidden, Ph.D.* *Associate Professor of Biostatistics* *University of California, San Francisco*
10:20–10:35 a.m.	**Break**

10:35–10:55 a.m.	**FHI: Phase 2 Effectiveness and Extended Safety Trial of Tenofovir to Prevent HIV Infection (Ghana, completed; Nigeria and Cameroon, halted)**
	Leigh Peterson, Ph.D. *Senior Scientist, Clinical Research Department* *Family Health International (FHI)*
10:55 a.m.–12:20 p.m.	**Q&A with PrEP Investigators**
12:20–12:50 p.m.	**Community Perspectives**
	Mitchell Warren *Executive Director* *AIDS Vaccine Advocacy Coalition*
	Lori Heise *Director* *Global Campaign for Microbicides*
12:50 p.m.	**Wrap Up and Adjourn**

MEETING TWO

April 19, 2007
London

April 19, 2007

8:30–8:40 a.m.	**Welcome and Overview**
	Stephen Lagakos, Ph.D. (Chair) *Professor of Biostatistics* *Department of Biostatistics* *Harvard School of Public Health*

Issues in Trial Design and Implementation

8:40–9:05 a.m.	**Site Preparedness and Implementation of Late-Stage HIV Prevention Efficacy Trials in Resource-Limited Settings** *Gita Ramjee, Ph.D.* *Director, HIV Prevention Unit* *South African Medical Research Council*
9:05–9:30 a.m.	**Context, Challenges, and New Ideas for HIV Prevention Trials** *Helen Rees, O.B.E.* *Executive Director, Reproductive Health and HIV Research Unit* *Department of Obstetrics and Gynecology* *University of the Witwatersrand* *Johannesburg, South Africa*
9:30–9:55 a.m.	**Accuracy of Self-Reported Sexual Behavior** *James J. Jaccard, Ph.D.* *Professor, Department of Psychology* *Florida International University*
9:55–10:10 a.m.	**Break**
10:10–10:35 a.m.	**Measurement of Adherence, Sexual Behavior, and Product Acceptability in MDP PRO 2000 Microbicide Trial** *Robert Pool, Ph.D.* *Senior Lecturer in Social Anthropology* *London School of Hygiene & Tropical Medicine*
10:35–11:00 a.m.	**Issues in Microbicide Trial Design, Monitoring, and Analysis** *Andrew Nunn, M.Sc.* *Associate Director, Clinical Trials Unit* *United Kingdom Medical Research Council*

11:00–11:25 a.m.	**Microbicide Product Development and Implications for Future Trials** *Robin Shattock, Ph.D.* *Reader in Cell Biology of Infection* *Department of Cellular and Molecular Medicine* *St. George's Hospital Medical School* *University of London*
11:25 a.m.–12:15 p.m.	**Panel Discussion**
12:15–1:00 p.m.	**Lunch**

Recent Late-Stage Non-Vaccine Biomedical HIV Prevention Trials

1:00–1:25 p.m.	**Male Circumcision to Prevent HIV Acquisition in Young Men in Kisumu, Kenya** *Kawango Agot, Ph.D., M.P.H.* *Coordinator and Coinvestigator, Universities of Nairobi, Illinois, and Manitoba (UNIM) Project* *Lumumba Health Center* *University of Nairobi*
1:25–1:50 p.m.	**Male Circumcision to Prevent HIV Acquisition and Transmission in Rakai, Uganda** *Maria J. Wawer, M.D., M.P.H.* *Professor, Department of Population, Family, and Reproductive Health* *Bloomberg School of Public Health* *Johns Hopkins University*
1:50–2:15 p.m.	**Lessons Learned from STD Treatment Trials for HIV Prevention** *Maria J. Wawer, M.D., M.P.H.* *Professor, Department of Population, Family, and Reproductive Health* *Bloomberg School of Public Health* *Johns Hopkins University*

2:15–2:40 p.m.	**Phase 3 Randomized, Placebo-Controlled Trial of HSV-2 Suppression to Prevent HIV Transmission Among HIV-Discordant Couples** *Connie Celum, M.D., M.P.H.* *Professor of Medicine and Adjunct Professor of Epidemiology* *Division of Allergy and Infectious Diseases* *School of Medicine* *University of Washington*
2:40–3:00 p.m.	**Break**
3:00–4:00 p.m.	**Panel Discussion**
4:00–4:30 p.m.	**The Latex Diaphragm to Prevent HIV Acquisition Among Women: A Female-Controlled Physical Barrier of the Cervix** *Nancy Padian, Ph.D., M.P.H. (by conference call)* *Executive Director, Women's Global Health Imperative* *Associate Director of Research, Global Health Sciences* *Professor, Departments of Obstetrics, Gynecology, and Reproductive Sciences* *University of California, San Francisco*
4:30–5:00 p.m.	**Key Summary Points and Discussion** *Kenneth H. Mayer, M.D.* *Professor of Medicine and Community Health* *Director, AIDS Program* *Brown University* *Attending Physician, Division of Infectious Diseases* *The Miriam Hospital, Providence, RI* *Research Medical Director* *Fenway Community Health, Boston*
5:00 p.m.	**Adjourn**

Appendix B

Acronyms

AIDS	acquired immunodeficiency syndrome
ANRS	Agence Nationale de Recherche sur le Sida (France)
ANVISA	Brazilian National Health Vigilance Agency
ART	antiretroviral therapy
AVAC	AIDS Vaccine Advocacy Coalition
CAPRISA	Centre for the AIDS Program of Research in South Africa
CDC	Centers for Disease Control and Prevention (U.S.)
CMED	Medicines Market Regulation Chamber
DMC	Data Monitoring Committee
DSMB	Data Safety Monitoring Board
EIA	enzyme immunoassay
ELISA	Enzyme-Linked ImmunoSorbent Assay
EMEA	European Agency for the Evaluation of Medicinal Products
FDA	Food and Drug Administration (U.S.)
FHI	Family Health International
HIV	human immunodeficiency virus
HPTN	HIV Prevention Trials Network
HSV	herpes simplex virus
HVTN	HIV Vaccine Trials Network
IAVI	International AIDS Vaccine Initiative
IND	Investigational New Drug application (to FDA, U.S.)
IOM	Institute of Medicine (U.S.)
IPM	International Partnership for Microbicides
ITT	intent-to-treat analysis
MCC	Medicines Control Council (South Africa)

MDP	Microbicides Development Programme
MRC	Medical Research Council
MTN	Microbicide Trial Network
NIAID	National Institute of Allergy and Infectious Diseases (U.S.)
NIH	National Institutes of Health (U.S.)
PEP	post-exposure prophylaxis
PI	principal investigator
PrEP	pre-exposure prophylaxis
STD	sexually transmitted disease
STI	sexually transmitted infection
TDF	tenofovir disoproxil fumarate
UNAIDS	The Joint United Nations Programme on HIV/AIDS
USAID	U.S. Agency for International Development
WHO	World Health Organization

Appendix C

Supporting Materials for Chapter 2

This appendix provides the supporting technical material for Chapter 2. This information includes the relationship between biological efficacy and effectiveness, approximations for the effects on sample size of incorrect assumptions about HIV incidence and the relative risk of an intervention, and the justification for the approximate formula for determining the relative size of those two factors.

RELATIONSHIP OF EFFECTIVENESS TO BIOLOGICAL EFFICACY AND ADHERENCE

The overall effectiveness of an intervention depends on its biological efficacy and the degree to which individuals adhere to the product's intended use. Nonadherence can be due to several factors. For example, individuals may never initiate the intervention, or they may be required to discontinue use of a product at some point because of a serious side effect, pregnancy, or other reason.

This section develops a simple approximation to illustrate how imperfect adherence dilutes the effect of an intervention. In this simple case, only a proportion, say f, of the individuals assigned to the intervention actually initiate it and use it as intended, while the remaining subjects never initiate the intervention.

Suppose that in the absence of an intervention, the incidence rate of HIV infection is I_0. Suppose also that the biological effect of the intervention, if it was initiated, reduced the incidence rate from I_0 to I_1. *Biologi-*

cal efficacy is defined as the proportionate reduction in the incidence rate associated with use of the intervention. That is,

$$Biological\ efficacy = 1 - \frac{I_1}{I_0} = 1 - r,$$

where $r = I_1 / I_0$. The quantity r is sometimes referred to as the relative risk, denoted RR.

Now consider the effectiveness of the intervention in a population of individuals where a proportion f use the intervention as intended, and as a result have incidence rate I_1. The remaining (in proportion 1 – f) do not initiate the intervention, and as a result have incidence rate I_0. We refer to f in this setting as the adherence rate. The incidence rate I in this population is a weighted average of the incidence rates I_0 and I_1:

$$I = frI_0 + (1 - f)I_0.$$

We define the effectiveness of the intervention to be the proportionate reduction in the incidence rate, when accounting for the possibility of imperfect adherence. That is, the *effectiveness* of the intervention is defined as

$$\begin{aligned} 1 - R &= 1 - \frac{I}{I_0} \\ &= 1 - (fr + 1 - f) \\ &= (1 - r)f. \end{aligned}$$

That is,

$$Effectiveness = Biological\ Efficacy \times Adherence\ Rate. \tag{1}$$

Thus the effectiveness of an intervention depends on both its biological efficacy and the adherence rate.

IMPACT OF ERRORS IN ASSUMPTIONS ON REQUIRED SAMPLE SIZE

This section discusses the impact on sample size requirements of errors in estimating two critical factors: the incidence rate of HIV infection in the control group, and the relative risk of the intervention.

Impact of the HIV Incidence Rate on Required Sample Size

Consider a two-arm randomized intervention trial with equal numbers of subjects on each arm. Suppose that the number of events (infections), X_1, in the control group has a Poisson distribution with expectation $I\ T$, where I is the HIV incidence rate and T is the total person-years of follow-up in the control group. Similarly, assume that the number of events in the intervention group has a Poisson distribution with mean $(I\ R\ T)$, where R is the relative risk of the intervention.

We assume that the trial is designed with equal sample sizes and follow-up in the two groups, so that person-years are the same in each group. We are interested in testing the null hypothesis of no effect of the intervention: that is, $H_0{:}R = 1$. Investigators typically calculate sample size proceed by assuming a plausible a priori value for R, and then size the trial to have adequate power to detect that relative risk. The value of R is usually of sufficient public health significance to warrant adoption of the intervention in the community if the trial demonstrates efficacy.

As discussed by Cox and Hinkley (1974), it is appropriate to condition on the total number of events ($D = X_1 + X_2$). Conditional on D, we have X_1~binomial(D, p), where $p = 1/(1 + R)$. Thus, the problem of determining the sample size for the two-arm trial is essentially equivalent to finding the sample size in a one-sample binomial situation.

Accordingly, the number of required events D depends only on the Type 1 error rate α, and on the power β to detect a specified relative risk R (see Breslow and Day, 1987, p. 282). We denote D, the required number of events, by the function $g\ (R, \alpha, \beta)$.

Suppose we initially assume that the incidence in the control group is I_1. Then, because the expected number of events is equal to the person-time per group (T) multiplied by $I_1\ (1 + R)$, the person-time of follow-up that is needed is

$$\frac{g(\alpha, \beta, R)}{I_1(1+R)}.$$

However, suppose that the true HIV incidence rate in the control group is I_2 and not I_1. Then the person-time per group that would be required to have the power β to detect the relative risk R is actually

$$\frac{g(\alpha, \beta, R)}{I_2\left(1+R\right)}.$$

Taking the ratio of these last two equations, we see that the factor g (α,

β, $R)/(1 + R)$ cancels. Thus the ratio of person-time that is actually needed to that which was originally planned is I_1/I_2. That is, the person-time that is actually required to achieve the desired power is (I_1/I_2) times larger than originally planned. If the duration of follow-up is unchanged, then the required sample size is also (I_1/I_2) times larger than originally planned.

We illustrate this result with an example. Suppose the incidence rate is initially assumed to be 5 percent, but that it is actually only 4 percent. Then the study would require 25 percent more person-years ($I_1/I_2 = 1.25$) than originally planned to achieve the desired power. The increase in person-years can be achieved by increasing the sample size by 25 percent, increasing follow-up time by 25 percent, or through a combination of increases in follow-up duration and sample size.

For example, a 25 percent increase in person-years can be achieved by a 10 percent increase in sample size together with a 14 percent increase in duration of follow-up for each participant (that follows because $1.10 \times 1.14 = 1.25$). As shown in Chapter 2, the consequence of not modifying the sample size or planned duration of a trial in this setting is a reduction in the power of the trial to detect an intervention effect.

Impact of the Relative Risk on Required Sample Size

In this section we develop some simple approximations for the impact on the sample size of changes in the assumed relative risk. The required total number of events (D) for a two-sided test at level α, with power β to detect a relative risk of R is to a first approximation (see Breslow and Day, 1987, p. 282), is

$$D \approx \frac{\left(z_{\alpha/2} + z_{1-\beta}\right)^2 \left(1+R\right)^2}{\left(1-R\right)^2}, \tag{2}$$

where z_α is the α critical value of a standard normal.

Suppose a study is designed with an assumed HIV incidence rate of I_1 and power β to detect a relative risk R_1. Then the number of person-years T_1 (per group) needed to yield the expected number of events is obtained by dividing equation (2) by I_1 $(1+R)$.

However, suppose in fact that the true incidence rate and relative risk are I_2 and R_2, respectively. Then the ratio of the required person-time T_2 (per group) based on the correct specifications (I_2, R_2) to the person-time T_1 (per group) originally planned based on the incorrect assumptions (I_1, R_1) is

$$\frac{T_2}{T_1} \approx \left(\frac{I_1}{I_2}\right)\left(\frac{\left(1-R_1\right)^2}{\left(1-R_2\right)^2}\right)\left(\frac{\left(1+R_2\right)}{\left(1+R_1\right)}\right). \tag{3}$$

This equation can be further simplified if we ignore the last factor, yielding the following approximation:

$$\frac{T_2}{T_1} \approx \left(\frac{I_1}{I_2}\right)\left(\frac{(1-R_1)^2}{(1-R_2)^2}\right). \tag{4}$$

Thus, the ratio of the person-years that are actually required to those originally planned approximately varies inversely with the product of the ratio of incidence rates and the ratio of the square of the effectiveness parameters. The approximations leading to equations (3) and (4) are most accurate when the relative risks are near 1.

We illustrate these results with an example. Suppose the study was originally designed to detect an effectiveness of 0.3 (corresponding to a relative risk of 0.70), but that in fact the effectiveness is actually 0.2 (corresponding to a relative risk of 0.80). How much larger would the study need to be to detect this more modest effect with the same power as originally planned?

If all other factors remained unchanged, the person-years required would need to be at least about 2.25 times larger than originally planned (because $(0.3/0.2)^2 = 2.25$). (This calculation is based on equation 4. If a more precise calculation is desired, equation 3 could be used instead, which gives a factor of 2.38.) If no change is made to the duration of follow-up, then the sample size would need to be inflated by the factor 2.25 to achieve the needed increase in person-years.

Impact of Imperfect Adherence on Required Sample Size

The results in the preceding section can be used to illustrate the impact of imperfect adherence on the size of trials. As shown by equation 1, non-adherence dilutes the effectiveness of an intervention.

Suppose we design a trial to evaluate an intervention that is believed to have a biological efficacy $(1 - r)$. Suppose we also believe that the adherence rate can be expected to be about f_1. We design the trial to detect an effectiveness of $f_1 (1 - r)$ with a specified power. We then ask how sensitive the required size of the trial is to the assumed value of the adherence rate, all other things being equal (such as HIV incidence, study power, and biological efficacy).

That is, suppose we assume an adherence rate of f_2 instead of f_1. It follows from equation 4 that the ratio of person-years, if we assume an adherence rate of f_2 instead of f_1, is

$$\frac{T_2}{T_1} \approx \left(\frac{f_1}{f_2}\right)^2.$$

Thus, the ratio of required person-years varies inversely with the square of the ratio of the adherence rates.

For example, suppose a trial is designed with the expectation that the adherence rate for an intervention (such as a microbicide) is $f_1 = 0.90$. We ask how much larger the trial would have to be if the adherence rate is actually only $f_2 = 0.5$. We find that the person-years required would need to be 3.24 times larger (because $(0.9/0.5)^2 = 3.24$).

IMPACT OF MULTIPLE FACTORS

The required sample size for a trial can be sensitive to a small difference in a single key design parameter, such as the HIV incidence rate or the relative risk, as the preceding sections show. If there are small differences in both the actual incidence rate and the actual relative risk compared with the assumed rates, then these differences compound, and can result in large differences in the required sample sizes.

For example, suppose a trial is designed to detect an effectiveness of 0.30 based on an annual incidence rate of 0.05. If instead we assume an effectiveness of 0.25 based on an incidence rate of 0.04, we find that the trial would need to be approximately 1.8 times larger (because $(0.05/0.04)(3/0.2)^2 = 1.8$). Such sensitivity analyses of the trial size to multiple design parameters are important in assessing the feasibility of a trial and the likelihood of success.

JUSTIFICATION FOR THE APPROXIMATE FORMULA FOR DETERMINING THE RELATIVE SIZE OF EFFECTIVENESS AND EFFICACY TRIALS

As noted in Chapter 2, because of the lack of a validated surrogate endpoint for HIV infection for non-vaccine HIV prevention trials, a traditional efficacy trial and and an effectiveness trial differ in duration, the HIV incidence rate in the control group, and the relative risk of the intervention. For example, a trial that focuses on evaluating the biological efficacy of an intervention may follow a highly compliant population for a short period of time, whereas an effectiveness trial may follow a more heterogeneous population for a longer period of time.

The degree to which the risk-taking behavior of subjects changes during either trial may determine the HIV incidence rate in the control group. And the underlying incidence rate in the more compliant population could well be different from that in the more general population—either lower or higher.

The third factor, relative risk, may largely reflect adherence. Investigators might expect a population used in an efficacy trial to be more adherent than a population used in a longer effectiveness trial, though this may not always be the case, as Chapter 2 notes.

Table C-1 gives the approximate ratios in sample size of efficacy and effectiveness trials for different HIV incidence rates (I_1 and I_2) in the control group, relative risks (RR_1 and RR_2), and duration of the effectiveness trial (D_2). For all settings, the efficacy trial is of six months duration. In almost all settings, the sample size needed for the efficacy trial exceeds that of the effectiveness trial, in many cases by a factor of two or more. The efficacy trial is smaller only when its control-group incidence rate is substantially higher and the intervention effect is substantially stronger in the efficacy trial than in the effectiveness trial.

Let I_1 and I_2 be the HIV incidence rates in the control group for the two designs, and let R_1 and R_2 denote the corresponding relative risk of intervention: control. The ratio of the required person-years in the second trial compared with the first trial is approximately

$$\frac{T_2}{T_1} = \frac{I_1}{I_2}\left(\frac{1-R_1}{1-R_2}\right)^2.$$

Suppose the duration of follow-up of each participant in these trials is denoted d_1 for the first design and d_2 for the second design. Then the ratio of required sample sizes (n) for the two trial designs is approximately

$$\frac{n_2}{n_1} = \left(\frac{I_1}{I_2}\right)\left(\frac{1-R_1}{1-R_2}\right)^2\left(\frac{d_1}{d_2}\right).$$

Thus, the relative sample sizes approximately depend multiplicatively on the ratio of incidence rates, the ratio of the square of the effectiveness, and the relative duration of follow-up.

To illustrate, suppose investigators are considering two designs to evaluate a particular microbicide. The adherence rates in the first and second designs are 0.90 and 0.50, respectively. Assume that the biological efficacy of the microbicide is the same in the two designs. If follow-up (per person) were twice as long in the second design as in the first, the first design would require a larger sample size if $I_1/I_2 < 0.62$ (because $(0.5/0.9)^2 \times 2 = 0.62$).

Thus, in this example, if the HIV incidence rate in the control arm of the first design is smaller than that in the second design—in particular, less than 62 percent that in the second design—then the first design would require a larger sample size.

TABLE C-1 Relative Sample Sizes of Efficacy Trials to Effectiveness Trials for Varying Control Group HIV Incidence Rates, Relative Risks (RR), and Participant Follow-Up (in years)

Efficacy trial size			Effectiveness trial			Sample Ratio
Pt FU	Incidence	RR	Pt FU	Incidence	RR	
0.5	2%	0.4	4	4%	0.6	7.11
0.5			3			5.33
0.5			2			3.56
0.5		0.3	4		0.6	5.22
0.5			3			3.92
0.5			2			3.56
0.5	3%	0.4	4	4%	0.6	4.74
0.5			3			3.56
0.5			2			2.37
0.5		0.3	4		0.6	3.48
0.5			3			2.61
0.5			2			1.74
0.5	4%	0.3	4	4%	0.6	2.61
0.5			3			1.96
0.5			2			1.30
0.5		0.2	4		0.6	2.00
0.5			3			1.50
0.5			2			1.00
0.5	4%	0.4	4	4%	0.6	3.56
0.5			3			2.67
0.5			2			1.78
0.5		0.3	4		0.6	2.61
0.5			3			1.96
0.5			2			1.31
0.5	4%	0.4	4	3%	0.6	2.67
0.5			3			2.00
0.5			2			1.33
0.5		0.3	4		0.6	1.96
0.5			3			1.47
0.5			2			0.98
0.5	4%	0.3	4	2%	0.6	1.31
0.5			3			0.98
0.5			2			0.65
0.5		0.2	4		0.6	1.00
0.5			3			0.75
0.5			2			0.50

NOTE: Pt FU = participant follow-up.

REFERENCES

Breslow, N. E., and N. E. Day. 1987. Statistical methods in cancer research. International Agency for Research on Cancer workshop, May 25–27, 1983. *IARC Scientific Publications* (82):1-406.

Cox, D. R., and D. V. Hinkley. 1974. *Theoretical statistics*. Toronto: Chapman & Hall.

Appendix D

Methods for Analyzing Adherence

Adherence to product use and recommendations for safe sexual behavior form an important outcome of any HIV prevention intervention, and also impact the effectiveness of a new product. In Chapter 5, the committee explored the types of questions that analyses of adherence can answer. This section outlines methods for conducting these analyses, and their limitations, using two relatively simple examples: (1) comparing adherence patterns between two study arms, and (2) relating the effect of the intervention to adherence. Investigators can use similar approaches to compare behavior patterns among study arms or analyze adherence and behavior in more sophisticated ways.

COMPARING ADHERENCE PATTERNS BETWEEN STUDY ARMS

In this example, assume first that study staff record a summary adherence measure Y for each individual at every clinic visit, and that visits are scheduled at regular intervals, such as monthly. Let the value of Y for individual i at visit t be denoted Y_{it}. Our goal is to compare the longitudinal patterns of these measures between study arms, as a means of comparing the arms with respect to adherence.

The adherence measure obtained at each time point could be a count, such as the number of exposures to microbicide gel in the past week, or the number of days in the past week on which a participant took a PrEP dose. The adherence measure could also be an average, such as the percentage of coital acts during the past three days in which a participant used gel, or some other measure deemed relevant for the specific product. (For a discussion of summary measures used in randomized trials, see Vrijens and Goetghebeur, 1997.)

By modeling the expected adherence $E(Y_{it})$ as a function of time on study t, and possibly some baseline characteristics, say x_i, and a subject's randomized intervention, say r_i, investigators can perform an intent-to-treat analysis of repeated adherence measures, and learn how these measures differ between subpopulations identified through baseline covariates. For example, in the absence of dropouts (Vrijens and Goetghebeur, 1997), analysts could compare daily measures of compliance (as measured by Electronic Drug Monitoring) between study arms using a marginal model.

If some subjects never start their randomized intervention, or abandon it at some point during the study, investigators may first compare persistence between intervention arms, such as the percentage of "never takers," and time from randomization to dropout for those who initiate the intervention. If all randomized participants actually start their assigned intervention, this amounts to applying standard time-to-event analysis methods to the time at which participants discontinue the intervention. These event times are right-censored as of the time of HIV infection by the end of the study (following staggered entry), and possibly but not necessarily by pregnancy.

Under the "strong null hypothesis" that the randomized interventions are exchangeable (which means that subjects in both study arms are comparable in all respects), these censored times are equally distributed between arms. When persistence is an issue, investigators could begin their analysis of compliance patterns by modeling adherence measures from the actual start of product use until the observed time of discontinuation. Interpretation of the results would need to consider both analyses jointly.

Now consider the analysis of compliance, or product execution. Under the strong null hypothesis—that is, that the arms are indistinguishable—pregnancies, failure times, censoring times, and patterns of adherence are distributed equally between the study arms. Censoring and failure time are important here, because these determine how long we can observe compliance, and because compliance patterns may change over time. Indeed, more frequent sexual activity typically increases the risk of HIV, and hence can decrease the amount of time during which we observe compliance.

Similarly, pregnancy is an indicator of unprotected sex, which will also have an impact on "compliance," because subjects found to be pregnant are commonly taken off product. Whether compliance analyses censor pregnant women at this time, or rather insert zero measures or carry the last observation forward, the resulting patterns should remain similar between study arms under the strong null hypothesis. However, for both modeling and interpretation, it is usually preferable to censor compliance measures at the time the intervention is discontinued because of pregnancy.

Now consider a situation where participants' adherence over time is the same in the intervention and control arms, but where the intervention delays the time to HIV infection. Because good adherers in the intervention arm would tend to remain uninfected longer, a simple cross-sectional comparison of adherence rates at a specific time point would tend to show higher average adherence levels in the intervention arm. Indeed, the good adherers would tend to drop out sooner from the control arm owing to HIV infection, and thus would no longer be observed for adherence.

To retain an unbiased evaluation of adherence levels in each study arm, we would need to adjust for "dropout" related to adherence and sexual behavior. This is possible when the study collects information on time-varying confounders: that is, on subject-specific covariates that vary over time and predict both adherence and the risk of HIV infection. When clinic visits occur irregularly, investigators must similarly account for that in their analysis, as a time trend in adherence and behavior may well exist. (Hernan et al. [2002] explain how to account for dropout in a population-averaged marginal analysis. For other approaches, see, for instance, Little, 1995; Robins et al., 1995; and Molenberghs et al., 2004).

ANALYZING THE EFFECT OF ADHERENCE PATTERNS ON HIV INCIDENCE

Participants' adherence to an intervention and their sexual behavior may evolve over time in response to the perceived effects of the intervention. These two factors are naturally correlated with the risk of HIV infection, even in the absence of any direct biological effect of the intervention.

In a blinded trial, participants' level of adherence should not depend on the randomized study arm. Thus a comparison between arms of times to HIV infection, adjusted for a subject-specific adherence level, would yield an unbiased measure of the effectiveness of the intervention. Investigators can stratify the analysis on the summary adherence measure, or use it as a baseline covariate in a Cox regression analysis, to obtain adherence-adjusted hazard ratios. However, investigators need to use caution with summary measures that average adherence over different time periods for different subjects, as these could introduce confounding, especially when the intervention has a causal effect.

More generally, investigators may need to allow for an intervention effect that could change a person's adherence level. For instance, the COL-1492 study observed a larger incidence of genital lesions in the experimental arm. Such lesions could change future compliance in that arm. In that case, causal models of the effect of the intervention can enable randomization-based inference that allows for confounding between compliance and potential intervention-free response. (For examples of such methods, see Mark and Robins, 1993; White et al., 1999.)

Randomization-based causal analysis is conceptually simple. Investigators start by proposing a causal model for how a participant's intervention history influences the residual time to HIV infection. For example, for each woman in the intervention arm, let T_0 denote her unobserved potential time to HIV infection in the control arm. Consider further that her observed (constant) adherence level A to the experimental treatment is a driver of the causal effect of treatment.

Investigators could then postulate that her observed time to HIV infection in the treatment arm T relates to her potential treatment-free time T_0 through a function of treatment level A. For instance,

$$T = T_0 \times \exp(\beta A).$$

This model states that for an adherence level A = 100 percent in the treatment arm, the time to HIV infection is multiplied by a factor exp (β). Models following this principle are called "structural accelerated failure time models." They can also handle adherence levels that change over time (Greenland and Robins, 1994; Vandebosch et al., 2005). Similar models work on the hazard scale (Loeys et al., 2005).

The principle of randomization-based estimation works backward from this model, to allow for correlation between compliance and intervention-free response. In the intervention arm, investigators transform the observed time to HIV infection T via observed adherence A to the latent intervention-free time T_0 using a postulated parameter value β. The estimated value of β is found when the back-transformed times in the treatment arm coincide in distribution with the observed times T_0 in the control arm. This equality in distribution can be tested, for instance using a log rank test. Under the null hypothesis of no causal effect, $\beta = 0$ corresponds to no transformation of observed times and yields equal distributions.

REFERENCES

Greenland, S., and J. Robins. 1994. Invited commentary: Ecologic studies: Biases, misconceptions, and counterexamples. *American Journal of Epidemiology* 139(8):747-760.

Hernan, M. A., B. A. Brumback, and J. M. Robins. 2002. Estimating the causal effect of zidovudine on CD4 count with a marginal structural model for repeated measures. *Statistics in Medicine* 21(12):1689-1709.

Little, R. 1995. Modeling the drop-out mechanism in repeated-measures studies. *Journal of the American Statistical Association* 90(431):1112-1121.

Loeys, T., E. Goetghebeur, and A. Vandebosch. 2005. Causal proportional hazards models and time-constant exposure in randomized clinical trials. *Lifetime Data Analysis* 11(4):435-449.

Mark, S. D., and J. M. Robins. 1993. A method for the analysis of randomized trials with compliance information: An application to the multiple risk factor intervention trial. *Controlled Clinical Trials* 14(2):79-97.

Molenberghs, G., H. Thijs, I. Jansen, C. Beunckens, M. G. Kenward, C. Mallinckrodt, and R. J. Carroll. 2004. Analyzing incomplete longitudinal clinical trial data. *Biostatistics* 5(3):445-464.

Robins, J., A. Rotnitzky, and L. Zhao. 1995. Analysis of semiparametric regression-models for repeated outcomes in the presence of missing data. *Journal of the American Statistical Association* 90(429):106-121.

Vandebosch, A., E. Goetghebeur, and L. Van Damme. 2005. Structural accelerated failure time models for the effects of observed exposures on repeated events in a clinical trial. *Statistics in Medicine* 24(7):1029-1046.

Vrijens, B., and E. Goetghebeur. 1997. Comparing compliance patterns between randomized treatments. *Controlled Clinical Trials* 18(3):187-203.

White, I. R., A. G. Babiker, S. Walker, and J. H. Darbyshire. 1999. Randomization-based methods for correcting for treatment changes: Examples from the Concorde trial. *Statistics in Medicine* 18(19):2617-2634.

Appendix E

Committee Biographies

Stephen Lagakos, Ph.D. (*Chair*), is a Professor of Biostatistics and the Director of the Center for Biostatistics in AIDS Research at the Harvard School of Public Health. Dr. Lagakos' current research involves a variety of statistical issues arising in clinical trials and other longitudinal studies, with particular emphasis on statistical methods and analyses relating to HIV and other infectious diseases. From 1989 to 1996, he served as Director of the Statistical and Data Analysis Center at the AIDS Clinical Trials Group, and from 1999 to 2006 he served as Chair of the Department of Biostatistics at Harvard. Currently, Dr. Lagakos serves on the Senior Biomedical Research Service Credentials Committee at the U.S. Food and Drug Administration (FDA), and is on the Editorial Board (Statistical Consultant) at the *New England Journal of Medicine*. Since 2002 he has served as Associate Editor for the *Journal of the American Statistical Association*. Dr. Lagakos studied at Carnegie Mellon (B.S., Mathematics) and at George Washington University (M.P.H., Ph.D., Mathematical Statistics). In 2002 he was elected to the Institute of Medicine (IOM). He has served on a number of IOM studies, including the Committee on Reviewing the HIVNET 012 Perinatal HIV Prevention Study, Committee on Assessing the Need for Clinical Trials of Testosterone Replacement Therapy, the Roundtable for the Development of Drugs and Vaccines Against AIDS, and the Committee on Postmarket Surveillance of Pediatric Medical Devices.

Harvey J. Alter, M.D., is Chief of the Infectious Diseases Section and Associate Director for Research of the Department of Transfusion Medicine at the Warren Grant Magnuson Clinical Center of the National Institutes of

Health (NIH). He is also Clinical Professor of Medicine at Georgetown University in Washington, DC. Dr. Alter has devoted most of his research career to the study of blood-transmitted infections, particularly viral hepatitis. He was the principal investigator in the first study to biophysically characterize the "Australia antigen," which was later shown to be the envelope protein of the hepatitis B virus. He led the prospective studies that identified the clinical entity known as non-A, non-B hepatitis and confirmed that it was a transmissible agent. He was the principal investigator in sequential prospective studies of transfusion-associated hepatitis, which influenced national blood policy mandating donor-screening assays. Dr. Alter's unique, long-term prospective studies identified transfusion risks, as well as donor-screening measures to alleviate those risks, and measured the outcome of these interventions. After the cloning of the hepatitis C virus (HCV), he conducted the key study that established HCV as the major cause of transfusion-associated hepatitis and demonstrated the clinical efficacy of anti-HCV screening assays. For his contributions to the discovery of the non-A, non-B/hepatitis C virus, and for his vital role in reducing hepatitis risk and improving the safety of the blood supply, Dr. Alter has received many awards and other recognition, including the Clinical Lasker Award. Dr. Alter is an elected member of both the Institute of Medicine and the National Academy of Sciences.

Ronald Bayer, Ph.D., is a Professor at the Center for the History and Ethics of Public Health in the Department of Sociomedical Sciences at the Joseph F. Mailman School of Public Health, Columbia University. Prior to coming to Columbia, he was at the Hastings Center, a research institute devoted to the study of ethical issues in medicine and the life sciences. Dr. Bayer's research has examined ethical and policy issues in public health. His empirical work has focused especially on HIV/AIDS, tuberculosis, illicit drugs, and tobacco. His broader project is to develop an ethics of public health. He is an elected member of the Institute of Medicine, and has served on the Board on Population Health and Public Health Practice and several IOM committees addressing the social impact of AIDS, tuberculosis elimination, vaccine safety, smallpox vaccination, and the Ryan White CARE Act. He has published extensively on ethical issues raised by the HIV/AIDS epidemic, including books such as *Private Acts, Social Consequences: AIDS and the Politics of Public Health* (1989); *AIDS Doctors: Voices from the Epidemic* (2000, written with Gerald Oppenheimer), and *Mortal Secrets: Truth and Lies in the Age of AIDS* (2003, written with Robert Klitzman). Dr. Bayer holds a Ph.D. in political science from the University of Chicago.

Solomon Benatar, M.D., is Professor of Medicine at the University of Cape Town (1980–) and Founding Director of the University of Cape Town

Bioethics Centre (1992–). He was Professor and Chair of the University of Cape Town's Department of Internal Medicine and Chief Physician at Groote Schuur Hospital from 1980 to 1999. Other positions include Visiting Professor of Medical Ethics at the University College London Medical School (1997–), Visiting Professor in Public Health Sciences and Medicine at the University of Toronto (2000–), President of the International Association of Bioethics (2001–2003), and Chair of the South African National Health Research Ethics Committee (2001–2005). After graduating from the University of Cape Town in 1965, he trained in anesthetics and medicine in Cape Town and London. His academic interests include respiratory medicine, academic freedom, medical ethics and the humanities in medicine, human rights, health care systems, health economics, international research ethics, and global health. He has published more than 250 journal articles and book chapters on these topics. Dr. Benatar is a corresponding member of the National Academy of Sciences' Committee on Human Rights, and has been a member of several multidisciplinary, international research groups. During the 1994/95 academic year, he was a Fellow in the Program in Ethics and the Professions at Harvard University and Visiting Professor at Harvard Medical School. He has been an advisor to UNAIDS in Geneva and to Médecins Sans Frontières in Holland. He is currently an ethics consultant to the U.S. HIV Prevention Trials Network, Director of the International Research Ethics Network for Southern Africa (an NIH Fogarty International Center-funded capacity-building program) (2003–2010), and a member of the Canadian Institutes of Health Research Standing Committee on Ethics (2006–). He is an elected Foreign Member of the Institute of Medicine (IOM) and of the American Academy of Arts and Sciences, and served on the IOM Committee for Examining the Probable Consequences of Alternative Patterns of Widespread Antiretroviral Drug Use in Resource-Constrained Settings.

Ronald Brookmeyer, Ph.D., is Professor of Biostatistics and Chair of the M.P.H. program at the Johns Hopkins Bloomberg School of Public Health. Dr. Brookmeyer's research focuses on the development and application of statistical methods and models in epidemiology. A main theme of Dr. Brookmeyer's work concerns statistical approaches for estimating and forecasting disease incidence and prevalence to track the health of populations, and the analysis and interpretation of disease surveillance data. Dr. Brookmeyer's most recent research concerns statistical models for anthrax outbreaks and other bioterrorism threats. Dr. Brookmeyer has worked extensively on developing statistical methods in AIDS epidemiology, including methods for tracking the course of the HIV/AIDS epidemic. Dr. Brookmeyer is the coauthor of *AIDS Epidemiology: A Quantitative*

Approach. His publications and research interests in biostatistical methodology include topics in survival analysis, truncated data, epidemic models, epidemiological statistics, and multidimensional longitudinal data. Dr. Brookmeyer is a Fellow of the American Association for the Advancement of Science and the American Statistical Association. He is also the 2007 Chair of the Statistics Section of the American Association for the Advancement of Science. He received his undergraduate degree from Cooper Union College in New York City and a Ph.D. in Statistics from the University of Wisconsin. He has served on a number of IOM panels, including the Committee on Perinatal Transmission of HIV, the Panel on Needle Exchange and Bleach Distribution Programs, and the Panel on Statistical Issues in AIDS Research.

Carlos del Rio, M.D., is Professor of Medicine in the Division of Infectious Diseases at Emory University School of Medicine, and Vice Chair for Grady Affairs in the Department of Medicine. He is Director for Clinical Sciences and International Research of the Emory Center for AIDS Research, and Director of the Emory AIDS International Training and Research Program. Dr. del Rio is a native of Mexico, where he attended medical school at Universidad La Salle. He did his Internal Medicine and Infectious Diseases residencies at Emory University. In 1989 he returned to Mexico, where he was Executive Director of the National AIDS Council of Mexico (CONASIDA), the federal agency responsible for AIDS policy. In November 1996 he returned to Emory, where he has been involved in patient care, teaching, and research. Dr. del Rio's research interests include the epidemiology of opportunistic infections in HIV and other immune deficiencies; the epidemiology and transmission dynamics of HIV and other sexually transmitted diseases; and issues related to early diagnosis of HIV, access to care, and compliance with antiretrovirals. He is also an investigator for the Adult AIDS Clinical Trials Group and an investigator on HIV vaccine trials. Dr. del Rio is a Member of the Board of Directors of the International AIDS Society-USA; a member of the Monitoring of the AIDS Pandemic (MAP) Network; a member of the Education Committee of Infectious Diseases Society of America; Associate Editor of *AIDS Clinical Care* and *AIDS Research and Human Retroviruses;* and a member of the Editorial Board of *Journal of AIDS*, *Women, Children and HIV*, and *Global Public Health*. Dr. del Rio has been a member of the Centers for Disease Control and Prevention and Health Resources and Services Administration Advisory Committee on HIV and STD Prevention and Treatment (2000–2003), and a member of the IOM Committee on the Ryan White CARE Act: Data for Resource Allocation, Planning, and Evaluation. He has coauthored five books, 30 book chapters, and more than 100 scientific papers.

David Feigal, M.D., M.P.H., is Senior Vice President for Global Regulatory Affairs and Global Safety Surveillance for Élan Pharmaceuticals. Most recently, he was a partner in NDA Partners LLC, a product development consultancy to the biopharmaceutical and medical device industries. He has also held several senior positions at the FDA. He first joined the FDA in 1992, when he was recruited to head the HIV Division in the Center for Drug Evaluation and Research. He then served as Director of the Division of Anti-Infective Drug Products, Director of the Office of Drug Evaluation IV, Medical Deputy Director of the Center for Biologics Evaluation and Research, and Director for the Center for Device and Radiological Health. Dr. Feigal holds an M.D. from Stanford University and an M.P.H. from the University of California, Berkeley. He completed his Internal Medicine Residency at the University of California, Davis, and a Fellowship in Clinical Epidemiology at the University of California, San Francisco.

Els Goetghebeur, Ph.D., is Associate Professor in the Department of Applied Mathematics and Computer Science at Ghent University, Belgium, and Adjunct Associate Professor in the Department of Biostatistics of the Harvard School of Public Health. At Ghent University she chairs the Center for Statistics and directs the Advanced Master in Statistical Data Analysis. She started her career in the Clinical Trials Unit at the London School of Hygiene and Tropical Medicine, and has had a keen interest in clinical trials ever since. A research position linked to the Janssen Research Foundation and LUC in Belgium allowed her to develop statistical methods for handling partial compliance with randomized drug therapy. The study of causal inference and noncompliance in clinical trials became a long-term research interest. Dr. Goetghebeur has served on the Editorial Board of several international journals, currently *Statistical Methods in Medical Research* and *Lifetime Data Analysis*. She collaborates with colleagues locally and abroad on studies of the prevention and treatment of HIV and AIDS, among other areas. She currently serves as a Statistical Expert for the European Agency for the Evaluation of Medicinal Products (EMEA). Her publications and research focus on statistical methods for clinical trials, noncompliance, causal inference more generally, and survival analysis.

Laura A. Guay, M.D., is Associate Professor in the Department of Pathology and Pediatrics at the Johns Hopkins University School of Medicine (JHU) and a Pediatric Infectious Disease Specialist. She has conducted HIV research in Uganda in collaboration with faculty from the Makerere University School of Medicine since 1988, living onsite in Kampala for 11 of these years. Dr. Guay is currently principal investigator of the NIH Division of AIDS–sponsored HIV Prevention Trial Network and DAIDS Clinical Trial Network MU-JHU Unit in Kampala, Uganda. She has participated in the design, implementation, and analysis of several HIV perinatal prevention trials in women and children in Uganda. She is the study protocol chair of HPTN 027, the first clinical safety trial in Africa of a vaccine to prevent mother-to-child transmission (PMTCT) of HIV through breast-feeding, which began enrolling participants in October 2006. She is also Co-Chair of the HPTN 046 phase 3 Trial (to Determine the Efficacy and Safety of an Extended Regimen of Nevirapine in Infants Born to HIV Infected Women to Prevent Vertical HIV Transmission During Breast-feeding), and an investigator on a study of high-titer HIV immunoglobulin for prevention of HIV-1 infection in breast-feeding infants. Her research interests include pediatric HIV-1 infection, prevention of HIV transmission from mother to child, and primary HIV prevention in women. Dr. Guay has established a comprehensive maternal-child HIV study clinic and immunology laboratory capable of supporting phase 1–3 clinical trials. In addition to the research activities in Uganda, Dr. Guay was instrumental in establishing a PMTCT program in all prenatal clinics at Mulago Hospital, which provides free HIV testing, counseling, PMTCT services, and access to HIV care to more than 35,000 pregnant women each year. Previous work includes studies of the natural history of HIV-1 infection, the neurodevelopmental effects of HIV-1 infection, and methods for early diagnosis of HIV-1 infection in Ugandan children.

Sally Hodder, M.D., is Professor of Medicine, Director of HIV Programs, and Vice Chair of the Department of Medicine at the New Jersey Medical School of the University of Medicine and Dentistry of New Jersey. Dr. Hodder received her B.A. from Mount Holyoke College and her M.D. from Case Western Reserve University. After completing training in Internal Medicine and Infectious Diseases, she was a faculty member in the Department of Medicine, Division of Infectious Diseases, at University Hospitals of Cleveland and Case Western Reserve University School of Medicine. In 2001, she joined Bristol-Myers Squibb, and was Vice President of U.S. Virology Medical Affairs, overseeing more than 100 HIV clinical trials worldwide. In February 2005 she joined the Infectious Disease Division at New Jersey Medical School, and since that time has directed a large clinic for HIV-infected persons in Newark. She leads a group of investigators evaluating outcomes and complications of HIV-infected urban residents in greater Newark, and she has a particular interest in outcomes of HIV-infected women in the United States. She is also an investigator for the Adult AIDS Clinical Trials Group. Dr. Hodder has received numerous awards, and has served as a member of various committees, including the National Board of Medical Examiners and the HIV Forum. She has published in many scientific and medical journals.

Shabbar Jaffar, Ph.D., is a Reader in Epidemiology at the London School of Hygiene and Tropical Medicine (LSHTM). He has been based at LSHTM for more than 12 years, with more than 10 of those in the Infectious Disease Epidemiology Unit. Dr. Jaffar's main research area is HIV/AIDS. He is primary investigator of a large cluster-randomized trial comparing home-based and facility-based delivery of antitretroviral treatment in southeastern Uganda. That trial is also examining virological failure, cost effectiveness, and adherence. Dr. Jaffar has provided statistical and epidemiological support to a large trial of pneumococcal conjugate vaccine in Gambian infants, a school-randomized trial of an HIV prevention strategy in Zimbabwe, studies of severe malaria in children in Yemen, a birth cohort of rotavirus infections in India, and a trial of micronutrient-fortified complimentary feeding of children in an area of high HIV prevalence in Zambia. He has lived and worked in West Africa (The Gambia), Uganda, and South Africa.

Edward K. Kirumira, Ph.D., Chair of the Uganda National Academy of Science Forum on Health and Nutrition, is Dean of the Faculty of Social Sciences at Makerere University, Kampala, Uganda. He holds a Ph.D. from the Department of Sociology at the University of Copenhagen in conjunction with Harvard University (Department of Population and International Health); an M.A. in Population Research from the Institute of Population Studies, Exeter University, UK; and a B.A. in Sociology from Makerere University. He has worked extensively on various aspects of population, fertility, and health in the Ugandan context, with reference to the HIV/AIDS crisis in sub-Saharan Africa. He has participated in numerous international conferences. Dr. Kirumira has risen through the academic and administrative ranks from Teaching Assistant in the Sociology Department to the position of Professor and Dean. He has been an External Examiner and Visiting Professor at a number of international universities in Europe, Asia, and the United States. He is a member of various professional bodies, including the Population Association of Uganda, the Organization of Social Sciences Research in East and Southern Africa, and the International Union of the Scientific Study of Population. He is also a Council Member and Fellow of the Uganda National Academy of Sciences. Dr. Kirumira has published widely on population and development, reproductive health, sexuality, and HIV/AIDS.

George Rutherford, M.D., is Director of the Institute for Global Health, Salvatore Pablo Lucia Professor of Epidemiology, Preventive Medicine, and Pediatrics, and Vice Chair of the Department of Epidemiology and Biostatistics in the School of Medicine at the University of California, San Francisco (UCSF). He is also Adjunct Professor of Epidemiology and Health

Administration at the School of Public Health at the University of California, Berkeley. Educated at Stanford University and Duke University School of Medicine, Dr. Rutherford is board certified in Pediatrics and General Preventive Medicine and Public Health. Following training in Epidemiology in the Epidemic Intelligence Service of the U.S. Centers for Disease Control and Prevention (CDC), he spent his early professional career in public health practice, with primary emphasis on the epidemiology and control of communicable diseases. He has held a number of positions at public health agencies, including serving as the State Health Officer and State Epidemiologist for the California Department of Health Services, Director of the AIDS Office for the San Francisco Department of Public Health, and the Director of the Division of Immunizations for the New York City Department of Health. He also directs the Joint UCSF–University of California, Berkeley, Residency Program in Public Health and General Preventive Medicine and the International Core for the Center for AIDS Prevention Studies. He is also Coordinating Editor of the Cochrane Collaborative Review Group on HIV Infection and AIDS at UCSF. His current research interests include the epidemiology and control of HIV infection and AIDS-related opportunistic infections (especially in developing countries), the prevention of coccidioidomycosis, sexually transmitted disease control in California, pediatric vaccination policy, the role of public health in managed care, evidence-based public health practice, the epidemiology and control of tuberculosis in California, emerging infectious diseases, and bioterrorism. Dr. Rutherford currently chairs the American Academy of Pediatrics Section on Epidemiology, and the California Tuberculosis Elimination Advisory Committee. Dr. Rutherford has served on a number of IOM committees, including the Committee on the Ryan White CARE Act: Data for Allocation, Planning, and Evaluation; the Committee on the Review of HIVNET 012 Perinatal HIV Prevention Study; and the Committee on Gulf War and Health: Review of the Medical Literature Relative to Gulf War Veterans' Health. He currently chairs the Committee on Gulf War and Health: Traumatic Brain Injuries.

Olive Shisana, M.A., Sc.D., holds a Doctor of Science from the Johns Hopkins University School of Public Health in Baltimore. She was accepted into Johns Hopkins University's society of scholars programme in 1999 for outstanding contribution to public health. Dr. Shisana is currently the President and Chief Executive Officer of the South African Human Sciences Research Council (HSRC). She previously served as Executive Director of a South African national research programme on social aspects of HIV/AIDS and health at the HSRC, the founder of the program. Prior to that she served as Professor of Health Systems at the National School of Public Health at the Medical University of Southern Africa, where she was a leading founder of a postgraduate diploma on the management of HIV/AIDS in the world of work, launched by the South African Deputy President in 2001. Before this appointment, she served as Executive Director of Family and Community Health at the World Health Organization in Geneva. In the latter portfolio, she established the WHO HIV/AIDS/STI initiative, reviving the role of WHO in this area, becoming a founding member of the Partnership on AIDS in Africa. Prior to this appointment she served as Director General of South Africa's postapartheid government, the first African and the first woman to hold the post. She has written among other subjects on HIV/AIDS, including the subject on AIDS: a human security issue, gender, HIV among health workers and educators. She was a principal investigator on the Mandela/HSRC study of HIV/AIDS, which is the first systematic national HIV/AIDS prevalence, behavioral risks, and mass media impact survey. She was also principal investigator of the 2005 HIV prevalence, incidence, and behaviour population-based survey in South Africa, and currently is the coprincipal of the same repeat survey for 2008. She was also the principal investigator of a survey of HIV prevalence among health workers and ambulatory and hospitalized patients in South Africa and also examined the impact of HIV/AIDS on South Africa's health care system. She also was a principal investigator on the national study on HIV/AIDS among public educators in South Africa. Dr. Shisana serves on the Board of the Nelson Mandela "46664" HIV/AIDS campaign and the Emory Global Health Institute Board. She also chaired the 2007 South African AIDS conference, which attracted people from 60 countries, adding to the 4,000-strong South African participants.

Gina Wingood, Sc.D., M.P.H., is the Agnes Moore Endowed Faculty in HIV/AIDS Research; Director of the Social and Behavioral Sciences Core, Center for AIDS Research; and Associate Professor in the Rollins School of Public Health at Emory University. Dr. Wingood serves as the principal investigator on several NIH-funded R01/U10 HIV prevention trials designed to reduce high-risk sexual behavior and sexually transmitted infections among women and heterosexual couples. Dr. Wingood also serves as the Director of a study funded by the National Institute of Allergy and Infectious Diseases to reduce high-risk sexual behaviors and HIV incidence among Xhosa-speaking women in South Africa. Dr. Wingood has published several CDC-defined evidence-based HIV prevention interventions for women, which CDC is disseminating nationally. Dr. Wingood is also known for applying the Theory of Gender and Power, a social-structural theory that examines the factors that increase women's vulnerability to HIV. She received her Sc.D. from Harvard University School of Public Health (1995) and an M.P.H. from University of California, Berkeley (1990).